Issues in Health Policy

Selections from *The CQ Researcher*

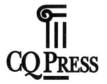

CQ PRESS

A Division of Congressional Quarterly Inc.
Washington, D.C.

CQ Press
A Division of Congressional Quarterly Inc.
1414 22nd Street, N.W.
Washington, D.C. 20037

(202) 822-1475; (800) 638-1710

www.cqpress.com

Printed and bound in the United States of America

05 04 03 02 01   5 4 3 2 1

☾ The paper used in this publication meets the minimum requirements of the American National Standard for Information Sciences—Permanence of Paper for Printed Library Materials, ANSI Z39.48-1992.

A CQ Press College Division Publication

Director	Brenda Carter
Acquisitions editor	Charisse Kiino
Managing editor	Ann Davies
Assistant Editor	Amy Briggs
Production editor	Belinda Josey
Composition	Paul Cederborg
Cover designer	Dennis Anderson
Indexer	Enid Zafran
Print buyer	Liza Sanchez
Sales	James Headley

Library of Congress Cataloging-in-Publication Data

Issues in health policy : selections from the CQ researcher.
    p. cm.
  Includes bibliographical references and index.
  ISBN 1-56802-633-1 (pbk. : alk. paper)
    1. Medical policy—United States. 2. Medical policy. I. CQ researcher.

RA395.A3 I864 2001
362.1'0973—dc21

                          00-065982

Contents

Annotated Table of Contents

The 12 *CQ Researcher* articles reprinted in this book have been reproduced essentially as they appeared when first published. In a few cases in which important new developments have occurred since an article first came out, these developments are mentioned in the following overviews, which highlight the principal issues that are examined.

ILLNESS, TREATMENT AND HEALTH POLICY

Alzheimer's Disease

Alzheimer's disease has been described as health care's "ticking time bomb." The degenerative disease slowly destroys the brain's ability to remember, reason or control simple bodily functions like swallowing food. While scientists have found compelling evidence suggesting possible causes, they still don't have a cure or a generally accepted way to screen for the disease. With the number of Americans age 65 and over expected to more than double by 2030, health-care experts are bracing for a surge of new cases that could devastate families psychologically and economically and strain the nation's health-care system. Researchers are hoping a series of new treatments may delay the onset of symptoms. But some experts say progress hinges on Congress providing more research funding.

Obesity and Health

Bad eating habits, a sedentary lifestyle and ever-larger portions of food have conspired to make the United States the fattest nation on Earth. The National Institutes of Health estimates that 97 million American adults — 55 percent of the adult population — now are overweight or obese. Public health officials say that weight problems often lead to chronic diseases, such as diabetes and high blood pressure, and contribute to as many as 300,000 deaths annually. Dieting and more exercise are the two most obvious solutions. But many Americans who lack the time or will are turning to medically assisted weight loss and diet drugs that promise to melt away pounds without significant lifestyle changes. Few of the drugs have been rigorously tested, and some have proven dangerous.

Childhood Depression

White, middle-class boys vented their anger — and some say their depression — by committing mass murders at several suburban schools in recent years. Depression, which in boys can manifest itself as hostility and violence, is not only increasing but is also appearing in younger and younger children, some mental health specialists warn. Many experts argue for more school-based counselors, because untreated depression can disrupt a child's life or even lead to suicide. Others worry about the implications of providing mental health services in schools. Meanwhile, antidepressant prescriptions for youngsters have skyrocketed in recent years, raising concern that they are being overprescribed for children, sometimes without accompanying talk therapy.

Asthma Epidemic

Asthma, a chronic breathing disorder, is rapidly increasing in the United States and many other industrialized countries. Asthma affects more than 17 million Americans, including more than 5.3 million youngsters, and the incidence rate has nearly doubled since 1982. Experts disagree about the causes of the epidemic-like increase, but many now believe the most important factors are indoor air contaminants that trigger the allergic reaction associated with asthma attacks. Medications can relieve asthma symptoms and control the inflammation of the airways that causes asthma, but asthma advocates say some doctors are not aggressive enough in prescribing treatments. Meanwhile, researchers are looking for more effective treatments and trying to determine the origins of the disease in hope of finding a cure.

Vaccine Controversies

Immunization rates are at all-time highs, and once-dreaded childhood diseases like polio and diphtheria are at or near record lows. But growing numbers of parents and a small group of scientists question the safety of some vaccines, claiming they can cause severe adverse reactions. They also contend that vaccines shouldn't be mandatory for illnesses like chickenpox and hepatitis B — which are mild or rare in children — and that tests on the vaccines have been inadequate. In addition, some scientists say that producing genetically engineered vaccines without knowing the long-term side effects is foolhardy. But drugmakers and health officials say there is no proof of a causal relationship between vaccinations and severe adverse reactions and that maintaining public health demands widespread mandatory immunization.

POLICY IN A MANAGED–CARE ENVIRONMENT

Patients' Rights

The continuing growth of managed-care health plans is provoking a powerful backlash. Many patients say managed care makes it harder simply to see a doctor, let alone get insurance coverage for needed treatment. Doctors are also chafing under restrictions that limit the way they treat patients. The managed-care industry insists, however, that it is improving the quality of health care and slowing the rise in costs. More than 30 states have passed laws strengthening patients' rights in dealing with insurers. Congress continues to consider imposing new regulations on managed-care companies. Patient and consumer groups are pushing for reforms as part of so-called Patients' Bill of Rights legislation, but insurers' and employers' groups warn that the result may be higher premiums and more uninsured workers.

Managing Managed Care

The managed-care industry succeeded in holding down health costs for most of the 1990s but has come under unprecedented attack from critics, who charge that HMOs and similar plans have seriously compromised the quality of care by excessively focusing on their bottom lines. With public frustration building, lawmakers are proposing a variety of regulatory remedies to rein in the power of health insurers to make critical care decisions. Reform advocates say the proposals would empower consumers and allow doctors to deliver patient care without interference. But managed-care advocates contend that the proposals would succeed only in driving up the cost of health coverage. The net result, they say, would be more uninsured people and bigger bills for working Americans.

Medical Mistakes

Many more patients are hurt by medical mistakes than hospitals ever acknowledge. In fact, a recent report by the Institute of Medicine confirms what medical experts have long known: Medical errors kill more people every year than AIDS, breast cancer or car crashes. The IOM says that encouraging doctors to admit their mistakes could help hospitals prevent future errors. In February 2000, President Clinton urged the states to require the reporting of medical errors. But medical lobbyists and consumers are at odds over how public the reports should be. Consumer advocates and large employers, including General Motors, say hospitals should be required to report their mistakes publicly. But hospitals and doctors want their identities protected to avoid malpractice suits and to encourage candor.

THE FUTURE OF HEALTH POLICY

Embryo Research

The use of embryos and aborted fetuses in scientific research is again under scrutiny, thanks to the landmark isolation of primordial human embryonic stem cells. These "master cells" are capable of evolving into virtually every kind of tissue in the body and could be the key to cures for conditions such as Parkinson's disease and diabetes. They also offer a never-before-seen glimpse into the earliest stages of human development. But anti-abortion groups and other critics contend the privately funded work runs counter to a 1995 congressional ban on embryo research and want to bar taxpayer money from subsidizing the research, regardless of the potential benefits. Congress and the National Institutes of Health are trying to devise new guidelines and sidestep political minefields.

Human Genome Research

Deciphering most of the human genome — the collection of some 100,000 genes that contain the operating instructions for the human body — is expected to enable doctors to diagnose many diseases from a patient's genetic profile and treat or even prevent diseases by targeting the underlying genetic flaws. But revealing the genome's secrets also poses a host of legal and ethical concerns, including whether genetic information should be patented or kept in the public domain. Critics also worry about potential privacy violations, discrimination by insurers or employers seeking to exclude the genetically "flawed" and the psychological impact of genetic testing for incurable diseases.

Global AIDS Crisis

An estimated 34 million people around the world have AIDS or the HIV virus. Most of the victims are from the developing world, two-thirds of them from Africa. Many experts say the United States and other Western nations aren't doing enough to help. In particular, they fault drug companies for pricing AIDS drugs far out of the reach of Third World nations. Drugmakers say that they are helping, but they argue that expensive drugs won't do much good in countries that lack adequate hospitals and other health-care infrastructure. Experts also disagree over the best way to prevent the disease from spreading. Some advocate distributing condoms and promoting safe sex. But others say that only encourages promiscuous behavior and that health workers should stress sexual abstinence.

Computers and Medicine

Health-care providers, insurers, drug companies, and research institutions have initiated a massive transformation from a paper-based health-care system to one that increasingly relies on computers and the Internet. In addition, parents can download information from medical Web sites and fill prescriptions on-line. But experts say that the large-scale collection of patient information in cyberspace raises questions about access to the data. The privacy concerns are at the center of a broader debate over regulating the Internet. Many politicians, consumer groups, and regulators are calling for new security standards and guidelines for proper conduct in cyberspace. Meanwhile, the federal government is expected to release guidelines on access to medical databases.

Preface

Should vaccinations be mandatory for all children in the United States? Could Internet access to computerized health information compromise patient privacy? Is the spread of AIDS in the developing world a threat to the U.S.? From patients to practitioners to policymakers, everyone has a stake in the answers to these questions. But there are no easy answers, and *Issues in Health Policy* does not take sides or champion a particular perspective. Instead, balanced accounts allow instructors and students to thoroughly and fairly explore opposing sides of today's health care policy debates. In such areas as disease treatment and prevention, health care delivery systems, ethical dilemmas facing the medical and political communities and the effects of new technologies on health care policy, students will be challenged to weigh in and form their own opinions on these important issues.

This reader is a compilation of 12 recent articles from *The CQ Researcher*, a weekly policy brief that brings into focus the often complicated and controversial issues on the public agenda. *The CQ Researcher* makes complex issues easy to understand. Difficult concepts are not oversimplified but are explained in plain English. Offering in-depth, objective and forward-looking reporting on a specific topic, each selection chronicles and analyzes past legislative and judicial actions in addition to current and possible future maneuvering. *Issues in Health Policy* is designed to encourage discussion, to help readers think critically and actively about these vital issues and to facilitate future research. Adding color and depth to the study of the policy process, real-world examples give a flavor of the substantive detail in a variety of policy areas while showing how policy making at all levels of government—federal, state and local—affects students' lives and futures.

This collection is organized into three subject areas that cover a wide range of important health policy concerns. The pieces were chosen with an eye toward exposing students to a wide range of subjects, from the specific effects of illness and treatment to broader problems posed by health care delivery systems. We believe the volume will function as an attractive supplement for courses in health policy found in political science departments, policy and public administration programs and schools of public health.

The CQ Researcher

The CQ Researcher was founded in 1923 under a different moniker: *Editorial Research Reports*. ERR was sold primarily to newspapers, which used it as a research tool. The magazine was given its current name and a design overhaul in 1991. Today, *The CQ Researcher* is still sold to many newspapers, some of which reprint all or part of each issue. But the audience for the magazine has shifted significantly over the years, and today many more libraries subscribe. Students, not journalists, are now the primary audience for *The CQ Researcher*.

People who write for the *Researcher* often compare the experience to that of drafting a college term paper. Indeed, there are many similarities. Each article is as long as many term papers—running about 11,000 words—and is written by one person, without any significant outside help. Like students, staff writers begin the creative process by choosing a topic. Working with the publication's editors, the writer comes up with a subject that has public policy implications and for which there is at least some controversy. After a topic is set, the writer embarks on a week or two of intense research. Articles are clipped, books ordered and information gathered from a variety of sources, including interest groups, universities and the government. Once a writer feels well informed about the subject, he or she begins a series of interviews with experts—academics, officials, lobbyists and people actually working in the field. Each piece usually requires a minimum of ten to fifteen interviews. Some especially complicated subjects call for more. After much reading and interviewing, the writer begins to put the article together.

Chapter Format

Each issue of the *Researcher*, and therefore each selection in this book, is structured in the same way, beginning with an overview of the topic. This introductory section briefly touches on the areas that will be explored in greater detail in the rest of the chapter.

Following the introduction is a section that chronicles the important debates currently going on in the field. The section is structured around a number of questions, known as "issue questions," such as "Is the use of stem cells from embryos morally or ethically wrong?" or

"Could a surge of new Alzheimer's cases bankrupt the Medicare and Medicaid systems?" This section is the core of each selection: the questions raised are often highly controversial and usually the object of much argument among those who work and think in the field. Hence, the answers provided by the writer are never conclusive. Instead, each answer details the range of opinion within the field.

Following these questions and answers is the "Background" section, which provides a history of the issue being examined. This look back includes important legislative and executive actions and court decisions from the past. Readers will be able to see how current policy has evolved.

An examination of existing policy (under the heading "Current Situation") follows the background section. Each "Current Situation" provides an overview of important developments that were occurring when the article was published.

Each selection concludes with an "Outlook" section, which gives a sense of what might happen in the near future. This part looks at whether there are any new regulations afoot, anticipates court rulings and considers possible legislative initiatives.

All selections contain other regular features to augment the main text. Each selection has two or three sidebars that examine issues related to the topic. An "At Issue" page from two outside experts provides opposing answers to a relevant question. Also included are a chronology, which cites important dates and events, and an annotated bibliography, which details some of the sources used by the author of each article.

Acknowledgments

We wish to thank the many people who were so helpful in making this collection a reality. First is Tom Colin, editor of *The CQ Researcher*, who gave us his enthusiastic support and cooperation as we developed this collection. He and his talented staff of editors have amassed a first-class library of *Researcher* articles, and we are privileged to have access to that rich cache. We also thankfully acknowledge the advice and feedback from the scholars who commented on our plans for the volume. In particular, we thank David Sloane and LaVonna Blair at the University of Southern California, Sunday E. Ubokudom at the University of Toledo, Kay Hofer at Southwest Texas State University, Jonathan W. Engel at Seton Hall University, Lorrie Clemo at the State University of New York at Oswego and Jacqueline Angel at the University of Texas at Austin.

Some readers of this collection may be learning about *The CQ Researcher* for the first time. We expect that many readers will want regular access to this excellent weekly research tool. Anyone interested in subscription information or a no-obligation free trial of the *Researcher* can contact Congressional Quarterly at www.cq.com; at (800) 432-2250, ext. 279; or at (202) 887-6279.

We hope that you are as pleased with *Issues in Health Policy* as we are. We welcome your feedback and suggestions for future editions. Please direct comments to Charisse Kiino, in care of CQ Press, 1414 22nd Street, N.W., Washington, D.C. 20037, or by email at ckiino@cq.com.

—The Editors of CQ Press

1 Alzheimer's Disease

ADRIEL BETTELHEIM

Day after day, Cary Henderson felt Alzheimer's disease slowly stripping away his memory and intellect. So in the first years after he was diagnosed, the former history professor took special pleasure in doing the simple things he had once taken for granted: watching Duke University basketball on television, listening to his favorite symphonies, walking his beloved Yorkshire terrier.

But Henderson's inability to do simple day-to-day tasks frequently brought on panic and despair, like the time he couldn't remember how to use a can opener.

"My dog, precious little dog, of course, has to eat once in awhile and my wife was sleeping and I don't know how to open the can of dog food," Henderson recalled in a tape-recorded journal he kept at the beginning of his illness. *(See story, p. 4.)* "So the best I could do was to try to dig a hole, make a little perforation and see if I could extend the side of it — and it was something like a panic. . . . I had to find some way to get the doggie some food, but this was one of those things that you get into if you're going to have a life with Alzheimer's. . . . Maybe my wife, one of these hours, will be feeling better and she can really open the can. Right now the doggie seems to be in fairly good shape. I'm not too sure I am."

Experiences like the ones Henderson described are only the beginning of an irreversible slide into helplessness that ultimately robs Alzheimer's patients of the ability to walk, speak, eat solid food and even control their bladders.

It's a slide scientists and policy-makers say could become increasingly commonplace in the next century. With aging baby boomers expected to more than double the population of Ameri-

From *The CQ Researcher,*
May 15, 1998.

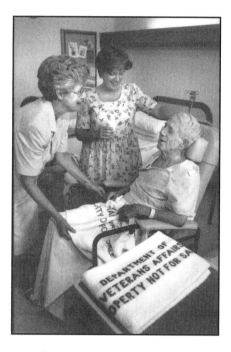

cans 65 and older by 2030, many experts are predicting a surge of new Alzheimer's cases that could psychologically and economically devastate families and strain the nation's health-care system.

An estimated 4 million Americans now suffer from some form of Alzheimer's. The General Accounting Office (GAO) estimates that after age 65, the prevalence of the disease in men and women doubles every five years. The Alzheimer's Association, a Chicago-based advocacy group for victims of the disease and their families, projects the total number of cases will reach 14 million by 2050 unless a cure is found.

Such an increase could bring about a significant financial squeeze for health care in the new millennium. The average annual cost of caring for Alzheimer's patients at home now stands at about $12,500. The annual bill for nursing-home care ranges from $42,000 to $70,000 in urban and suburban areas. With many Alzheimer's patients living 10 or more years after the initial diagnosis, families frequently exhaust most of their savings on medical care, even if they get

home-care benefits and other aid from Medicare, the federal-state health-care program for the elderly. Taxpayers then must step in and pay their future bills through Medicaid, the health-care program for the poor. [1]

"The only way we are truly going to save Medicare from bankruptcy when the baby boomers retire is to reduce the length and incidence of expensive illnesses like Alzheimer's," says Sen. Tom Harkin, D-Iowa, who contends Congress should head off what he calls "a ticking time bomb" by spending more to find a cure for the disease.

The Alzheimer's Association is lobbying Congress to spend $100 million more on Alzheimer's research next year to fund clinical trials on new treatments. The federal government has earmarked $349.2 million on preventing the disease this year, making Alzheimer's the fourth-most-funded affliction after cancer, HIV/AIDS and heart disease. *(See graph, p. 6.)*

However, many observers say Alzheimer's is only a small piece of a much larger health-care riddle and dismiss predictions it will single-handedly bankrupt entitlement programs. They say rising general health-care costs and the growing number of retirees in the coming decades are a far greater threat to the solvency of Medicare and Medicaid than any single disease.

"Projections of the frequency of a disease 30 years from now should be taken with a grain of salt," says Gail Wilensky, chairman of the federal Physician Payment Review Commission and a former deputy assistant to the president for policy development in the Bush administration. "We don't know how the frequency of other diseases will rise or fall, and how that will affect longevity. And even though medical research has brought increased longevity and quality-of-life improvements, it's difficult to prove it has saved us a lot of money."

The new concerns about Alzheimer's

Alzheimer's Cases Could Skyrocket

The number of Alzheimer's victims in the United States could skyrocket after 2030, when the first baby boomers hit age 85. People over 85 face the greatest risk of being incapacitated by Alzheimer's and needing long-term nursing care. About 4 million Americans are now afflicted with the disease.

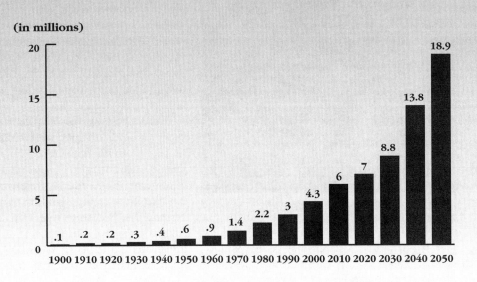

Americans age 85 and over

(in millions)

1900 .1, 1910 .2, 1920 .2, 1930 .3, 1940 .4, 1950 .6, 1960 .9, 1970 1.4, 1980 2.2, 1990 3, 2000 4.3, 2010 6, 2020 7, 2030 8.8, 2040 13.8, 2050 18.9

Source: "Report to Congress on the Scientific Opportunities for Developing Treatments for Alzheimer's Disease," June 1995; U.S. Census Bureau

breakdown of the brain chemical acetylcholine observed in Alzheimer's patients, though neither can restore memory or reverse the disease's pattern of killing brain cells.

There are no tests that can reliably predict who among the general population has Alzheimer's. Even the apparently straightforward act of estimating how many people have the condition has proven dicey because there's no single definition of Alzheimer's and the disease sometimes occurs in tandem with strokes and other neurological disorders.

Perhaps most ominously, Alzheimer's still suffers from the image of being an old person's disease. The commonly held, if rarely expressed, view is that devoting more money and effort to curing the disease will only prolong the life of very elderly people a few more years. Put another way: if you don't die of complications from Alzheimer's, you'll still die of something else. Even former President Ronald Reagan's 1994 announcement that he had the early stages of the disease didn't prompt a flood of new money for finding a cure.

"There's definitely some ageism at work," says John Morris, professor of neurology and co-director of the Alzheimer's disease research center at Washington University School of Medicine in St. Louis. "We kind of anticipate people are going to slip a bit in their older years, and we tolerate it until we

come at a time when significant advances in aging research are offering new hopes of finding a cure, or at least of forestalling symptoms. Scientists over the last decade have identified genetic mutations on four human chromosomes that can make a person more predisposed to Alzheimer's, providing important clues for how to detect the illness in its earliest stages.

Several promising therapies are also being tested, including administering megadoses of the anti-oxidant vitamin E to slow the progression of the disease. Other potential treatments include the use of estrogen replacement in postmenopausal women and administering anti-inflammatory drugs. [2]

"I'm very optimistic that in 10 years

we will be able to significantly alter the course of the disease," says Zaven Khachaturian, a Maryland neurobiologist and former director of Alzheimer's research at the National Institutes of Health. "It's more of a technical problem than a conceptual one; the key is finding a way to detect it early, years before the first symptoms are seen."

But such optimism is tempered by the vexing nature of the disease, which researchers admit they still aren't close to fully understanding. Despite federal expenditures of more than $3 billion on Alzheimer's research since 1976 scientists only have been able to develop two drugs approved by the Food and Drug Administration to treat the disease. Both have been found to temporarily delay the fast

have to provide care or there are be-havioral complications. As more baby boomers get older, we ought to find a way to indicate where the normal aging process differs from early dementia and build more interest."

Alzheimer's slowly robs memory and judgment through a still-unexplained pro-cess that kills neurons in the brain. The disease gets its name from Alois Alzheimer, a German neuropathologist who first observed severe memory lapses, paranoia and anxiety in a 51-year-old fe-male patient. When she died in 1906, Alzheimer examined her brain and found lesions and abnormal deposits of a sticky plaque outside and around the nerve cells. Masses of tangled fibers lined the inside of the cells. Even today, doc-tors rarely can make a definite diagnosis of Alzheimer's until an autopsy turns up those hallmarks of the dis-ease. However, they believe the disease can eat away at the brain for 20 years or longer before the first symp-toms of memory loss are noticed.

Despite the way it physically ravages the brain, Alzheimer's doesn't actually kill its victims. Patients can live 20 years or longer after an initial diagnosis, slowly losing the ability to carry out everyday tasks like reading a book or eating a meal. Sometimes they undergo significant personality changes, wander aimlessly and can turn violent. The patients often die of pneu-monia or other complications from their weakened condition.

The effects of the disease are nearly as devastating on the families of victims, who frequently move in with ailing loved ones only to watch their personalities and cognitive abili-ties slip away. Donna Lyttle, a Queens, N.Y., health-care program manager, moved in with her 76-year-old widowed mother, who has suf-fered from Alzheimer's for 11 years, instead of sending her to a nursing home. She spends evenings trying to make some contact.

"To look at her you'd think she's the picture of health, but there's just no response," says Lyttle, who esti-mates her mother's care costs $25,000 to $30,000 annually. "I talk to her and say, 'This is Donna,' and she looks at you like somewhere in the back of her mind she's seen the face before.

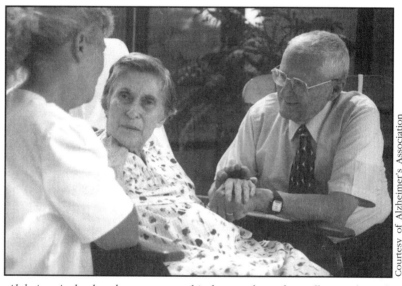

Alzheimer's slowly robs memory and judgment through a still-unexplained process that kills neurons in the brain.

Courtesy of Alzheimer's Association

But it's a distant look."

As scientists try to better under-stand the disease, and public policy experts debate how it will affect health-care in the 21st century, here are some questions they are asking:

Could a surge of new Alzheimer's cases bankrupt the Medicare and Medicaid programs?

What happened to Lynda Gormus of Richmond, Va., illustrates what some say is a looming crisis in long-term health care.

Gormus' 85-year-old father died in 1992 after an 11-year battle with Alzheimer's that exhausted most of the middle-class family's savings. Her 80-year-old mother now suffers from Parkinson's disease, seizures and a brain tumor. Gormus is trying to sell her parents' house to pay her mother's medical bills, which she says total about $2,100 a month. In the mean-time, she's negotiated a reduced-pay-ment schedule with the assisted-liv-ing center where her mother resides.

"Just dealing with the emotional part of it is tough, but it's real scary how quickly the funds go down," says Gormus, who works part time. "You think that you're not going to have problems, that old age is a way down the road. Then something like this happens, and the funds just aren't there."

The Gormus' story illustrates a perilous cycle in which mil-lions of Americans outlive their ability to take care of them-selves. Those with chronic conditions like Alzheimer's have to pay the majority of their long-term care costs out of pocket before they become poor enough to qualify for Medicaid. Their grown children often help pay the bills but, in the process, deplete their own savings. [3]

Medical care for Alzheimer's pa-tients typically is more expensive than for the elderly without cognitive prob-lems. Alzheimer's patients have trouble following directions for tak-ing medication, requiring nurses or other specialized care. Those who suffer from acute illnesses like heart

An Alzheimer's Journal

Familiar places like one's own home become foreign and difficult to navigate. A family get-together turns into a confusing jumble of sounds. There's a nagging fear of being belittled or cheated. Everyday items like eyeglasses are always being misplaced.

Alzheimer's patients experience such frustrations as the disease begins to eat away at their cognitive skills.

To help others understand their frustration and despair, social workers at the Duke University Center for Aging in Durham, N.C., asked some patients to keep journals during the early stages of the disease.

Cary Henderson, a former American history professor at James Madison University in Harrisonburg, Va., was diagnosed with Alzheimer's when he was 55. His physician first thought he had a rare disorder that can cause Alzheimer's-related symptoms but can be surgically corrected. Henderson's wife, Ruth, feared otherwise. At her urging, the neurologist removed a tiny amount of his brain tissue and performed a biopsy, confirming her suspicions. Henderson, thus, is one of the few living patients with an absolutely confirmed case of the disease.

Henderson kept his tape-recorded journal in 1991 and 1992, when he was in his early 60s. Portions of the journal were transcribed by Ruth and published in "The Caregiver," the newsletter of the Duke Family Support Program, in 1994. Henderson today is in the late stages of Alzheimer's and lives in an assisted-living facility. His complete journal will appear as a book, *Partial View*, to be published this fall by Southern Methodist University Press. Following are excerpts:

"Being dense is a very big part of Alzheimer's. And forgetting things. Although I'm not as bad as I sometimes am, it comes and goes. It's a very come-and-go disease. When I make a real blunder, I tend to get defensive about it — a sense of shame for not knowing what I should have known and for not being able to think things and see things that I saw several years ago when I was a normal person. But everybody by this time knows I'm not a normal person, and I'm quite aware of that.

"Whenever there's a gathering of people, it seems, at least in my mind, to be a lot of confusion. I just feel the need for quiet. I have to acknowledge the fact that for somebody like me, and I assume it's true of a lot of people with Alzheimer's, I can only think of one thing at a time. And large gatherings, whatever they may be, are very hard to understand. I really never quite know what is going on. As I've said before, I have not the vaguest idea about time, and after being a professor of history for 31 years, it's kind of weird to think I no longer have a sense of time and sense of change.

"With Alzheimer's you just know you're going to forget things, and it's impossible to put things where you can't forget them because people like me can always find a place to lose things, and we have to flurry all over the house to figure where in the heck I left whatever it was ... It's usually my glasses. No matter where I put my glasses, they don't seem to be in the right place at the right time. You've got to have a sense of humor in this kind of business, and I think it's interesting how many places I can find to lose things.

"With Alzheimer's people, there's no such thing as having a day which is like another day. Every day is separate, and you don't know what's going to happen in any one day or any other thing like that. It's as if every day you have never seen anything before like what you're seeing right now. It just never will be the same again. But you can't beat Mother Nature.

"One of the things, I guess, people like myself with Alzheimer's put up with is the fact that other people have to put up with us. I think this disease does make us kind of irrational — and sometimes it's out of fear and sometimes it's being left out of things ... I do think it's bad that we sometimes become almost afraid of ourselves and almost afraid of our caregivers and family ... I think for a lot of us the feeling of being cheated or belittled and somehow made jokes of, I think that's the one thing that is among the worst things about Alzheimer's.

"We have some music to start off with today. This is Mahler's 'Resurrection Symphony,' which I dearly love. It's a little bit loud, but sometimes, I actually feel that way. I want to shout. I want to raise some hell. I want to be somebody I'm not."

disease frequently are unable to detail their full medical histories to doctors, creating the need for expensive batteries of tests. The federal Health Care Financing Administration (HCFA) estimates per capita Medicare expenditures for Alzheimer's patients stand at $7,682, compared with $4,524 for non-Alzheimer's recipients. [4]

But Medicare and private insurance only cover a fraction of health-care costs for Alzheimer's sufferers. The federal program, created in 1965 to provide medical care for the aged, is heavily weighted to providing acute care. It doesn't pay for the long-term care that many Alzheimer's patients require unless there is a coexisting medical condition. Medicaid comes to the rescue if a patient is at least 65, blind or disabled and meets strict income and asset limitations. But that means the patient first must turn over a significant part of his life savings to the nursing home or other qualified care facility.

Demographics suggest the problem will only get worse in the next century. The U.S. Census Bureau estimates the number of Americans 85 and over, who are at the greatest risk of needing long-term care for Alzheimer's, will rise from 3 million in 1990 to 4.3 million by the turn of the century. By 2030, the number of the nation's "oldest old" citizens will total 8.8 million, and by 2050 the number will rise to 18.9 million.

"We're confronting this [flood of new cases] for the first time," says Stephen McConnell, vice president for public policy at the Alzheimer's Association. "At the turn of the century, life expectancy was in the mid-40s. One of the benefits of the advances in health-care and modern technology is people are living longer. The downside is we have diseases like Alzheimer's to contend with."

Congress spent much of 1995 and 1996 debating how to solve the problems with Medicaid and Medicare spending to head off a financial squeeze, proposing a series of measures that would affect long-term care for the elderly. One controversial proposal passed in 1996 and since changed would have made it a federal crime for the elderly to give away assets or personal property in order to become eligible for Medicaid—a proposal derided by critics as the "Send grandma to jail" law. [5]

More recently, Congress made sweeping changes to Medicare, encouraging the elderly to enroll in health maintenance organizations and other health plans like those offered by employers. Policy-makers also considered reducing payments to doctors and hospitals, increasing beneficiary cost-sharing and offering new alternatives to financing health-care, such as private medical savings accounts.

Joshua Wiener, a long-term care specialist with the Urban Institute's Health Policy Center in Washington, is skeptical of claims that more Alzheimer's cases will cripple the health-care system. He estimates inflation-adjusted spending on

long-term care will roughly double from 1993 and 2018, from $75.5 billion to $168.2 billion, adjusted for inflation. But assuming modest economic growth, that will only account for about 2.2 percent of the gross domestic product.

"It's a sizable increase, but I don't know if it's the end of civilization as we know it," Wiener says. "Long-term care for the Alzheimer's caseload would be easily manageable. The problem really is that Social Security and Medicare are also looking for additional revenues to help the same population—the elderly. Long-term care may be the last straw that breaks the camel's back."

Guy King, former chief actuary for HCFA, which administers Medicare and Medicaid, agrees. King says the Medicare program has already factored in rapidly aging baby boomers and projections of future Alzheimer's cases. The far bigger threat to the program's solvency is rising health-care costs and the growing number of retirees by the end of the next decade, King and others say.

King says Medicaid will be under more pressure from future Alzheimer's cases, though current projections only predict the state of the program five years ahead. "One of the problems with baby boomers is they have very low savings rates, in comparison to previous generations," King says. "It's going to be a problem, and the burden will fall on the program and their relatives."

Buying private long-term care insurance may be an option. The policies are expensive and aren't suited for everyone. But proponents say they can protect one's life savings if an Alzheimer's patient needs expensive care at home or in a nursing home. Employers have traditionally been reluctant to offer new long-term insurance because they already face millions of dollars of unfunded pension benefits.

Terms and prices of the private policies vary widely, and more than 100 companies sell them. The terms range from one year to as long as the patient needs. Coverage usually

specifies nursing home-care, home care or assisted living facilities, with comprehensive coverage, offering a choice of care arrangements, costing more. They also have significant deductible payments, meaning the policyholder will have to pay for a certain number of days of long-term care before the insurance kicks in.

Stephen Moses, spokesman for LTC Inc., a Seattle company that markets long-term care insurance, offers an example of a typical policy that costs $2,376 a year. A healthy 69-year-old man would get $96 a day for assisted living or $120 a day for nursing home care for four years (on average, people die 2 $\frac{1}{2}$ years after entering nursing homes). The plan has 5 percent inflation protection but the policyholder has to pay the cost of the first 100 days of long-term care himself, or $12,000 to $15,000 out of pocket. [6]

Health economist Wilensky says it's worthwhile for people to save their money or buy long-term care insurance in a society where personal savings are low. However, she notes, "It's tricky to get people to focus on something 10 to 20 years down the road, unless they're already focused on the problem because they have a relative with Alzheimer's."

Are researchers close to finding an effective treatment for Alzheimer's disease?

Until the 1960s, scientists viewed Alzheimer's disease as one of those unexplained byproducts of aging — if they thought about the disease at all. There was understandably little cause for concern. At the time Alzheimer made his first diagnosis, only one in 25 Americans lived beyond 65.

But increasing life expectancy and rapid advances in molecular biology in the 1970s allowed scientists to begin to understand the biological underpinnings of the disease. Research is now progressing in several directions: un-

Research Funding a Recent Phenomenon

Scientific breakthroughs and increased public awareness led the federal government to begin funding Alzheimer's research in the 1970s. Today it is the fourth most funded affliction, after cancer, HIV/AIDS and heart disease.

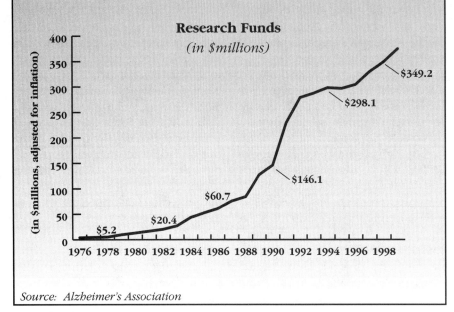

Research Funds
(in $millions)

$349.2

$298.1

$146.1

$60.7

$20.4

$5.2

Source: Alzheimer's Association

derstanding how mutant genes make some people predisposed to the disease; finding ways to slow the progression of its symptoms; and trying to identify precisely when Alzheimer's first begins in the brain.

"We have to work on all these different avenues at once because we don't know which will lead fastest to a cure," says Marcelle Morrison-Bogorad, associate director of the neuroscience of aging program at the National Institute on Aging in Bethesda, Md. "We understand how the liver and heart work, but the brain is so incredibly complex that if we waited to know every little bit before we tried to slow the progression of the disease, the public wouldn't thank us."

On the genetics front, researchers over the last six years have identified a series of mutations on genes that are believed to make a person more susceptible to the disease, though the presence of one doesn't always give rise to the condition. The presence of a num-

ber of biological markers has led some to speculate Alzheimer's actually may not be a single disease but a group of closely related disorders.

One important development came in 1992 when biologists at Duke University in Durham, N.C., identified a variant of the gene responsible for creating the chemical apolipoprotein in patients who developed the most common form of "late-onset" Alzheimer's. Apolipoprotein normally carries blood cholesterol throughout the body. But researchers believe the suspect gene, known as apoE4, may contribute to the buildup of the abnormal protein plaques that strangle brain cells in Alzheimer's patients. The gene also may lower the age at which patients begin to suffer the onset of the disease. ApoE4 is found in about 40 percent of all late-onset Alzheimer's cases. [7]

Genetic screening for the mutation could someday help scientists find people with markers for the disease

to include in clinical trials of new drugs. Indeed, a simple blood test can turn up the presence of apoE4 or two other common Alzheimer's-related mutations. But some researchers say there's little point to screening until a preventive treatment for Alzheimer's is available. Moreover, testing could cause unintended harm, exposing those who test positive to discrimination in obtaining insurance or healthcare and causing unnecessary anxiety in people who have the gene but don't develop the disease. The American Association for Geriatric Psychiatry, the Alzheimer's Association and the American Geriatrics Society issued a consensus statement last year, declaring testing may not prove useful in diagnosing dementia patients. [8]

The difficulty of linking the disease with a single gene was illustrated in March, when researchers at Columbia University in New York examined different ethnic and racial groups' chances of getting the disease. The team reported blacks and Hispanics who carry the apoE4 gene are about as likely as whites to get the disease by the time they reach age 90. But blacks without the suspect gene are at four times the risk of contracting Alzheimer's, and Hispanics who lack the gene variation are at more than twice the risk. The findings suggest other genes or environmental circumstances are at work in minority populations. [9]

While researchers sort out various risk factors, they also are looking for new ways to forestall symptoms of the disease. Most involve shoring up brain cells by boosting their energy or blood supply with commonly used substances. Most of the agents have already been approved by the FDA for use in humans, making the treatment much cheaper than developing completely new drugs.

The most battle-tested regimen so far may be the anti-oxidant vitamin E, given alone in 2,000-unit megadoses

Mystery of "Hexed" Russian Villagers Solved

Most Alzheimer's patients develop the so-called "late-onset" form of the disease, which strikes at random in people age 65 and over. But there are scattered cases of a faster-spreading version that can develop in individuals as young as their mid-30s and appears to run in families.

Scientists over the last six years have pinpointed mutations on any one of three genes that, if present in an individual, almost always result in familial, or early-onset, Alzheimer's. The high predictability gives researchers an unusual opportunity to explore how the disease manifests itself in the brain and how genes may affect when a person develops symptoms.

"The reason we focus on it is because [the high predictability makes it] the path of least resistance," says Gerard Schellenberg, a geneticist at the Veterans Affairs Medical Center in Seattle, who helped discover the genetic links. "People get it early in life and usually die before there are complications from other chronic diseases; the mechanism for the disease is basically the same as late-onset Alzheimer's."

Researchers at the University of Washington began to explore the condition in the mid-1980s after discovering it in five families that all traced their ancestry to ethnic Germans who settled in Russia's Volga Valley in the 18th century. Some of the families emigrated to the United States between 1870 and 1920.

Descendents told researchers that residents in the Volga villages of Walter and Frank were said to be bewitched, hexed or possessed. Follow-up studies on four more families with identical ties led the Washington researchers to conclude the "hexing" was evidence of Alzheimer's-like dementia. The geneticists said the villages likely experienced a "founder effect" — essentially all of the residents were distant blood relatives who inherited an Alzheimer's gene from some unknown common ancestor who lived centuries ago.

"Germans from Russia as a group aren't any more predisposed to Alzheimer's than anyone else," says University of Washington neurologist Tom Bird. "But people from these two villages were essentially all distant cousins with a predisposition for the trait."

Similar cases have turned up elsewhere, such as the small farming community of Harvey, in New Brunswick, Canada. Barb Hatfield, 42, grew up in the town and lost her mother to Alzheimer's-related symptoms when she was 56. Hatfield's maternal grandmother, three maternal aunts and an uncle also died from the disease. Some of her mother's first cousins now suffer from Alzheimer's.

"My mom would never talk about it. She literally would only say, 'She lost her mind' and that was the end of the conversation," Hatfield recalled.[1] "I can remember many times wishing it was some normal disease like cancer or something. This was something nobody understood."

The suspect mutations linked to the condition arise in the genes that code for the proteins presinilin 1 and 2 and amyloid precursor protein. Carriers of the mutation for presinilin 1 and amyloid precursor protein are practically guaranteed to get Alzheimer's before they turn 60, Schellenberg says.

People carrying the mutation for presinilin 2 tend to develop Alzheimer's at middle age but sometimes don't develop the condition until well into their 70s. Scientists want to study the gene more to understand how chemical changes may influence when the disease strikes.

Early-onset Alzheimer's is a particularly cruel version of the disease that strikes in the prime of life and moves quickly, destroying brain cells and leading to patient deaths in six to eight years, compared with 10 or more years in late-onset Alzheimer's.

Some researchers have used gene coding for the amyloid precursor protein to breed laboratory mice with the mutation causing early-onset symptoms. The animals have provided convenient models for observing when the characteristic Alzheimer's plaques form in brains and how they kill neurons.

"We're much closer to finding a cure," said Linda Nee, a geneticist at the National Institutes of Health, who has studied the New Brunswick villagers. "We've come light years from where we started because the technology has improved so much."[2]

---

[1] Quoted in Chris Morris, "Family Curse Key to Medical Mystery? Village's High Incidence of Alzheimer's Leads to Major Study," *Toronto Star*, March 27, 1998, p. F6.

[2] *Ibid.*

---

or in combination with selegiline, a prescription drug used to treat Parkinson's disease. A research team led by Mary Sano, a biologist at Columbia University's College of Physicians and Surgeons in New York, conducted clinical trials on 341 patients and reported last year that memory loss and cognitive problems were slowed by about seven months in test groups of patients who took the drugs compared with those who received no medicine.[10]

The results could explain how antioxidants like vitamin E and selegiline eradicate toxic substances known as "free radicals" that contribute to the breakdown of brain cells. However, the drugs didn't improve patients' scores on cognitive tests as compared with untreated patients. Skeptics said the treatment may only have affected patients' behavior but not the underlying disease.

Another prospective treatment is estrogen, a hormone credited with helping prevent heart disease and osteoporosis that also can influence the levels and function of several brain chemicals—seratonin, dopamine and acetylcholine—linked to Alzheimer's.

Scientists at Johns Hopkins University in Baltimore and the National Institute on Aging reported last year that estrogen-replacement therapy halved the risk of Alzheimer's in a control group of 472 menopausal and post-menopausal women that was observed over 16 years. But researchers still don't know how the hormone affects memory or what effect decades of missing estrogen has on the female body, let alone the brain.

The therapy also can present dangerous side effects, such as increased risk of stroke. Richard Mayeux, professor of neurology, psychiatry and public health at Columbia University, regards the hormone as an "effective primary or secondary treatment" that, taken in conjunction with other drugs, acts as a kind of nerve-growth factor that makes neurons survive better and longer. [11]

Clinicians have also reported success administering regular doses of ibuprofen and other anti-inflammatory drugs on Alzheimer's patients to improve blood flow in the brain. Even the plant extract Ginkgo biloba has been shown to have some therapeutic effects in limited clinical trials and has been approved for the treatment of dementia in Germany.

Scientists acknowledge that knowing Alzheimer's symptoms without knowing the true cause of the disease makes their efforts look somewhat scattershot and uncoordinated. But neurobiologist Khachaturian draws comparisons to early efforts to treat polio in the 1940s and '50s. The first treatments for the disabling disease centered around providing care and easing pain. Only later did research lead to a vaccine that finally eliminated the disease.

"As scientists develop new drugs, they pursue leads that will shed light on the causes of the disease," he says. "You can always look at the empty portion of the glass, but I prefer to look at the current situation more positively. It's half full."

Should Congress and the White House earmark more money for Alzheimer's research?

"I cannot bear to see anyone I love go through this ever again," David Hyde Pierce, who stars as Dr. Niles Crane in the television show "Frasier," told a House Appropriations subcommittee in January, as he recalled how his grandfather succumbed to Alzheimer's. "If we do not find a way to prevent it soon, Alzheimer's will be the epidemic of the 21st century." [12]

Pierce was one of 20 witnesses to come before the panel, seeking more money for various scientific research and education programs. In what has become a familiar Washington scene, celebrities with personal connections to diseases join forces with advocacy groups to lobby Congress to earmark funds for certain afflictions in annual spending bills.

Pierce and the Alzheimer's Association are pressing for $100 million more in research money in fiscal 1999. It would mark the first significant increase in Alzheimer's funding since 1991, when annual spending jumped 57 percent, to $229.8 million. That increase was largely due to the efforts of a lawmaker with a personal connection to the disease — former Sen. Mark O. Hatfield, R-Ore., then ranking Republican on the powerful Senate Appropriations Committee, whose father died of Alzheimer's-related complications.

Alzheimer's research funding has increased modestly since then, despite wider public awareness of disease after former President Reagan's announcement that he had the condition. The current $349.2 million funding level lags well behind the approximately $1 billion spent annually on heart disease and $1.5 billion a year spent on HIV/

AIDS. Cancer research receives by far the largest targeted spending — approximately $3.1 billion a year. [13]

Congress in recent years has been reluctant to target certain diseases over others, preferring to let NIH make the choices. Most lawmakers, aware there isn't enough money to please everyone, don't want to risk appearing insensitive to certain groups of chronic disease sufferers.

"Congress' role has been one of appropriation and oversight, not micromanagement of disease research," says Rep. John Edward Porter, R-Ill., chairman of the House Appropriations Subcommittee on Labor, Health and Human Services and Education to which Pierce delivered his testimony.

Porter and others opposing earmarks for specific diseases argue that NIH administrators closest to the labs are in the best position to decide how money should be spent. Targeting more money toward a specific disease also ignores the interdisciplinary nature of research, they say. For instance, research on infectious particles called prions that have been linked to so-called "mad cow" disease also are shedding new light on brain damage in Alzheimer's and may provide a foundation for new drugs.

But other lawmakers say Congress should play a greater role in dictating basic research priorities. A few like Rep. Ernest Istook, R-Okla., have openly criticized NIH for playing politics and spending heavily on HIV/AIDS research while not devoting more resources to conditions with higher incidence, including cancer, Alzheimer's and heart disease.

"Whether you analyze it by the number of patients, a per death basis, a cost-per-patient basis or any other common-sense way, our research dollars are not being spent where they could do the most good," Istook says. [14]

Harkin, whose home state of Iowa

has one of the largest percentages of residents 85 and over, takes a different tack, saying spending more on new Alzheimer's treatments like vitamin E will save money decades later. Harkin cites studies by the American Federation for Aging Research showing that delaying the onset of Alzheimer's even five years could save as much as $260 billion in health-care costs each year. In contrast, a clinical trial on a promising drug costs $1-$2 million.

"For years, the focus of research has been to identify a cure or a way to prevent [Alzheimer's]. Delaying the onset holds great hope and could bring more immediate results than traditional means," Harkin says.

But the notion of bigger research budgets and targeted spending doesn't sit well with everyone. Daniel Callahan, director of international programs at the Hastings Center, a bioethics think tank in Garrison, N.Y., argues American society and the medical industry are on an endless quest to conquer all diseases and should recognize the finiteness of the human condition. The more progress that is made against disorders that strike earlier in life, the harder it will be to tackle those that emerge at later ages, he says.

"We can shuffle the causes of death, and we can live longer in the process. But death is still waiting in hiding for all of us, eventually to make its appearance," Callahan writes in his new book, *False Hopes: Why America's Quest for Perfect Health Is a Recipe for Failure*. Chronic diseases, such as cancer, heart disease, Alzheimer's and kidney failure, "will continue to take thousands of lives. In the diseases of aging, we seem to be up against some formidable biological barriers." ∎

BACKGROUND

An Ancient Evil

Alzheimer's disease is hardly a new condition. The ancient Greeks and Romans occasionally described symptoms resembling Alzheimer's and other forms of dementia. Among the chroniclers was the Greek playwright Sophocles, who in the fifth century B.C. observed: "All evils are ingrained in long old age, with vanished, useless actions, empty thoughts."

Centuries later, William Shakespeare wrote about very old age as a time of

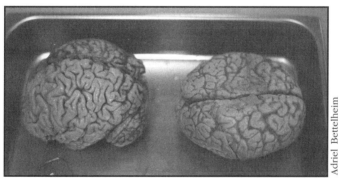

The brain of an Alzheimer's victim, left, shows marked atrophying compared with a normal brain. (Oregon Brain Bank, Oregon Health Sciences University; National Museum of Health and Medicine, Armed Forces Institute of Pathology)

Adriel Bettelheim

"second childishness and mere oblivion." Toward the end of the play, Shakespeare's King Lear laments to his daughter Cordelia: "I am a very foolish fond old man/Fourscore and upward, not an hour more or less/And, to deal plainly/I fear I am not in my perfect mind."

Though symptoms were easily noticed, few people bothered to explore the causes of dementia, often assuming it was an irreversible consequence of aging and "hardening of the arteries." Additionally, so few people lived to the age at which dementia of the Alzheimer's type

usually strikes that the disorder rated scant public attention.

That began to change in the mid-1800s, when British psychiatrist James Pritchard outlined stages in the progression of dementia, from memory impairment to the loss of reason, incomprehension and the loss of instinctive action. French psychiatrist Jean Etienne Dominique Esquirol coined the term "senile dementia" in 1838, writing in his book *Des Maladies Mentales* that the disease progresses slowly, weakening sensations and slowly robbing sufferers of their impulses and will.

Alzheimer's Discovery

The disease finally received a name and a firm definition of the symptoms in November 1906, when German neuropathologist Alzheimer described the case of a 51-year-old female patient to a meeting of the South West Germany Society of Neurologists. The woman, known as Auguste D., suffered from fits of paranoid jealousy, anxiety and disturbing memory lapses. Alzheimer tracked her condition for four years and, upon her death, autopsied her brain tissue, finding the distinctive lesions that are now a telltale sign of the disease.

Some of Alzheimer's contemporaries suspected he misdiagnosed Auguste D., and that she instead suffered from a rare metabolic disorder called metachromatic leukodystrophy. Earlier this year, scientists uncovered slides containing long-lost samples of her brain tissue in a basement at the University of Munich and retested them. They confirmed she, indeed, suffered from classic Alzheimer's. [15]

Because Alzheimer's patient was relatively young, most of the scientific community dismissed his report on Auguste D. as a rare case of pre-senile dementia and forgot about it. Interest was rekindled only after British researchers in the 1960s compared autopsied brain tissues from relatively young and elderly dementia sufferers and found in both the classic pathologic signs of the disease: plaques (the dense protein deposits that surround brain cells) and neurofibrillary tangles (the twisted strands inside the cells). The presence of the same abnormalities in two types of patients suggested the disease was more widespread than previously thought.

The physical scars come from the way the disease destroys neurons in parts of the brain that control memory. The damage occurs when neurons congregate and form protein masses called amyloids that are water-soluble in normal brains but undergo structural changes and can't be dissolved in Alzheimer's patients. The masses disrupt nerve cell functions and begin to cause symptoms such as the loss of short-term memory. Gradually the damage spreads to the cerebral cortex, which controls language and reasoning. As more nerve cells die, patients begin to lose their language skills and judgment and sometimes become easily agitated.

The deterioration of the brain is accompanied by a drop-off in the production of the neurotransmitter acetylcholine, which plays a key role in cognitive functioning. The two FDA-approved drugs that have been developed to combat Alzheimer's — tacrine (Cognex) and donepezil hydrochloride (Aricept) — can temporarily boost acetylcholine levels in mild to moderate cases, though they can't reverse the progression of the disease.

It's unclear whether the amyloid plaques actually cause Alzheimer's disease or result from some process in the development of the disease. Other possible causes, or contributing factors, include head injuries and abnormally high concentrations of calcium brought on by metabolic

Former President Ronald Reagan greets a visitor to the Ronald Reagan Presidential Library in July 1997, three years after he announced he had Alzheimer's.

imbalances. Recent research in Britain and Norway found groups of Alzheimer's patients had higher blood levels of the amino acid homocysteine — a condition that can be treated with a dietary supplement of folic acid and vitamin B12.

U.S. Launches Program

As the long-term implications of the disease became clear in the 1970s, federal officials realized that finding an effective treatment or cure should be made a priority. The National Institute on Aging launched an Alzheimer's program in 1978 and now devotes approximately half of its budget to improving screening for the disease and developing therapies.

Prompted by the federal effort, seven private caregiver organizations combined in 1980 to form the Alzheimer's Disease and Related Disorders Association, since renamed the Alzheimer's Association. The Chicago-based nonprofit has grown from a fledgling organization with an $85,000 annual budget into a prominent health-care lobbying group, with 200 chapters and a budget of nearly $100 million. It promotes scientific research and lobbies Congress for long-term health care, nursing home reform and respite care for family members of Alzheimer's victims.

Reagan's Dramatic Disclosure

The steadily building interest in Alzheimer's reached new heights on Nov. 5, 1994, when former President Ronald Reagan disclosed he had been diagnosed as suffering from early stages of the disease. Reagan, then 83, said the diagnosis indicated he had begun "the journey that will lead me into the sunset of my life."

In a handwritten letter released by his Los Angeles office, Reagan said he had experienced acute memory loss and other Alzheimer's symptoms for about a year. He said he decided to make his condition public to increase awareness of the disease. Reagan joined a list of high-profile

Chronology

1900s *The pathological signs of Alzheimer's disease in the human brain are described for the first time.*

November 1906
German neuropathologist Alois Alzheimer details his findings about the disease that now bears his name.

——— • ———

1970s *New research makes the American public aware that Alzheimer's is a disorder, not simply a natural part of the aging process.*

1976
British researchers report that levels of the neurotransmitter acetylcholine fall sharply in people with Alzheimer's disease. The National Institutes of Health (NIH) and other federal agencies with interest in the aging brain subsequently stress the importance of distinguishing between Alzheimer's and other forms of dementia.

——— • ———

1980s *Government funding of Alzheimer's research increases while various studies report progress establishing causes of the disease.*

1980
Families, physicians and health-care professionals across the country meet at NIH and form the Alzheimer's Disease and Related Disorders Association. The group, since renamed the Alzheimer's Association, is now based in Chicago.

October 1984
The National Institute on Aging (NIA) announces the establishment of five Alzheimer's disease research centers.

1986
President Ronald Reagan signs into law the Alzheimer's Disease and Related Dementias Services Research Act, which establishes a council on Alzheimer's disease in the U.S. Department of Health and Human Services.

November 1989
On the basis of a study of elderly people living in East Boston, Mass., the NIA estimates that 4 million Americans have some form of Alzheimer's — nearly twice the previous estimate.

——— • ———

1990s *New studies reveal Alzheimer's has multiple causes as public interest and research efforts intensify.*

1990
Congress approves a 57 percent funding increase for Alzheimer's research for fiscal 1991, to $229.8 million, as Sens. Mark O. Hatfield, R-Ore., and Tom Harkin, D-Iowa, argue the disease represents a looming public health crisis.

1992
Researchers at Duke University find an increased risk for the common "late-onset" Alzheimer's in patients over age 65 who inherit the apoE4 gene on chromosome 19. NIA-affiliated scientists also uncover evidence of a defective gene on chromosome 14 that leads to a rarer inherited form of Alzheimer's.

1993
The Food and Drug Administration approves the sale of tacrine (Cognex), the first prescription drug to treat early and middle stages of Alzheimer's. Congress creates the "Safe Return" program, a public-private effort to locate Alzheimer's patients who wander and become lost.

Nov. 5, 1994
Former President Ronald Reagan, 83, announces he has been diagnosed with Alzheimer's disease after suffering acute memory loss and other symptoms for about a year.

1996
The FDA approves donepezil hydrochloride (Aricept), another drug to treat Alzheimer's symptoms. An international panel of neuroscientists develops new guidelines for definitively diagnosing Alzheimer's at autopsy.

1997
Alzheimer's researchers report commonly available substances may delay the onset of Alzheimer's. Columbia University-led clinical trials show megadoses of vitamin E and the prescription drug seligiline can delay symptoms of Alzheimer's by about seven months. Johns Hopkins University researchers report a 16-year study shows estrogen may slow the disease in post-menopausal women.

1998
The Alzheimer's Association presses for a $100-million increase in funding for Alzheimer's research. NIA researchers focus on identifying people at risk of Alzheimer's before they develop any signs of the disease.

Sometimes It Isn't Alzheimer's

Alzheimer's disease is often confused with other neurological conditions that also cause memory loss and behavioral changes and impair reasoning. Doctors must administer a battery of physical and mental tests and consult with family members before making a diagnosis. Conditions that cause Alzheimer's-like symptoms include:

Depression — A common affliction among the elderly, especially those with physical problems. Symptoms include sadness, inactivity, difficulty thinking and concentrating and feelings of despair. Depressed persons often have trouble sleeping, experience changes in appetite, fatigue and agitation. Depression can often be treated with drugs such as Prozac that affect concentrations of brain chemicals known as neurotransmitters.

Delirium — A state of temporary but acute mental confusion that comes on suddenly. Symptoms may include anxiety, disorientation, tremors, hallucinations, delusions and incoherence. Delirium can occur in older persons who have short-term illnesses, heart or lung disease, long-term infections, poor nutrition or hormone disorders. Alcohol or drugs, including medications, also may cause confusion.

Parkinson's disease — A degenerative nerve disease that causes rhythmic tremors of the hands and other parts of the body, spastic motion of the eyelids and a bent-over posture. Patients have trouble walking and take slow, shuffling footsteps. More than a half-million Americans suffer from the condition, which is caused by a deficit of a chemical messenger in the brain called dopamine. Doses of the medication L-dopa can help, but they often lose their effectiveness over time.

Huntington's disease — An inherited brain disorder that leads to progressive deterioration of physical and mental capabilities. Symptoms include uncontrollable nervous movements of parts of the body, an abnormal gait, slurred speech, difficulty swallowing, cognitive difficulties and personality changes. The condition has been linked to a gene on chromosome 4.

Pick's disease — A relatively rare, hard-to-diagnose neurological disorder usually confined to the frontal lobes of the brain. Unlike Alzheimer's, the disease usually strikes people between ages 40 and 60, and death follows after five to six years. Another difference from Alzheimer's is that personality changes are observed before memory loss. New cases of Pick's are rare after 60.

Creutzfeldt-Jacob disease — A rare disorder caused by a viral-type organism called a prion. Onset typically takes place around age 50, with symptoms including personality changes, loss of coordination, dementia, muscle tremors and rigid posture. The loss of brain function with the telltale presence of lesions in cerebral tissue is similar to Alzheimer's but progresses faster. The disease can be caused by tissue transplants and also is believed to be heritable in some families.

Multi-infarct dementia — The second most common form of dementia in older persons, after Alzheimer's. Multi-infarct dementia is caused by a series of strokes that damage or destroy brain tissue. The strokes may be so tiny that the first few produce no observable symptoms. Gradually, victims may exhibit forgetfulness, incontinence and emotional problems and get lost in familiar places. Those most at-risk are between ages 60 and 75. Men are slightly more likely to develop the condition than women. High blood pressure, diabetes and high blood cholesterol are important risk factors.

Sources: National Institute on Aging, Alzheimer's Association.

---

victims that includes actress Rita Hayworth, humorist E. B. White, illustrator Norman Rockwell, former middleweight and welterweight boxing champion Sugar Ray Robinson and former Metropolitan Opera General Manager Sir Rudolf Bing.

"Unfortunately, as Alzheimer's disease progresses, the family often bears a heavy burden," Reagan wrote. "I only wish there was some way I could spare Nancy from this painful experience. When the time comes I am confident that with your help she will face it with faith and courage."

Dueling Statistics

Establishing reliable estimates of just how many people suffer from Alzheimer's has been problematic. Researchers in the 1970s and '80s relied on surveys of specialized-care facilities, psychiatric hospitals and nursing homes to arrive at a generally accepted population of 2 million to 2.5 million sufferers nationwide.

In 1989, a group of Boston-area researchers took a different approach, administering simple memory tests to 3,811 residents age 65 and over in the working-class community of East Boston. More elaborate clinical tests were then administered as a follow-up to 467 of the individuals to rule out other causes of mental impairment. After calculating the data, the researchers concluded that 10.3 percent of elderly East Boston residents probably had Alzheimer's disease.

By extrapolating the numbers to the entire United States, the researchers concluded the current Alzheimer's population stands at approximately 4 million patients, effectively doubling the accepted estimate. They further projected the number of Alzheimer's patients would rise to as high as 14.3 million by 2050, with the most significant increases coming in people age 85 and over. From 1980 to 2050, the researchers said the number of Alzheimer's patients in that age group would rise almost sevenfold, from 1.02 million to 7.07 million. [16]

The researchers cautioned that their numbers could be low because they only surveyed non-institutionalized people. But many public policy analysts and medical researchers embraced the study in succeeding years, crediting it with sounding the alarm about rising Alzheimer's caseloads. The National Institute on Aging, among others, began using the group's 4 million estimate of current patients.

"[The study is] likely to be disturbing to the general public, given the widespread fear of Alzheimer's disease, and should receive the careful attention of health planners and physicians: the fastest growing segment of our population is this same group of persons more than 85 years old," the *Journal of the American Medical Association* said in an editorial. [17]

Early this year, the U.S. General Accounting Office threw some cold water on the estimates after analyzing 18 published studies of Alzheimer's prevalence. Using a statistical analysis, the GAO concluded only 1.9 million Americans 65 and older suffered from some level of the disease. The agency said the population would likely rise to 2.1 million if one counted cases of Alzheimer's combined with other dementia and instances where some patients slipped through the screening process.

The National Institute on Aging dis-puted the numbers, saying the GAO relied on 15 studies of Alzheimer's patients outside of the United States that may have used different diagnostic criteria. Institute director Richard Hodes said NIH was trying to arrive at accurate estimates of its own, including studies of various racial and ethnic minority populations that have largely been left out of earlier surveys.

"An accurate estimate of Alzheimer's prevalence in the U.S. is important, but it is even more important that policy-makers and public health officials improve their understanding of the differences in prevalence among populations in the U.S.," Hodes says. ■

Researchers in Boston estimate there are now 4 million Alzheimer's sufferers in the United States and could be 14 million by 2050.

Courtesy of Alzheimer's Association

CURRENT SITUATION

Diagnosing Dementia

How does one establish whether a person has Alzheimer's disease? Short of directly obtaining a sample of brain tissue, clinicians have to rely on memory tests, physical evaluations and personal accounts from patients' relatives. There is no widely accepted screening test in use for the general population.

A group of Vermont psychologists is trying to change that with a seven-minute word-and-picture test they claim is 90 percent accurate in identifying patients with early Alzheimer's. The results of a study of the test given to 120 people were published in March in the *Archives of Neurology*. [18]

"The judgment we can make is that someone is performing in a way that is entirely normal or that they have a dementia characteristic of Alzheimer's disease," says Paul Solomon, co-director of the Southwestern Vermont Medical Center memory clinic and a psychologist at Williams College in Williamstown, Mass.

The study involved 60 patients who had been referred to the Vermont clinic because of a suspected problem and 60 people with no known memory problems. Examiners who administered the test — consisting of four short quizzes and a clock test — did not know which patients had memory problems. The test correctly identified 13 of 13 patients known to have early Alzheimer's. A follow-up study on another 800 people has shown similarly encouraging results but has yet to be published, according to Solomon.

The quizzes examine a patient's ability to recall sets of flash cards in 16 different categories just moments after they are displayed. Patients who can't recall everything are provided with reminder words as prompts. The reminders help non-Alzheimer's patients but don't help people with the disease. Patients are also asked to draw a clock face with all 12 numbers in the proper place, and to arrange the hands to show the time of 20 minutes to four. Patients with memory problems will leave out numbers or arrange the hands incorrectly.

Researchers say such tests could be useful diagnostic tools if they can be proven to work consistently on very large populations. But they note the new test can't distinguish between Alzheimer's patients and people who suffer memory lapses from other diseases — and have to be tested on much larger populations to be validated. "None of the existing tests, to my mind, can reliably predict who has Alzheimer's," says Washington University neurologist Morris.

The difficulty of assessing who has the disease can also be compounded by cultural attitudes toward mental illness in some ethnic groups. Sue Levkoff, associate professor in the department of social medicine at Harvard University Medical School, spent four years studying how African-American, Latino and Asian communities in Boston dealt with Alzheimer's-like dementia. Many resisted seeking medical care for ailing relatives, regarding Alzheimer's and similar diseases as a normal product of aging.

"There's a certain inability to admit there's a problem that could require someone to go to a nursing home," Levkoff says. "There are communities [particularly Asian and His-

panic] where not directly caring for family is viewed as a stigma."

Ethnic Differences in Seeking Treatment

Levkoff says she found different rationalizations for not seeking medical help. Some Chinese families she studied believe the body is something akin to a machine, and parts naturally begin to break down. Latinos were more apt to view the condition as the outcome of failings, such as the family not treating the

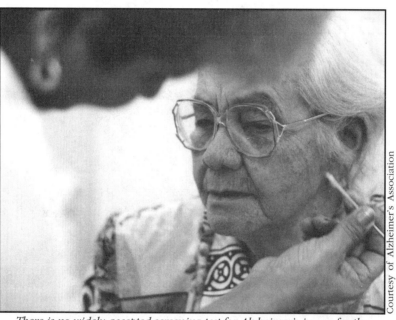

There is no widely accepted screening test for Alzheimer's in use for the general population. Clinicians have to rely on memory tests, physical evaluations and personal accounts from patients' relatives.

Courtesy of Alzheimer's Association

mother well. African-Americans tended to turn to the Bible, though they didn't necessarily seek out support from their church. Most of the time, a doctor's visit was only considered after patients began to display disturbing behavioral problems.

Science is gradually providing more precise ways to diagnose the disease, even though the most advanced imaging techniques still can't turn up the characteristic plaques and tangles that reside deep in the brain.

Investigators at the General Clinical Research Center at the New England Medical Center in Boston have used magnetic-resonance imaging to diagnose older patients with Alzheimer's by looking for lower blood volume in parts of their brains.

Other physicians are focusing on brain structures that can be damaged by the disease in its early stages. Johns Hopkins University researchers have used CT scans to show a relationship between a decline in cognitive functions in Alzheimer's patients and enlargement of the suprasellar cistern, a fluid-filled area in the base of the brain.

A study at the National Institute on Aging is using another radiological technique, positron emission tomography, to assess how early plaques and tangles can be detected in the brain. Researchers have used a small group of Down's syndrome patients, ages 32 to 61, because their affliction often leads to Alzheimer's-like symptoms after middle age.

The aging institute's Morrison-Bogorad says such work may eventually pinpoint exactly when Alzheimer's begins to physically manifest itself. Because the disease can go undetected for decades, finding a precise biological starting point could allow doctors to begin administering drugs to delay symptoms.

"If you want to have healthy aging, we have to understand where unhealthy aging begins," Morrison-Bogorad says. "It's like digging the first dike as the waves start lapping over the wall, you try to slow the progression." ∎

At Issue:

Should Congress earmark research funds for specific diseases like Alzheimer's?

M. MARSEL MESULAM
Director, Alzheimer's Disease Program, Northwestern University School of Medicine

TESTIMONY BEFORE APPROPRIATIONS SUBCOMMITTEE ON LABOR, HEALTH AND HUMAN SERVICES AND EDUCATION, APRIL 17, 1997.

*a*s you have heard in previous testimony from [National Institutes of Health Director Harold] Varmus and others, Alzheimer's disease is very common and very costly, both in terms of human suffering and in health-care spending. Its annual cost, borne primarily by families, is already a staggering $100 billion. Each year an effective treatment is delayed, another 400,000 Americans are stricken. The only hope for reversing this trend lies in research.

Basic research supported by this subcommittee in the past has opened the door to several promising developments. We now have two drugs to aid in treating the symptoms of Alzheimer's disease, and at least eight others are undergoing clinical trials. The real breakthroughs will come when science comes up with drugs that can disarm the trigger that kills nerve cells in the brain of patients with Alzheimer's disease.

Alzheimer's can last 15 years, yet we still do not have tests that can definitively diagnose the disease in a living patient. The development of a diagnostic test remains a high priority.

The changes in the brain that lead up to Alzheimer's may begin 10 to 20 years before they cause observable changes in memory and behavior. If we could detect the disease at the very beginning and then find a way to slow its progression by as little as five years, the number of people who show the symptoms of Alzheimer's disease would be cut in half and society would save $50 billion annually. . . .

Lastly, we still know very little about this disease in African-American and Hispanic populations. We must fund research and outreach programs that examine any special features that may need specific interventions.

Clearly, Mr. Chairman, how quickly we overcome these challenges depends in large measure on how much this subcommittee invests in Alzheimer's research. . . . We have the know-how. We have the research infrastructure. We have shown a willingness to make the most of scarce resources by collaborating with one another. And we have momentum on our side. . . .

We urge this subcommittee to appropriate a minimum of $355 million for Alzheimer's research at NIH and $10 million to [the Health Resources and Services Administration] to enable more states to reach underserved populations.

REP. JOHN EDWARD PORTER, R-ILL.
Chairman, Appropriations Subcommittee on Labor, Health and Human Services and Education

*t*here is a serious and growing threat to biomedical research within Congress: a well-intended but extremely ill-advised effort to allocate specific amounts within the federal budget for research into specific diseases. This practice, commonly known as "earmarking," substitutes political decisions for scientific judgment.

In my view, this would be a tragic mistake. To understand why, we must examine the history and methods of [National Institutes of Health]-funded research.

From the inception of NIH 50 years ago to the present, Congress' role has been one of appropriation and oversight, not micro-management of disease research. We in Congress are responsible for the bottom line and for determining how much we can allocate to NIH and its 18 separate institutes in any given year. We do not — and neither does NIH — fund by disease. Once funds have been allocated by institute, proposals seeking funding for research are considered by professional peer-review groups composed of accomplished investigators who evaluate applications for scientific merit. In determining research priorities, NIH also consults with a broad range of advisory groups, including health advocacy and research organizations. The result is a wide range of research conducted not at NIH's Bethesda campus but principally at academic research institutions throughout the United States.

In June, I invited Dr. Harold Varmus, director of NIH, to testify before my subcommittee and explain in greater detail how these funding decisions are made. His presentation and responses to members' questions were enlightening, and he outlined important reasons why funding is not allocated on a disease-specific basis. . . .

Varmus noted that "no disease is confined to one institute, and no institute is confined to a specific disease . . . hence distribution of funds is usually an inadequate measure of support for research on a specific disease. We know from repeated experience that research aimed in one direction frequently provides benefits in an unexpected direction."

In other words, biomedical research is serendipitous. Research on a cancer-related issue may yield a breakthrough on Parkinson's disease; an AIDS research project may lead to new ways to treat diabetes. As Varmus put it, "It is therefore crucial that the system for allocating NIH funds be sufficiently flexible to accommodate a new proposal with an important, imaginative idea, regardless of the category to which it might be assigned."

FOR MORE INFORMATION

Alzheimer's Association, 919 N. Michigan Ave., Suite 1000, Chicago, Ill. 60611-1676; (800) 272-3900; www.alz.org. A nationwide advocacy group for Alzheimer's patients and their families that lobbies Congress and provides information on types of care available.

Alzheimer's Disease Education and Referral Center, P.O. Box 8250, Silver Spring, Md. 20907-8250; (800) 438-4380; www.alzheimers.org. The center is the National Institute on Aging's clearinghouse for information on Alzheimer's and related disorders.

American Association of Retired Persons, 601 E St. N.W., Washington, D.C. 20049; 1-800-424-3410; www.aarp.org. The AARP offers consultation and information to consumers on long-term care and provides extensive references on specific caregiving and housing needs.

Health Care Financing Administration, 7500 Security Boulevard, Baltimore, Md. 21244; (410) 786-3000; www.hcfa.gov. This agency of the Department of Health and Human Services administers the Medicare and Medicaid programs and operates a center for long-term care that monitors compliance of nursing homes with federal standards.

The National Council on the Aging, 409 Third St. S.W., Washington, D.C. 20024; (202) 479-1200; www.ncoa.org. This advocacy group for the elderly monitors legislation and regulations governing long-term care.

OUTLOOK

Focus on Benefits

Policy-makers in March began to explore how chronic diseases like Alzheimer's will affect baby boomers when a bipartisan commission on the future of Medicare held the first of a yearlong series of meetings. The commission, authorized by the 1997 balanced-budget act and appointed by Congress and President Clinton, has until March 1, 1999, to recommend how to keep the health-care system solvent and meet the projected increase in elderly patients.

Few expect the panel to order radical changes. But the commission — consisting of members of Congress, public-policy experts and health-care professionals—is expected to modify the Medicare benefit package and try to coordinate the program with Medicaid and long-term service providers.

"Millions more Medicare recipients will depend on long-term care (in the next century) than today," says Sen. John B. Breaux, D-La., chairman of the commission. "It is necessary to look at and evaluate the effects these strains on our health-care system will have on individuals' and families' pocketbooks." [19]

One key issue for Alzheimer's patients is whether the panel tightens eligibility for home health benefits. Many early and middle-stage Alzheimer's patients get subsidized care at home but still attend adult day-care programs at nearby hospitals. However, some Alzheimer's advocates report patients are being denied home care if they leave their house for periods of time. "The explosive growth in home care is making this a big focus of proposed changes," says health economist Wilensky.

Meanwhile, some members of Congress are taking up the Alzheimer's Association's call for more money for research. Sens. Arlen Specter, R-Pa., and Harkin have introduced a resolution calling on the Senate Budget Committee to make room in the fiscal 1999 budget resolution for a $2 billion increase in funding for NIH — $860 million more than the increase proposed by President Clinton. Sixty-four senators and House members — including House Speaker Newt Gingrich, R-Ga. — separately have endorsed the call to increase Alzheimer's research funding by $100 million.

If more money does come, it will likely help fund additional clinical trials on vitamin E and its ability to delay the onset of Alzheimer's symptoms. The National Institute on Aging wants to test the agent on people with mild cognitive impairment — a common precursor to Alzheimer's — to see whether it can reduce the number of people who would otherwise progress to more advanced stages of the disease.

Ultimately, researchers hope to identify people at risk before they show any signs of the disease and treat them with drugs that can halt development of clinical Alzheimer's. The search for more Alzheimer's genes continues, as well, providing new opportunities for studying cellular events that may lead to the disease. A team of University of Pittsburgh geneticists reported in March that people with a particular variant of the gene that controls production of the enzyme bleomycin hydrolase appear to have twice the risk of developing the disease. [20]

Research isn't confined to Alzheimer's victims. Recent studies have documented the mental and physical toll the disease has left on family members of Alzheimer's patients. Ohio State University biologists have documented how caregivers under stress are more vulnerable to diseases like influenza. This year, Stanford University psychologists reported a greater incidence of high blood pressure and racing hearts in women, rather then men, caring for parents with Alzheimer's, Parkinson's disease and strokes. Daughters tended to show more resentment, anger and a sense of being trapped, while wives tended to have a greater sense of duty about caring for their husbands. [21]

The National Institutes of Health is in the midst of a five-year study to develop and test new ways for families and friends to manage daily activities and stresses of caring for Alzheimer's victims. That's some comfort to Donna Lyttle, the Queens, N.Y. woman who cares for her ailing mother at home and often ponders the ravages of the disease.

"It's almost as if you can't understand it unless you're actually experiencing it," she says. "You think how this person had so much life and was always on the go, and now you realize this just isn't a quality life." ∎

Notes

[1] Many of the national cost estimates of caring for Alzheimer's patients are derived from a 1993 study of patient care in Northern California and adjusted for inflation and regional differences. See Dorothy P. Rice et al., "The Economic Burden Of Alzheimer's Disease Care," *Health Affairs*, summer 1993, pp. 164-176.

[2] See Richard Hodes, "Meeting the Challenges of an Aging Population," *Academic Medicine*, October 1997, pp. 892-893.

[3] For background, see "Caring for the Elderly," *The CQ Researcher*, Feb. 20, 1998, pp. 145-168.

[4] See Franklin Eppig and John Poisal, "Mental Health of Medicare Beneficiaries: 1995," *Health Care Financing Review*, spring 1997, pp. 207-210.

[5] Congress rewrote the law to target lawyers or accountants who advise the elderly to give away their assets to become eligible for Medicaid.

[6] Quoted in Michael Vitez, "The High Cost of Living Longer," *Philadelphia Inquirer*, March 16, 1998, p. A1.

[7] See National Institute on Aging, "Progress Report on Alzheimer's Disease, 1997," National Institutes of Health Publication No. 97-4014, pp. 7-28.

[8] See Gary Small et al., "Diagnosis and Treatment of Alzheimer's Disease and Related Disorders," *Journal of the American Medical Association*, Oct. 22/29, 1997, pp. 1363-1371.

[9] See Brigid Schulte, "African-Americans, Hispanics At Greater Risk of Alzheimer's," *Knight-Ridder Tribune News Service*, March 11, 1998.

[10] See Mary Sano et al., "A Controlled Trial of Selegiline, Alpha-Tocopherol or Both as Treatment for Alzheimer's Disease," with accompanying editorial, *The New England Journal of Medicine*, April 24, 1997, pp. 1216-1245.

[11] See Jamie Talan, "The Memory Molecule? Studies of Estrogen Intensify, Look Encouraging," *Newsday*, Oct. 21, 1997, p. C5.

[12] See Ruth Larson, " 'Boomer' Numbers Fuel Plea for Funds; Alzheimer's Gets Attention on Hill," *Washington Times*, Jan. 30, 1998, p. A6.

[13] A separate category of Alzheimer's spending is the "Safe Return" program, created by Congress in 1993 to assist in the timely return of Alzheimer's patients who wander and become lost. The program — operated by the Alzheimer's Association with money from the U.S. Justice Department and Janssen Research Foundation — provides identification tags for patients and training for police and emergency personnel to recognize and assist them. President Clinton requested $900,000 for the program in his fiscal 1999 budget, the same amount as 1998. Congress will take up the request later this spring.

[14] Weekly column to constituents, June 9, 1997.

[15] See Martin Enserink "First Alzheimer's Diagnosis Confirmed," *Science*, March 27, 1998, p. 2037.

[16] See Denis A. Evans et al. "Estimated Prevalence of Alzheimer's Disease in the United States," *Milbank Quarterly*, Vol. 68, No. 2, 1990.

[17] Quoted from "Alzheimer's Disease in the Community," *Journal of the American Medical Association*, Nov. 10, 1989, p. 2591.

[18] See "Quick Screening Test Developed for Alzheimer's," The Associated Press, March 13, 1998.

[19] Testimony before the Senate Special Committee on Aging, March 9, 1998.

[20] See Charles Henderson, "Another Gene Discovered To Be Associated With Alzheimer's," *Gene Therapy Weekly*, March 16, 1998.

[21] See "Stress on Caregivers Measured," *UPI Science News*, March 27, 1998.

Bibliography

Selected Sources Used

Books

Mace, Nancy, and Peter Rabins, *The 36-Hour Day*, The Johns Hopkins University Press, 1991 (revised edition).
Two psychiatrists explain in exhaustive detail what it's like to live with an Alzheimer's patient and what steps prospective caregivers should be prepared to take when the disease strikes a loved one.

Field, Marilyn, and Christine Cassel, eds., *Approaching Death: Improving Care at the End of Life*, National Academy Press, 1997.
A National Academy of Sciences committee of health, legal and public-policy experts offers perspectives on how Americans die and the dimensions of caring at, the end of life.

Rowe, John, and Robert Kahn, *Successful Aging*, Pantheon, 1998.
The president of Mount Sinai Hospital and School of Medicine in New York and a former psychology professor at the University of Michigan assert that far too many assumptions about the elderly are based on people who were sick or in institutions. They note that in many people ages 74-81, short-term memory loss doesn't lead to mental decline or Alzheimer's.

Articles

Wilcock, Gordon, "Current Approaches to the Treatment of Alzheimer's Disease," *Neurodegeneration*, Vol. 5, 1996, pp. 505-509.
A British neurologist provides a well-organized overview of current strategies for forestalling the symptoms of Alzheimer's.

Evans, Denis, et al., "Estimated Prevalence of Alzheimer's Disease in the United States, *The Milbank Quarterly*, Vol. 68, No. 2, 1990, pp. 267-287.
The authors detail a Harvard Medical School study of elderly residents in East Boston, Mass., that prompted the National Institutes of Health and others to revise upward the estimate of the number of Alzheimer's cases in the United States.

Gladwell, Malcolm, "The Alzheimer's Strain: How to Accommodate Too Many Patients," *The New Yorker*, Oct. 20 & 27, 1997, pp. 125-139.
Gladwell describes how dementia specialists at a Pennsylvania long-term care group designed a safe, familiar facility in which Alzheimer's patients could freely wander around without being a threat to themselves.

Rovner, Sandy, "An Alzheimer's Journal," *Washington Post health section*, March 29, 1994, pp. 1-15.
Rovner profiles Cary Henderson, a former American history professor at James Madison University, who kept a journal during the early stages of Alzheimer's disease.

Vitez, Michael, "Life's Last Chapter: How Well Will We Care?" *Philadelphia Inquirer*, March 15-18, 1998.
A Pulitzer Prize-winning reporter examines the economic and societal issues surrounding care for the frail elderly, including Alzheimer's patients, in a four-part series.

Reports and Studies

Alzheimer's Disease: Estimates of Prevalence in the United States, U.S. General Accounting Office, GAO/HEHS-98-16, January 1998.
The GAO, the investigative arm of Congress, reviewed 18 studies of the prevalence of Alzheimer's disease and arrived at a conservative estimate that the disease affects at least 1.9 million Americans.

National Institute on Aging, *Alzheimer's Disease: Unraveling the Mystery*, 1995, National Institutes of Health Publication No. 95-3782, U.S. Government Printing Office.
This booklet for people interested in Alzheimer's research includes basic definitions, the search for causes, research on diagnosis and possible treatments.

Advisory Panel on Alzheimer's Disease, *Alzheimer's Disease and Related Dementias: Acute and Long-Term Care Services*, 1996, National Institutes of Health Publication No. 96-4136, U.S. Government Printing Office.
An advisory panel to the U.S. Department of Health and Human Services delivers a sometimes critical assessment of the health-care system's ability to provide long-term care to Alzheimer's patients.

2 Obesity and Health

The line at a Washington, D.C., Burger King stretches 20-deep most weekday lunch hours as office workers and tourists belly up for fare like the $4.19 "Whopper value meal": a husky hamburger with all the trimmings, French fries and a soft drink.

Few pay attention to a nutrition chart posted near the counter that reveals the combination has up to 1,340 calories — about two-thirds of the calories most adults need in a day.

Down the block, a Chinese restaurant serves up mountainous portions of kung pao chicken and steamed rice — a popular peanut-garnished dish packed with some 1,620 calories and almost twice the recommended daily allowance of fat.

If those options seem too rich, there's always a tuna fish sandwich. But even that old standby has hidden perils. A typical serving weighs 11 ounces, nearly three times the recommended serving size, as defined by the Food and Drug Administration (FDA). Total calories: 720.

With fast-food restaurants everywhere, it's no wonder that finding ample portions of inexpensive, tasty food is something most Americans take for granted. But researchers say the bounty is contributing to an alarming outbreak of obesity that has transformed the United States into the fattest nation on Earth.[1]

In 1998, the National Institutes of Health (NIH) released new dietary guidelines that concluded 97 million American adults — 55 percent of the population — are either overweight or obese, based on a measurement known as body mass index (BMI). In the early 1960s, the number was about 43 percent. The standard medical definition of obesity is weighing at least 20 percent more than ideal

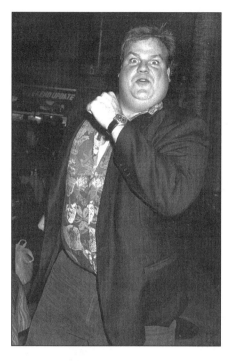

body weight.[2]

Numerous studies conclude that excess fat makes it more likely that a person will develop chronic disorders, such as diabetes, high blood pressure, arthritis and elevated levels of blood cholesterol. The NIH estimates that total costs attributable to obesity-related disease now approach $100 billion annually. Officials say obesity contributes to as many as 300,000 deaths each year.

"People come out of a fast-food restaurant feeling satisfied. They can't project 15 years ahead, when everything hits hard and they have a heart attack or come down with diabetes or cancer," says F. Xavier Pi-Sunyer, director of the obesity research center at St. Luke's-Roosevelt Hospital Center in New York City and chairman of the panel that developed the NIH guidelines.

Food intake is only part of the problem. Americans also are less physically active than ever, choosing to drive short distances instead of walking and to ride elevators and escalators rather than climb stairs.

Many spend their workdays at desks, cut off from virtually all physical activity. In their free time, one in four admits to being completely sedentary, and 40 percent rarely exercise.

Similar patterns are observed abroad, particularly in Western Europe. But while people there may, in fact, consume more fat in their diets, health experts say they also tend to eat more balanced meals, snack less and walk or bicycle during the day. Obesity rates in England, France and the Netherlands are not as bad as those in the United States, according to the World Health Organization.[3]

"All of these changes in physical activity and diet that promote weight gain have kind of made us like rats in a cage," says Donald Hensrud, a preventive medicine and nutrition specialist at the Mayo Clinic in Rochester, Minn. "It's a problem affecting the broad population that requires an effective solution."

Self-restraint and more exercise are the two most obvious remedies. But many Americans who lack the time or will are turning to medically assisted weight loss and diet drugs that promise slimmer bodies without major lifestyle changes. Dozens of pharmaceutical and biotechnology companies are developing agents that can block the absorption of fats in the intestines or affect brain chemistry to change the body's perception of hunger.

Market analysts conservatively estimate a product that's proven truly safe could generate sales of $5 billion per year. By contrast, a blockbuster drug to treat common conditions like stomach distress and ulcers rarely generates more than $1 billion in annual sales. To date, however, most diet drugs have only been shown to be temporarily effective, and some have proven dangerous.

The risks were illustrated when the medications fenfluramine

From *The CQ Researcher*, January 15, 1999.

A Nation of Heavyweights?

More than half of all U.S. adults — 97 million Americans — are either overweight or obese, according to National Institutes of Health dietary guidelines. In the early 1960s, 43 percent were overweight.

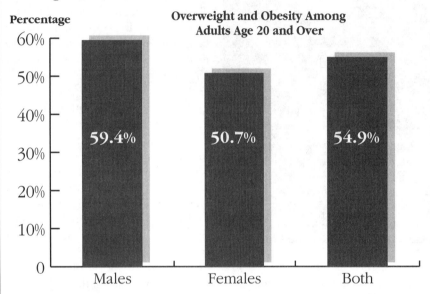

Overweight and Obesity Among Adults Age 20 and Over

- Males: 59.4%
- Females: 50.7%
- Both: 54.9%

Sources: National Health and Nutrition Examination Surveys, 1988-1994; National Institutes of Health, 1998.

(Pondimin) and dexfenfluramine (Redux) were pulled from the market in 1997 after they were linked to potentially lethal heart-valve damage in some patients. More than 18 million prescriptions for the popular combination treatment fen-phen (of which fenfluramine is the "fen") and Redux were written between 1992 and 1997.[4]

"There are a lot of people walking around with very mild valvular disease" who don't know it, says Hensrud, noting that some studies show the longer patients took Redux or fen-phen, the more likely they were to develop valve problems.

Phentermine, the second half of the fen-phen combination, remains available and is occasionally prescribed for weight loss in tandem with the popular anti-depressant Prozac. The practice isn't approved by the FDA, and Hensrud says there is no scientific evidence to justify the combination.

In the long run, drug companies hope to take advantage of recent research showing there are various genetic routes to becoming overweight. The public was captivated by the 1994 discovery of a mouse gene that produced a protein called leptin that was capable of regulating body weight. A similar pathway was subsequently found in humans. But while at least nine human chromosomal regions are now linked to body fat and weight, researchers caution they know of no "magic bullet" to losing weight, such as shutting off a single, key gene.

Experts also don't know the precise way excess fat gives rise to conditions like diabetes. They think it may be related to visceral fat, a type of fat cell that is highly active

metabolically. Visceral fat discharges fatty acids and other harmful components into blood vessels, which eventually deliver them to the liver and other vital organs. However, the relationship between visceral fat and total body fat is still unknown; some adults have large quantities of visceral fat but aren't obese.

Though obesity is, first and foremost, a medical issue, it has strong emotional and societal consequences, as well. Various studies suggest fat people lack self-esteem and are less likely to marry and achieve professional success. The prevalence of obesity also hits particularly hard in minority communities — especially among African-Americans — who often have lower household incomes and rely more on cheap foods that are high in fat.

Millions of Americans place losing weight at or near the top of their New Year's resolutions after overindulging during the holiday season. Many buy nutritional supplements or sign up for diet plans that promise quick results but don't always promote the long-term behavioral changes health professionals insist are necessary to keep the pounds off.[5]

Some observers believe eating has gone beyond being a necessity to become a form of psychological release in our fast-paced society. Peter Stearns, a social historian at Carnegie Mellon University in Pittsburgh, says increased stress at home and at work — arising from broad changes like corporate downsizing and single-parenting — have conspired to make people snack more, even if they know it's unhealthy.

"We're increasingly defying eating rules that we know are good for us and saying, 'My life is hard enough,'" says Stearns, author of the recent book *Fat History*. "In general, Americans probably don't like their bodies as much today as they did 20 years ago, and that's a sad commentary."

How the Body Controls Weight

The body's internal weight-control system reacts to exercise, diet and other external factors and influences how much fat is stored. Eating a piece of food (1) prompts a gene-based response in which the fat cells secrete a hormone called leptin (2). Leptin signals the brain that the body absorbed more fat (3). The brain then calls for a decrease in food intake and an increase in metabolism (4). The system can be unbalanced by excessive or not enough food intake, overexercise and other extremes.

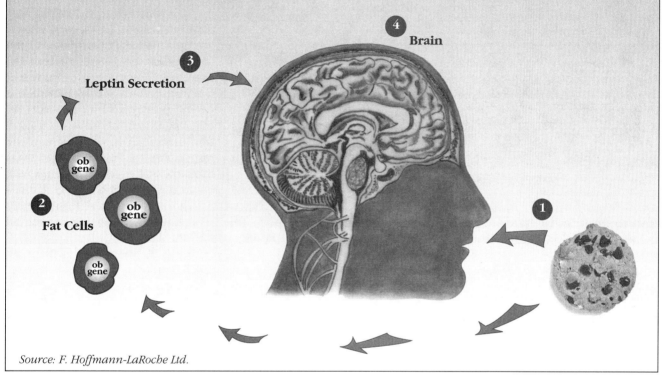

Source: F. Hoffmann-LaRoche Ltd.

Debra James/Angela S. Dixon

Although they may feel bad about their figures, Americans often can't rely on government and private health plans for obesity treatment. Insurers have traditionally viewed obesity as a behavioral problem and declined to provide full coverage for weight loss unless there is a concurrent obesity-related disease. Doctors who help patients lose weight say they often have to seek reimbursement from private insurance plans by treating high blood pressure or some other "co-morbid condition."

Similar criteria are found on the federal level. Medicare and Medicaid don't cover obesity treatments. The Social Security Administration is currently proposing to delete obesity from its listing of impairments under which individuals can file for disability insurance.

Obesity also doesn't rank particularly high in the federal health research portfolio. The NIH spends approximately $100 million per year studying causes and treatments for obesity. But that is dwarfed by the $1 billion spent each year on heart disease, or the $3.1 billion in targeted annual spending for cancer research.[6]

Some health professionals are aggressively advancing the notion that obesity is a widespread, chronic disease. Three years ago, former Surgeon General C. Everett Koop launched Shape Up America!, a physical-fitness campaign, asserting obesity is the nation's No. 2 cause of death, behind smoking. Others contend the figure has been exaggerated, and the disease claims inflated. The respected *New England Journal of Medicine* last year questioned the obesity-as-a-disease model, arguing obesity appears to be more of a symptom in many people.

While the debate rages, the diet industry is trying to settle longstanding questions about its business practices. Well-established weight-loss programs, including Weight Watchers and Jenny Craig, have heeded warnings from the Federal Trade Commission (FTC) and agreed to new standards that will restrict the claims they can make in advertisements. The FTC has long questioned the truthfulness

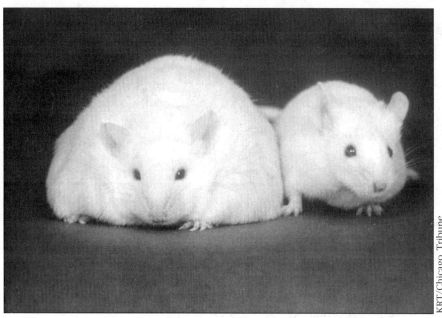

The mouse on the left became obese due to a genetic defect that caused it to store too much fat.

KRT/Chicago Tribune

of some companies' claims, and filed a series of false advertising complaints over the past decade.

The FDA, meanwhile, is devising new guidelines for dietary supplements and foods fortified with nutrients and minerals. Many of the products claim to fight high cholesterol and other obesity-related symptoms but aren't regulated in the same fashion as drugs or food additives, such as artificial sweeteners.[7]

Advocates for the obese say the moves may help raise consumer awareness and discourage unscrupulous promoters from preying on overweight Americans. They add the actions also may raise general awareness of obesity — a condition they contend is so universal, it doesn't elicit much sympathy.

"The death rate from obesity is probably equal to the premature deaths from smoking . . . but there's no evil enemy here to fight against, like the tobacco companies," says Morgan Downey, executive director of the American Obesity Association, a Washington-based group that lobbies Congress for more money for

obesity research. "It's a powerful disease that's been avoided by policymakers."

As Americans keep putting on the pounds, here are some questions being asked:

Should drugs be used to treat obesity?

Sheila Hammond used the popular drug combination fen-phen to shed 73 pounds from her 300-pound frame before the product was pulled from the market in 1997.

The 43-year-old woman from Placentia, Calif., gained 83 pounds over the next four and a half months and finally enrolled in a Weight Watchers program to try to regain control through diet and exercise. Despite concerns about the health effects of diet drugs, Hammond continues to look to the pills for hope.

"When you get to the point where you can't fit into anything and you're not mobile, you're just desperate," Hammond says. "I had people calling me, saying, 'You're going to have this heart problem.' But when you're that obese, you don't care."[8]

Part of the worry about diet drugs is that they are frequently misused. Some of the medications were originally developed for other medical conditions and now are sold on the black market or dispensed to people who only need to lose a few pounds. Many affect the central nervous system and can pose other health risks that don't become apparent until they have been taken over several years. [9]

The situation is partly due to the vagaries of the U.S. drug-approval process. Once the FDA approves a medication for a specific disorder, it can be prescribed by physicians for other purposes, known as "off-label use." But the FDA, which is primarily responsible for bringing new drugs to market, often can't keep up with all the new uses of old drugs and has to rely on drugmakers to file yearly reports with any new information on the drugs.[10]

The FDA approved phentermine and fenfluramine as short-term appetite suppressants in 1959 and 1973, respectively, but never approved their use together. Despite this, doctors noticed the combination helped many people lose weight and wrote more than 7 million prescriptions per year by 1997. It was only after medical technicians at a clinic in Fargo, N.D., began noticing heart valve problems in patients, and the Mayo Clinic conducted follow-up studies, that the FDA pressured drugmakers to recall the products.

The NIH obesity guidelines issued last June state it's appropriate to use drugs that have been specifically approved for long-term weight loss. NIH recommends medications for people whose initial BMI is 30 or higher — for instance, someone who is 5-foot-6 and weighs 185 pounds or more. Overweight patients with other health problems, such as diabetes or high blood pressure, can be treated with drugs if their BMI is 27 or higher — that is, someone who is 5-foot-6 and weighs 167 pounds or more, the guidelines state.*

Anyone with a BMI of 25 or above is regarded as overweight. Anyone with a BMI of 30 or above is regarded as obese. (*See chart, p. 24.*)

To date, the FDA has only approved one drug that has been tested specifically for long-term weight loss Sibutramine (Meridia) — developed by Knoll Pharmaceutical Co., the Mount Olive, N.J.-based subsidiary of the German conglomerate BASF AG — was first introduced as an antidepressant a decade ago. It failed to help patients get over depression. But researchers noticed they lost weight because the drug increases levels of the brain chemicals serotonin and norepinephrine, which have an effect on appetite and feeling satisfied.

Subsequent clinical trials of 6,000 people who were treated with sibutramine showed they achieved a 5-10 percent reduction in body weight. The company recently launched a television and print advertising campaign and estimates global sales to peak at $400-$500 million per year.

The Swiss pharmaceutical company F. Hoffmann-LaRoche Ltd. has spent two decades developing another diet drug, Xenecal, that is expected to win FDA approval early this year. The drug works through an entirely different process, blocking an enzyme in the intestines that breaks down fats and allows them to be digested. Studies show people who take the drug absorb about one-third less fat. The drug already is on the market in parts of Asia and in Europe, where the British press dubbed it "Viagra for fatties."

But even the new drugs are raising concerns about possible side effects. A small number of patients taking Meridia experienced a substantial in-

---

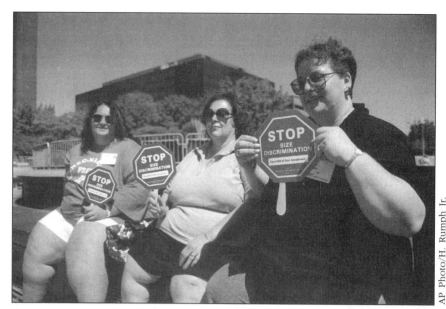

The National Association to Advance Fat Acceptance held a rally in Philadelphia in July 1997 to protest size discrimination.

crease in blood pressure. As a result, doctors have to monitor all patients taking the drug. Xenical received heightened scrutiny after women taking the drug in clinical trials appeared to have elevated incidence of breast cancer. Hoffmann-LaRoche presented evidence suggesting this was coincidence, and the FDA has signaled its intention to give the drug its okay. Still, doctors are expected to be cautious in prescribing it.

"I'm not for or against using drugs for weight loss, but you need reasonable safety data," says Pi-Sunyer of St. Luke's-Roosevelt Hospital Center. "One has to remember there is no [diet] drug on the market that has been tested for longer than one year" and shown to work.

Is obesity influenced by our genes?

When the Washington-based Coalition for Excess Weight Risk Education surveyed obesity rates in 33 cities in 1997, there were a variety of explanations for why certain towns fared particularly badly.

New Orleans, which topped the list, has moist weather that discour-

ages exercise and a profusion of rich local delicacies like gumbo, fried shellfish and bread pudding. People in New York and Cleveland generally eat too much high-fat ethnic cuisine. Residents of Washington, D.C., work long hours and, as a result, seem to always be eating on the run.

Another factor not mentioned and not linked to the environment could be a hormone that emanates from fat tissue called leptin.

Since scientists in the 1950s developed strains of inbred mice with inherited defects that caused them to store too much fat, researchers have probed the precise role genetics plays in weight control. In 1994, a team at Rockefeller University in New York made a breakthrough, succeeding in isolating the mutation that caused the inbred mice to become extremely obese. The discovery enabled them to uncover a gene for obesity and its human counterpart.[11] The gene secreted a hormone that was called leptin — from the Greek *leptos*, meaning thin — which signals the brain when to stop eating.

The discovery raised hopes that researchers eventually would be able

---

To compute your BMI without a chart, divide your weight in pounds by your height in inches squared, then multiply by 704.5.

What's Your BMI?

The body mass index (BMI) is used to assess if a person is healthy, overweight or obese. New National Institutes of Health guidelines warn that a BMI over 27 is cause for concern and could lead to serious chronic conditions such as diabetes and heart disease. A BMI under 25 is regarded as healthy.

To use the table, find your height in the left-hand column and move across to your weight. The number at the top of the column is your BMI.

Body Mass Index													
19	**20**	**21**	**22**	**23**	**24**	**25**	**26**	**27**	**28**	**29**	**30**	**31**	**32**
Height (inches)					Weight (pounds)								
59" 94	99	104	109	114	119	124	128	133	138	143	148	153	158
60" 97	102	107	112	118	123	128	133	138	145	148	153	158	163
61" 100	106	111	116	122	127	132	137	143	148	153	158	164	169
62" 104	109	115	120	126	131	136	142	147	153	158	164	169	175
63" 107	113	118	124	130	135	141	146	152	158	163	169	175	180
64" 110	116	122	128	134	140	145	151	157	163	169	174	180	186
65" 114	120	126	132	138	144	150	156	162	168	174	180	186	192
66" 118	124	130	136	142	148	155	161	167	173	179	185	192	198
67" 121	127	134	140	146	153	159	166	172	178	185	191	198	204
68" 125	131	138	144	151	158	164	171	177	184	190	197	203	210
69" 128	135	142	149	155	162	169	176	182	189	196	203	209	216
70" 132	139	146	153	160	167	174	181	188	195	202	209	216	222
71" 136	143	150	157	165	172	179	186	193	200	208	215	222	229
72" 140	147	154	162	169	177	184	191	199	206	213	221	228	235
73" 144	151	159	166	174	182	189	197	204	212	219	227	235	242
74" 148	155	163	171	179	186	194	202	210	218	225	233	241	249
75" 152	160	168	176	184	192	200	208	216	224	232	240	248	256

Source: National Heart, Lung and Blood Institute, National Institutes of Health

abnormality in their weight regulation system," says Michael Schwartz, associate professor of medicine at the University of Washington School of Medicine and Puget Sound Veterans Affairs Health Care System in Seattle.

Schwartz likens controlling body weight to controlling blood pressure. Just as the body adjusts blood pressure to stay constant with different physical activities and stimuli, its internal weight-control system limits the effects diet, exercise and other environmental factors have on how much fat is stored. If we get depressed and eat a slice of chocolate cake to cheer up, the fat cells secrete leptin, signaling the brain that the body has more fat. The brain then calls for a decrease in food intake and an increase in metabolism. (*See diagram, p. 21.*)[12]

The Thousand Oaks, Calif.-based biotechnology company Amgen Inc. is trying to apply the leptin discovery by injecting the hormone in overweight patients. Last summer researchers at Tufts University and the New England Medical Center in Boston succeeded in causing obese people recruited for a small clinical trial to lose an average of 16 pounds after they received high doses of the hormone.[13]

But scientists are still learning about other signaling pathways that control body weight. Researchers at the University of California-Davis, Duke University Medical Center in Durham, N.C., and France's Centre National de la Recherche Scientifique have identified another gene called UCP2 that plays a role in burning excess calories in the diet as surplus body heat, before the calories can be stored as fat. This could explain why certain people can eat whatever they want and never get fat. Further studies could lead to treatments that increase expression of the gene in overweight people and help them burn off more calories.[14]

to chemically tinker with people's DNA to alter leptin levels and help them melt away excess pounds. Subsequent research has shown weight regulation to be a far more complex interaction between biology and the environment. Just how much a part our genes play is influencing ongoing research into obesity — and the debate over whether the condition should even be regarded as a disease.

"While some people are born to become obese, most people experience weight gain because of a slight

Scientists at the Joslin Diabetes Center in Boston recently isolated a substance called melanin-concentrating hormone, which they believe increases the urge to eat, unlike leptin. Mice missing the gene that makes the hormone eat about 12 percent less than normal mice and seem to burn off more of their calories. The researchers say the hormone could be a target of new diet drugs.

While gene-based obesity treatments could tap into a vast market, some experts believe they don't address the fundamental cause of the problem. These experts contend America's weight gain is, first and foremost, the product of a culture that places too much emphasis on quantity and consumption. Put another way, overeating may be more a function of society than a clinical condition.

Supporting evidence comes from an NIH study of Arizona's Pima Indian tribe, which has such a high incidence of obesity that the average male tribe member has an 80 percent chance of becoming diabetic before age 55. Researchers believe the Indians at one time evolved "thrifty" fat genes as a mechanism to conserve fat and survive famine and droughts in the desert.

After World War II, the tribe abandoned its traditional foods of cactus buds, honey mesquite, mule deer, beans and squash, and began to eat like other Americans. The thrifty fat genes became a liability, storing excessive amounts of fat instead of metabolizing it. Now, tribe members can't appear to stop themselves from eating their way to illness.[15]

Other studies suggest there are strong psychological links to overeating. A London study in 1995 found fat people underestimated their food intake as much as 50 percent, especially when reporting high-calorie foods. Researchers say they don't know if their subjects were simply lying or subconsciously omitting items. [16]

"To combat the epidemic of obesity, we must first cure the environment," James Hill, director of the Colorado Clinical Nutrition Research Unit at the University of Colorado, wrote in *Science* magazine last May. "Our genes have not changed substantially during the past two decades. The culprit is an environment which promotes behaviors that cause obesity."

Are the new weight guidelines unreasonable?

At 6-foot-5 and 250 pounds, strapping baseball home run king Mark McGwire hardly looks like a candidate for a fat farm. And yet according to the new NIH obesity guidelines, McGwire is overweight, bordering on obese, with a BMI approaching 30.

He's not the only elite athlete to be technically overweight. Denver Broncos quarterback John Elway, Utah Jazz power forward Karl Malone and Baltimore Orioles infielder Cal Ripken Jr. each have BMIs of 27, while Olympic skier Picabo Street has a BMI of 25.

The release of the guidelines has triggered a debate in the health-care community over whether the government is promoting one-size-fits-all diagnoses. More broadly, some are questioning whether the medical establishment is unfairly stigmatizing people who aren't seriously overweight and making them more likely to seek out diet remedies.

"This is a society that is obsessed with thinness. Now we have the federal government adding their prestige to this mania," Barbara Moore, president of Shape Up America!, said after release of the guidelines. She and Koop unsuccessfully urged NIH to relax the definition of overweight, arguing it would confuse the public and make some people forgo increased exercise for more serious remedies like diet drugs.

The NIH guidelines are intended to replace the weight charts produced by the Metropolitan Life Insurance Co. in the 1950s, which set desirable weights for men and women based on the size of their body frames. The desirable weights were intended to give insurers guidelines for what constitutes a healthy person, but were not intended as a criterion for those who needed medical help. They translated to a BMI of 20-25 in men, and 19-26 for women.

The new federal guidelines expanded the definition of overweight to include everyone with a BMI of 25 or above. That made 29 million more adults who thought they were healthy fall into that category. But obesity experts acknowledge some of these people have muscular bodies or other physical characteristics that put them at that level, but who aren't actually carrying excess fat. Most acknowledge the potential for serious health problems really increases when a person's BMI exceeds 27.[17]

Pi-Sunyer, who headed the NIH panel that developed the guidelines, defends the BMI calculation, saying it helps primary care physicians understand where health risks are when evaluating patients. The guidelines are based on statistical calculations for weights at which risk of heart disease, high blood pressure, stroke and diabetes have been shown to increase.

"Most Americans associate obesity with cosmetic appearances. We need to educate them about the serious health consequences," Pi-Sunyer says.

But physicians, dietitians and other health professionals remain divided over whether obesity gives rise to health problems or is a disease in itself. The FDA and leading drugmakers view obesity as a chronic disease, and the World Health Organization terms the current conditions an "epidemic." Koop has repeatedly

Coping With Fast Food

Fast food is often deemed the single biggest reason Americans are overweight. Nutritional analyses show many items, indeed, are higher in calories, sodium, fat and cholesterol. But experts note that doesn't necessarily mean fast food is bad, only that people should take care to fit the items into balanced, healthy diets.

One way is by ordering more carefully. A growing number of establishments have noticed that consumers are more health-conscious and are tailoring their menus accordingly. The experts say ordering burgers and sandwiches without mayonnaise, focusing on smaller portions or opting for items like chili or a salad as a side dish, can cut caloric intake, fat and cholesterol without completely sacrificing enjoyment.

The Minnesota Attorney General's Office offers examples in its guide "Fast Food Facts," which tracks the nutritional value of menu items in the most popular fast food restaurants. The guide reveals a combination meal from KFC consisting of two pieces of fried chicken (breast and wing), a buttermilk biscuit, mashed potatoes and gravy, corn-on-the-cob and a 16-ounce soda has 1,232 calories, 57 grams of fat, 157 milligrams of cholesterol and 2,276 milligrams of sodium. That's all the sodium one needs in a day, and more than half of the calories, fat and cholesterol.

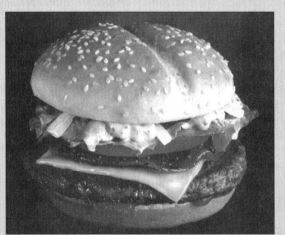

Contrast that with an alternative consisting of a wing, mashed potatoes and gravy, cole slaw and a 16-ounce diet soda. The healthier selection has only 373 calories, 19 grams of fat, 46 milligrams of cholesterol and 943 milligrams of sodium.

Similar savings can be achieved with a traditional meal of burgers and fries. A quarter-pound cheeseburger, large fries and 16-ounce soda from McDonald's has 1,166 calories, 51 grams of fat, 95 milligrams of cholesterol and 1,450 milligrams of sodium. That's about half the calories, one-third of the cholesterol and all of the fat and sodium one needs daily.

Contrast that to ordering a plain McDonald's hamburger, small fries and a 16-ounce diet soda. The combination has 481 calories, 19 grams of fat, 30 milligrams of cholesterol and 665 milligrams of sodium.

Some fast food items can't be slimmed down. The fragrant Cinnabon cinnamon rolls that have become staples of shopping malls and airports feature margarine and cream-cheese frosting over dough — a combination that totals 670 calories, the equivalent of three Pepperidge Farm cinnamon rolls.

A single slice of original cheesecake from the popular restaurant chain The Cheesecake Factory totals 710 calories. The Center for Science in the Public Interest, a Washington consumer advocacy group known for aggressive critiques of restaurant food, says its nutritional analysis shows the cheesecake slice has the same amount of saturated fat as a Pizza Hut Personal Pan Pepperoni Pizza and two Dairy Queen Banana Splits.

Large portions also distort fast food calorie counts. Most fruit and spice muffins found in delicatessens or restaurants weigh 4 ounces or more and have upward of 430 calories, depending on the flavor. The Center for Science says that's double the FDA's "official serving" of 2 ounces, which would total 190 calories.

"The food industry is selling food in larger portions," says Marion Nestle, chairman of New York University's Department of Nutrition and Food Studies. "It's a great sales technique. People buy larger sizes because they perceive them as food value. If they're going to spend all this money on food, especially in a restaurant, they figure they might as well get a lot to eat."[1]

Though most appear happy with the big portions, a few people are mounting a backlash against convenience food. A group of left-leaning European gourmets founded a movement known as Slow Food in the late 1980s that emphasizes simple, natural foods — slices of mozzarella cheese, fresh tomatoes, ripe olives and homemade jams — over heavily processed, mass-marketed items.

The movement — which preaches eating better-balanced meals, sometimes over a couple of hours — publishes cookbooks and guides to food, wine and travel from its headquarters south of Turin, Italy. While it doesn't depict itself as strictly a healthy alternative, the movement is gaining followers throughout Europe and North and South America.

"We're fast losing our grasp on the real things in life," says member Darina Allen, who runs the Ballymaloe Cookery School in Ireland.[2]

---

[1] For background, see "Supersize Food, Supersize People," *Nutrition Action*, July/August 1998.

[2] Quoted in John-Thor Dahlburg, "Cooking Up a Reply to Big Mac," *Los Angeles Times*, Nov. 18, 1998, p. A1.

described the condition as "a major public health threat" resulting in about 300,000 lives lost each year. The figures are based on a review of death records filed in 1990 published in the *Journal of the American Medical Association* and would make obesity the second leading killer of Americans, behind smoking.

Others believe obesity is a behavioral symptom that gives rise to diseases that kill people. A 1997 study by the Dallas-based Cooper Institute for Aerobics Research found thin people who don't exercise were more likely to die prematurely than overweight people who exercise regularly. Other studies have indicated the correlation between high BMIs and risk of death declines steadily with age until about 74 years, after which there appears to be no connection at all. The conclusion: Our behavior has more impact on our mortality and the diseases we contract than our body size.[18]

The New England Journal of Medicine weighed in on the debate with a strongly worded Jan. 1, 1998, editorial, charging the obesity-as-disease model was a symptom of "political correctness" on the part of the medical establishment. It termed losing weight "an ill-fated New Year's Resolution."

"[The] medical campaign against obesity may have to do with a tendency to medicalize behavior we do not approve of," wrote Journal editors Jerome Kassirer and Marcia Angell. "It seems that obese people can be criticized with impunity, because the critics are merely trying to help them."[19]

The back-and-forth is more than an arcane academic debate for Sally Smith, executive director of the National Association to Advance Fat Acceptance. The Sacramento, Calif., group consists of members who typically weigh 250 to 300 pounds and tries to help them overcome the shame they've been taught to feel about their condition.

Smith says doctors and dietitians fretting about how to make fat people thin reinforces obese people's sense of failure. Instead, she promotes making people feel better about their condition, then helping them integrate more healthy diets and exercise into their lifestyles.

"A lot of this obesity research is valid, but what they do with the information is disturbing," Smith says. "Instead of treating obesity as a symptom or disease, we think of it as a physical characteristic. The key is self-esteem and making people think it's worthwhile to take care of themselves. Then, you can give them information about how diet and exercise helps." ■

BACKGROUND

From Feast to Famine

Americans always have been hearty eaters. The earliest settlers in the New World found ample supplies of wild game, particularly turkey, bear and venison. Native Americans taught the newcomers to grow potatoes, pumpkins, beans and corn. By the mid-1700s, most cabins had adjoining plots of land to grow a variety of crops and grains.

The main meal on a typical 18th-century day might have consisted of pork and hominy, corn pone and johnnycake (a cornmeal cake), brown bread and fried bear meat or venison. In the evening, there was cornmeal mush flavored with milk, molasses, bear oil or the gravy of fried meat. On special occasions, such as a house-raising or a harvest day, pot pies were baked.[20]

Such a daily menu probably was the nutritional equivalent of several of today's fast food meals. But most Americans weren't overweight or obese because they were spending their days burning off thousands of calories doing manual labor. A predominantly agricultural lifestyle necessitated big meals with energy-rich foods, particularly English-style breakfasts with several different kinds of meat.

Not that there weren't early signs of trouble. Many Americans suffered gastric distress from meals that were heavy on pork and other meats and low in fiber. One of the first to notice was Sylvester Graham, an eccentric New England health fanatic, who believed only bread, vegetables and water should be consumed. Graham expounded his theories walking the streets of Northampton, Mass., in the 1840s, sometimes only clad in a bathrobe. His promotion of more natural foods prepared at home left a lasting legacy in the graham cracker.

By the middle of the 19th century, vegetarianism and temperance became mainstream lifestyles as many Americans tried to regulate their bodily functions to achieve better health. Meats, spices and coffee were blamed for overstimulating the digestive tract and even promoting sexual dysfunction. In Battle Creek, Mich., a colony of Seventh-day Adventists — barred from eating animals for religious reasons — founded a dietary institute that came to be headed by the puritanical John Harvey Kellogg.

Kellogg believed poor nutrition caused every ill and tried to develop bran-rich vegetarian foods and palatable coffee substitutes. On one occasion, Kellogg accidentally left grain out overnight in his experimental kitchen. The next morning, he passed the grain through rollers, creating the world's first cereal flakes. Kellogg's younger brother William recognized the potential and eventually mass-marketed the product, forever changing the way Americans eat breakfast.

Advances in Science

Not everyone bought into Kellogg's program. By the end of the 19th century, Gilded Age industrialists were eating freely and parading their girth from restaurant to restaurant as a sign of status. "Diamond Jim" Brady was among the most conspicuous, consuming dinners that included a dozen oysters, assorted crabs and terrapin soup, a porterhouse steak, numerous side dishes and boxes of candy, all washed down with vast quantities of orange juice — reportedly his favorite beverage. Another prominent figure was William Howard Taft — the 27th president and, later, chief justice of the United States — who tipped the scales at 361 pounds.

By the beginning of the 20th century, scientists were beginning to understand the connections between excess fat and health problems. Rabbits fed a diet of meat, whole milk and eggs developed fatty deposits on the walls of their arteries that constricted blood flow. In 1913, scientists identified the substance responsible for the deposits and called it cholesterol. [21]

In 1916, the U.S. government began publishing food guides. The Department of Agriculture's "Food Guide for Young Children" focused on choosing enough of the kinds of foods to provide nutrients for good health. Later guides, such as "Basic Seven" in 1946 and "Basic Four" in 1958, reflected a fine-tuning of the science of nutrition. But it wasn't until the 1960s that the research indicated a direct connection between excessive consumption of fats, cholesterol and sodium and the risk of heart disease, high blood pressure and other chronic conditions.

Meanwhile, new innovations were changing America's eating habits. Until the 1920s, most people's diets were tied to seasonal harvests, even though refrigeration and canning preserved some foods. In 1924, Clarence Birdseye perfected a method for quick-freezing foods under high pressure. Birdseye noticed that fish, meats and vegetables could be preserved in such a fashion while working as a government naturalist in the Arctic. His boxed frozen products soon allowed many Americans to enjoy more types of food year-round.

Another significant development came out of World War II research on microwaves. In 1940, an electrical engineer at Raytheon Co. named Percy Spencer demonstrated to colleagues how the radiation could make food molecules vibrate, creating friction and heat. Spencer held a bag of corn kernels in front of one microwave generator, causing them to explode into popcorn. The development led to the microwave oven, which by the 1970s was greatly reducing the time necessary for food preparation — and contributing to more eating on the run.

Fast-Food Flood

Most experts believe America's weight problem began to get out of hand in the late 1970s. Fast food establishments started competing with each other by offering larger portions, and food manufacturers rolled out a new generation of prepared foods that were tasty and, not surprisingly, high in fat. Americans found the increased variety and larger portions irresistible — even as their lifestyle was becoming more sedentary with the advent of computers, remote controls and other gadgetry.

"Overconsumption of certain dietary components is now a major concern for Americans," Koop wrote in the 1988 "Surgeon General's Report on Nutrition and Health," the government's first formal recognition of the role of diet in certain chronic diseases.

The following year, the National Research Council (NRC) recommended that Americans eat less fat and more fruits, vegetables and complex carbohydrates. The NRC report stated that individuals need to devote more time and attention to their daily diets, and health professionals would have to assist the public in diet planning. [22]

Government figures from three National Health and Nutrition Examination Surveys (NHANES) indicate that the prevalence of obesity in the population increased about 9 percent from 1980 to 1994. Curiously, Americans at the same time heeded some dietary warnings, cutting down on consumption of red meats and eating more fruits and vegetables.

Why did obesity rise just as Americans appeared to be more concerned about nutrition? Dietitians believe people increased their caloric intake by eating more fast food, convenience dishes and low fat products that weren't totally free of calories. The average daily caloric intake recorded by NHANES III for adults ages 20-74 was 2,200 in 1988-1991, compared with 1,969 in 1976-1980. The average total number of grams of fat consumed daily also increased to 85.6 from 81.

Statistics from the U.S. Department of Agriculture's Economic Research Service provide a more detailed picture. The service measures food consumption from year-to-year in many categories. It cautions that the data may overstate what is actually eaten because it does not account for waste. But, assuming the nation isn't wast-

Chronology

1900s-1940s

The effect of calories and fat on weight becomes known, while technology makes more food choices available to Americans.

1900
Illustrator Charles Dana Gibson's images of an elegant woman with an hourglass figure begin appearing in *Harper's* and *Collier's Weekly.* "The Gibson Girl" becomes an archetype of American femininity and pinup art.

1916
The nation's first nutritional guide, "Food Guide for Children," is developed by the U.S. Department of Agriculture.

1924
American biologist Clarence Birdseye perfects a process for quick-freezing fish, meats and vegetables under high pressure. Frozen foods greatly expand Americans' diets and make them less dependent on seasonal harvests.

1935
Cornell University researcher Clyde McCay demonstrates that rats on low-calorie, nutritionally dense diets live twice as long as rats allowed to eat freely.

1940
Percy Spencer, an electrical engineer at Raytheon Co., begins to adapt microwave technology to create a new kind of oven, enabling Americans to prepare meals in minutes.

1948
Esther Manz of Milwaukee starts the first diet club, called Take Off Pounds Sensibly (TOPS), after shedding 45 pounds during a year of supportive weekly meetings with friends.

———— • ————

1950s-1960s

The weight-loss movement gains momentum, raising concerns about the effectiveness of some diet programs and the use of drugs by dieters.

1950
Slenderella salons use vibrating tables and diets to promote weight loss. The fad lasts five years.

1960
The Mead Johnson drug company introduces Metrecal, the first liquid diet product. Overeaters Anonymous is established for compulsive eaters along the lines of Alcoholics Anonymous.

1963
Jean Nidetch, an overweight woman from Brooklyn, N.Y., starts Weight Watchers.

1967
Wispy British model Twiggy (Lesley Hornby) creates a fashion sensation upon her arrival in the United States and popularizes being skinny.

1968
Susanna McBee, a slender *Life* magazine reporter, documents how she received prescriptions for diet pills from every one of 10 doctors she visited on an undercover assignment. The story helps expose the amphetamine-based diet pill scandal.

1970s-1990s

As Americans continue to grapple with their weight, new obesity findings emerge.

1979
The Metropolitan Life Insurance Co. revises its weight tables, making "ideal" weights 10-15 pounds heavier than in the original table, developed in 1959.

1993
The Federal Trade Commission announces it is investigating weight-loss claims by five top diet companies. The Department of Agriculture reports that virtually all school lunches served under the federally funded school-lunch program exceed recommended fat levels.

1994
Researchers at Rockefeller University discover a mouse gene and its human counterpart that appear to cause obesity.

1996
The Food and Drug Administration (FDA) approves the synthetic fat olestra, which becomes a popular snack food additive because it is not absorbed in the intestines.

1997
The FDA issues a public health advisory after evidence surfaces that the popular diet drugs fenfluramine and dexfenfluramine caused heart valve damage.

1998
New National Institutes of Health guidelines for obesity indicate that 97 million American adults are overweight or obese.

ing any more food than it did two decades ago, trends indicate Americans are generally eating more of everything.

For instance, the average American more than doubled annual consumption of cheese (excluding full-skim, cottage, pot and baker's cheese), from 11.4 pounds in 1970 to 28 pounds in 1997. Most of the extra amount is found in pizzas and microwavable side dishes, such as broccoli with cheese and scalloped potatoes.

Consumption of fats (including butter, margarine, salad and cooking oils) also rose, from 52.6 pounds per person in 1970 to 65.6 pounds per person in 1997. Larger soft-drink servings (the FDA defines an official serving as 8 ounces, but machines now routinely dispense 20-ounce plastic bottles) helped drive up per-capita consumption of caloric sweeteners from 122.3 pounds per year in 1970 to 154.1 pounds per year in 1997. Comparable data on low-calorie sweeteners found in diet drinks is unavailable.

On the other hand, Americans are eating more fruits and vegetables. Total consumption of the two food categories rose from 564.4 pounds per person in 1970 to 704.7 pounds per person in 1997. And admonitions to eat more pasta and grains also are having an effect. Consumption of flour and cereal products rose from 135.6 pounds per person in 1970 to 200.1 pounds per person in 1997.

Some surveys suggest Americans will continue to eat more — and with less concern about possible health effects. After a decade of health consciousness, trend trackers sense that Americans at the millennium gradually are relaxing, but not abandoning, their nutritional values. Some have grown disillusioned with low-fat foods that don't have enough flavor, others are tired of grueling exercise to take pounds off.[23] The effects are seen in the resurgence of

higher-end steakouses and other establishments serving large cuts of red meat.

The research firm Yankelovich Partners conducts an annual survey of 2,500 consumers. The firm's researchers have noticed the number responding who say their weight concerns them has steadily declined since the mid-1990s. When asked what they most want to do next year, the majority say have more fun.

"They're saying, 'I need pleasure, I want pleasure, I deserve it, without apologies to myself or anybody else,' " says Yankelovich partner Barbara Caplan. ■

CURRENT SITUATION

Crackdown on Diet Ads

Approximately 8 million Americans join weight-loss programs each year. But the diet regimens have been frequent targets of criticism and legal complaints charging the companies don't fully disclose costs, potential health risks and success rates.

For most of the 1990s, the Federal Trade Commission (FTC) has pursued a crackdown on the advertising claims of several plans, saying they are unsubstantiated and, in some cases, deceptive. In 1997, two of the largest plans — Jenny Craig International Inc. and H. J. Heinz's Weight Watchers International Inc. — settled deceptive advertising complaints without admitting wrongdoing or paying fines. The firms had been criticized for using glowing testimonials about weight loss and promot-

ing their low registration fees without mentioning the cost of foods participants must buy. The tab for food can be as high as $100 per week.[24]

Last November, the regulators' actions culminated in a disclosure agreement in which the largest weight-loss firms agreed to tell customers the total costs they can expect to pay for products and services. The firms — which include Jenny Craig, Weight Watchers and Slim Fast Foods Co. — refused to disclose how much weight their customers lost and kept off, saying it was too difficult to profile a "typical" member and define what an effective weight treatment would be for such a person.

The agreement, which is expected to be finalized this year, brings the diet plans more in line with the strict disclosure rules in effect for hospital-based weight-loss programs. But some consumer groups criticized the FTC for declining to issue rules and, effectively, asking the industry to regulate itself.

"We just want up-front information so consumers can know about the effectiveness of a program," says Michael Jacobson, executive director of the Center for Science in the Public Interest, a Washington-based consumer advocacy group. "Regulators should develop standards on the costs of the programs and the quality of the staffing."

FTC officials say they hope the diet plans will eventually provide information about how much weight customers kept off.

The actions against the plans are only part of regulators' efforts to establish broader ground rules for the diet industry. The FTC also is targeting dietary supplements that advertise health benefits without necessarily providing scientific evidence to back up the claims. The supplement industry has annual sales of more than $12 billion, with about half coming from vitamins and min-

Are the New Higher-Fat Diets Safe?

For more than a decade, nutritionists and U.S. public health officials have told dieters to cut back on fat and protein and eat more carbohydrates. The "heart healthy" formula has virtually become conventional wisdom and filled American larders with boxes of pasta and low-fat foods.

But some of the most popular diet books on the market are challenging that notion. Authors are recommending that people eat more eggs, nuts, cheese, butter and red meat and eschew servings of rice, potatoes, certain breads and other carbohydrates.

Why the discrepancy? It all has to do with how diet influences the body's hormones, they say. Popular diets such as *The Zone* and *Sugar Busters!* contend that an overabundance of carbohydrates in the diet forces the body to produce insulin, which promotes fat storage. Reducing reliance on carbohydrates and eating more red meat and other often-proscribed foods can even out the imbalance, they say. Other diets promoting similar theories include *Protein Power* and *Dr. Atkins' New Diet Revolution.*

The theories have drawn some sharp criticism from dietitians and physicians but proven a commercial success. More than 1.5 million copies of *The Zone* have been printed since Massachusetts biochemist Barry Sears devised the plan in 1995. Perhaps the most controversial aspect of the regimen is Sears' contention that it can bring about a state of "superhealth" in people and help fight the effects of cancer, AIDS and heart disease.

"Living in the Zone is the best revenge against cancer," Sears writes in one passage. "The best weapons in the war against cancer aren't pills or potions, or magic herbs, or gruesome anticancer treatments . . . . [It is] the food you put in your mouth." [1]

Sears cites anecdotal evidence of elite athletes who've benefited from his plan, including members of the NCAA champion Stanford University women's swim team. The foods he recommends tend to be rich in fiber, which can reduce the risk of some cancers and improve control of blood sugar.

However, critics say there's little solid science backing up Sears' claims, other than a single 1956 study published in the British medical journal *Lancet.* The editors of the University of California at Berkeley "Wellness Letter" last year termed Sears' diet "a zone where you don't need to go," noting there is no evidence that high insulin levels make you fat. They also criticized implications that the

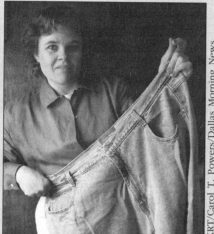

Nutritionists and diet promoters disagree over whether popular diets can achieve significant weight loss.

KRT/Carol T. Powers/Dallas Morning News

diet can reverse cancer, AIDS and other chronic diseases.

"Such claims create false hopes for sick people. His biochemical claims sound impressive, but are unfounded and oversimplified," the editors wrote. [2]

Similar controversy swirls around *Sugar Busters!*, a diet developed by a group of New Orleans doctors and business executives. Sales of the self-help book have exceeded 1 million since 1995, bolstered by an NBC "Dateline" segment last June. [3]

Sugar Busters! operates on a general thesis similar to The Zone and contends sugar is toxic and should be reduced significantly from the diet. The plan breaks down foods into "Acceptable" and "Foods to Avoid" categories and says it's okay to eat anything in the acceptable column without measuring amounts or worrying about calories.

Most of the acceptable foods would pass muster with any dietitian: lean beef, skinless chicken or turkey, most fruits and vegetables, olive oil and pure fruit jelly and peanut butter, as long as sugar isn't added.

But the foods to avoid include such often-recommended items as potatoes, white rice, corn, carrots, beets and anything with refined sugar, which includes most processed foods, and sugar-free ice cream and yogurt. The diet also shuns fruits with high sugar content, such as bananas, pineapple and watermelon. [4]

The authors say different food products are broken down at different speeds, meaning quickly digested carbohydrates on their "avoid" list are broken down into a lot of glucose at once. That forces the pancreas to produce more insulin than the body needs, they argue, slowing down the mechanism for burning fat.

Critics say the *Sugar Busters!* authors primarily rely on anecdotal data instead of solid scientific studies. Stephen Clement, a Georgetown University endocrinologist, warns that diets that recommend avoiding one type of food such as sugar often prompt people to overcompensate by eating other things. Clement adds higher-fat diets like Sugar Busters! can also make insulin levels rise.

[1] See Barry Sears, *Enter The Zone* (1995), pp. 170-172.

[2] For background, see Karen Goldberg Goff, "Figuring Out The Zone," *The Washington Times,* June 28, 1998, p. C9.

[3] For background, see H. Leighton Steward et al. *Sugar Busters!* (1995).

[4] For background, see Judith Weinraub, "Losing Weight The Sugar Busters Way," *The Washington Post,* Nov. 11, 1998, p. E1.

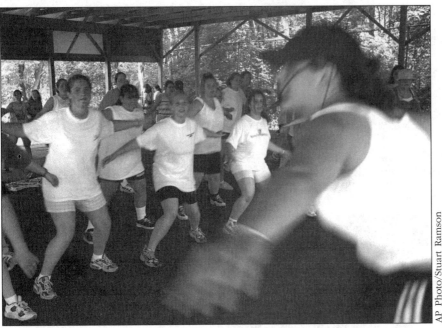

AP Photo/Stuart Ramson

It's aerobics time at Camp Shane in Ferndale, N.Y., one of several weight-loss camps for children scattered throughout the United States.

erals and another 33 percent from herbal and botanical products.[25]

The FTC has brought 60 cases against supplement manufacturers since the mid-1980s, most of which ended in consent decrees, in which the firms agreed to stop certain marketing practices without admitting wrongdoing. Now, regulators want rules that specifically address claims supplement manufacturers make. For instance, if ads touting a supplement mention it is used by four out of five heart specialists, the company must be able to support the statistic — and the implication that the product is good for the cardiovascular system.

The FDA separately is trying to develop ground rules for dietary supplements and other nutritional products. Supplements, such as garlic pills to lower cholesterol, receive much less FDA oversight than prescription drugs, and can go on the market without prior approval from the agency. The FDA does, however, conduct safety reviews on substances added to regular food, such as the fat substitute olestra and artificial sweet-

eners. In the gray area are so-called "functional foods" — foods with added nutrients or components to ward off diseases.

In what many view as a test case, the FDA in October charged Johnson & Johnson Co.'s new low-cholesterol Benecol margarine was illegal because it contained an unapproved food additive. The company responded that the active ingredients, a class of chemicals known as stanol esters, were supplements and didn't require the agency's blessing.[26]

Studies show Benecol lowered cholesterol at least 10 percent in test subjects. The company has given the FDA new scientific data and agreed to revise labeling. But many believe the FDA's final decision on just how to treat Benecol will affect a host of other products, including nutrition bars with the plant extract gingko biloba and orange juice fortified with calcium.

The FDA's legal ability to challenge advertising health claims for supplements was affirmed by the U.S. Supreme Court in December. The high court rejected a challenge from the Nutritional Health

Alliance — a group of manufacturers, retailers and consumers of supplements, who contended FDA regulations violate free-speech rights. A federal judge in New York and the 2nd U.S. Circuit Court of Appeals had ruled against the challengers, citing the need to protect consumers before any harm occurs. ■

OUTLOOK

Childhood Obesity

While public health officials bemoan the weight problems plaguing American adults, they say they are equally alarmed by the increased incidence of childhood obesity and the difficulties fat children have in overcoming their condition.

The percentage of overweight children 6-17 years of age has doubled in the United States since 1968. The most recent National Health and Nutrition Examination Survey found that one in five children in the United States was overweight. Studies also show up to 70 percent of overweight children ages 10-13 will be overweight or obese as adults.[27]

U.S. Surgeon General David Satcher told a recent U.S. Department of Agriculture conference on childhood obesity that the condition has reached "epidemic levels" and that government officials have been remiss in not addressing the problem.

"Today, we see a nation of young people seriously at risk of starting out obese and dooming themselves to the difficult task of overcoming a tough illness," Satcher said.[28]

Experts say there are a variety of factors involved, including increased consumption of fast food outside of the home. There also are distractions like television, video games and

At Issue:

Are medical researchers overemphasizing the health risks associated with being overweight?

NATIONAL ASSOCIATION TO ADVANCE FAT ACCEPTANCE

FROM "DISPELLING COMMON MYTHS ABOUT FAT PERSONS," ADAPTED FROM MATERIAL DEVELOPED BY CARRIE HEMMENWAY.

*t*he issue of fat and health is a complex one, with many factors to consider. Medical research has raised more questions than it has answered. It seems that while there are health risks associated with being fat, there are also some health benefits. It may be healthier to remain at a stable high weight than to yo-yo diet.

Added to questions raised by medical research, we also must consider that, in our society, it is very difficult for fat people to stay healthy and become fit. Due to prejudicial medical treatment and harassment by health care professionals, many fat people do not receive adequate preventative health care, and put off seeking treatment when there is a medical problem. In addition, many fat people do not feel comfortable participating in activities that would lead to a greater level of fitness. Due to the harassment they face, fat people rarely feel comfortable using public pools or health clubs, or participating in recreational exercise.

Given that permanent weight loss is elusive for most fat people, the issue of fat and health is irrelevant. The only true option available is to be as healthy as you can, regardless of your weight. (Often times the health issue serves as a smoke screen to justify denying fat people their civil rights. The assumption that fat people are unhealthy is often used to defend discrimination in employment, educational opportunities, housing and adoption privileges. Health issues should never supersede one's civil rights.). . .

The compulsive eater, whether fat or thin, is a person with an eating disorder. Simply being fat does not indicate the presence of an eating disorder. Studies which set out to prove that fat people eat more than thin people concluded that there is no measurable difference in the food consumption of fat and thin people. Compulsive dieters, who ignore their body's hunger messages, tend to become obsessed with food, and usually overeat after a round of dieting. . . .

Beauty is a learned concept, and the cultural norm of beauty changes over time. At the turn of the century, the leading sex symbol, Lillian Russell, weighed over 200 pounds. Marilyn Monroe would be considered "overweight" today. The media, advertisers and the diet industry tend to set the standard of beauty in today's society. We must remember that they are selling us dissatisfaction with our bodies in order to make a profit.

MICHAEL FUMENTO
A medical journalist and research fellow at the American Enterprise Institute

FROM THE FAT OF THE LAND, *BY MICHAEL FUMENTO, VIKING/PENGUIN BOOKS, © 1997.*

*s*ince 1959, data began to confirm earlier suspicions that obesity is harmful. That's when the first Build and Blood Pressure Study appeared. [It] found that . . . the fatter the person, the more likely the person was to die prematurely. By the time one reached 30 percent over recommended weight, there was a 42 percent greater chance of dying early. . . .

The second Build and Blood Pressure Study came out 20 years later and confirmed the findings of the first. Death rates increased steadily as weight increased, and went up steeply as the percentage over ideal weight increased. The 1979 study found that those least likely to die before their time were from 5 to 15 percent underweight. . . .

Traditionally obesity has been defined as 20 percent overweight, because it was thought you had to be carrying around that much extra poundage before health problems kicked in. This belief has now been shot to pieces by two major studies, one of Harvard male alumni that appeared in 1993 and one of female nurses that appeared in 1995. . . .

The Harvard study . . . made it clear that unless you are affecting your immediate health (such as some anorexics do) one cannot be too thin. It looked at almost 20,000 male Harvard alumni who graduated between 1916 and 1950. By 1988, almost 4,500 had died. The less the men weighed . . . the less likely they were to be among the dead. . . .

The Nurses' Health Study . . . was much larger than the study of Harvard men. It comprised 115,000 women and . . . excluded smokers. . . . It found that women who weighed about 15 percent less than the average American woman of the same height were least likely to die during the study. . . . Risk did not increase appreciably until the [Body Mass Index] surpassed 25, however. Since the average American woman is 5 feet 5 inches tall and weighs 150 to 160 pounds, the study indicates that the average woman weighs 30 pounds too many to have a full life expectancy. Those women in the lightest category (120 pounds or less) had the lowest death rates. . . .

Making yourself little but skin and bones is not healthy; being below average weight in a country where most people are overweight is healthy.

Reprinted by arrangement with Viking Penguin, a division of Penguin Putnam Inc.

Catering to Plus-Size Women

At Saks Fifth Avenue in New York, haute couture is no longer just for the svelte. An in-store boutique sells $250 skirts and $5,000 mink-trimmed coats from the designer Marina Rinaldi — in sizes from 10 to 22.

A recent advertising campaign for Just My Size, a lingerie line for plus-size women, states, "I am a sister. A daughter. A lover. I am not 100 pounds. I am not one-size-fits-all. I am a size 18. 20. SIZE 24. I am beautiful. I am over half the women in this country. I am not outside the norm."

The glossy women's magazines on newsstands include *Mode*, a 500,000-circulation publication that almost exclusively features plus-size models, and *Girl*, which is aimed at overweight teenagers.

Call it the revenge of the big people. Overweight Americans — once the target of pitches for fad diets and vibrating reduction beds — now are being courted by many of the world's leading designers, retailers and manufacturers. Kellogg's, Lazy Boy and The Body Shop, among others, have each crafted recent advertising campaigns built around greater acceptance of heavy people, often featuring plus-size models.

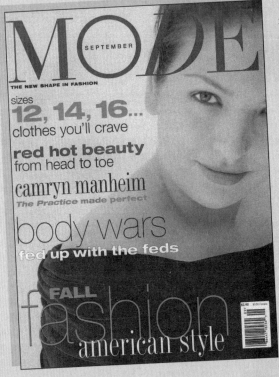

"It represents a major turnaround because, until a few years ago, you just didn't see anyone who wasn't a Christie Brinkley type in ads," says Sally Smith, executive director of the National Association to Advance Fat Acceptance. "This is a recognition that the average American woman doesn't look like the woman on the cover of *Vogue*. It's not shame-based anymore."

Most of the pitches are directed at plus-size women in their 30s and 40s, who are at a prime age for fashion shopping but complain they long had to choose from unattractive clothes. The marketing firm NPD Group estimates consumers buy $23 billion worth of women's apparel size 16 and above each year, accounting for more than one-quarter of all women's fashion sales. *Mode* estimates 62 percent of American women wear size 12 or above. [1]

The targeted advertising has made an overnight star of Emme Aronson, a 5-foot-11, 190-pound model who wears size 14 to 16 clothes. Aronson has appeared in ads for Hanes pantyhose and Liz Claiborne's plus-size line, Elizabeth. She also has written a book and hit the lecture circuit, emphasizing it's more important to be fit than obsess over one's weight.

While Aronson has had an impact on size acceptance, marketing to overweight people remains a delicate balancing act. Most heavy women still yearn to be thin and view their clothing sizes as a type of failure. Large men tend to be less appearance-conscious, and view excess weight as mainly a health issue.

Marina Rinaldi's ads in magazines and on billboards and bus stops carry the slogan "Style is not a size ... it's an attitude" but feature a slender model doing an acrobatic leap in her living room.

The Body Shop chain of fitness centers uses a more direct, self-empowering pitch, featuring an overweight mannequin with a slogan that reads "There are 3 billion women who don't look like supermodels, and eight who do."

The ads have proven so popular that the chain made posters of the mannequin, nicknamed "Ruby," because it is "Rubenesque." "Just as soon as a store gets some posters in, it sells out," says chain spokesman Randy Williamson.

[1] For background, see Margaret Webb Pressler, " 'Plus Size' Consumers Get Retailers' Attention," *The Washington Post*, Nov. 3, 1998, p. A1.

computers that cut down on physical activity and make kids skip meals. Children in poor, minority neighborhoods tend to be victimized by a lack of neighborhood recreation programs. William Dietz, director of the U.S. Centers for Disease Control and Prevention's Division of Nutrition, told the Agriculture Department conference that TV has changed national food consumption patterns. Dietz contends children are more likely to eat foods that are advertised, which tend to be higher in calories.

Regardless of the causes, experts say the health effects of childhood obesity are most clearly seen in the increased incidence of type II, or adult-onset, diabetes. Researchers have documented a fourfold increase in this kind of diabetes in children ages 10-14 since 1982, and note the onset of the condition was directly linked to obesity.

Diabetes affects about 16 million Americans and results in a breakdown in the body's system for absorbing sugar. Most children with the disease develop type I, or juvenile diabetes, in which the pancreas mysteriously stops producing insulin, a hormone that controls glucose use. In type II diabetes, the pancreas produces insulin, but the body's organs gradually grow resistant to it.

Obese children also are likely to develop other conditions. A long-running NIH study in Bogalusa, La., found children are likely to develop abnormally high blood sugar, blood pressure and blood fats, putting them at increased risk of long-term health problems.

Agriculture Secretary Dan Glickman says the government is taking steps to address the issue, such as reducing calories in school lunches to better meet dietary guidelines and providing nutrition education grants to give low-income families access to healthier diets.

"The simple fact is that more people die in the United States of too much food than of too little, and that the habits that lead to this epidemic become ingrained at an early age," Glickman says.

Researchers at Johns Hopkins University in Baltimore and Stanford University in Palo Alto, Calif., also have ongoing projects aimed at improving children's eating habits and cutting their BMI by reducing their TV-watching and computer-game playing. The Stanford researchers found they could cut BMI by half a unit in children who watched 25-33 percent less TV. One recommendation: Don't allow kids to have TV sets in their bedrooms.[29]

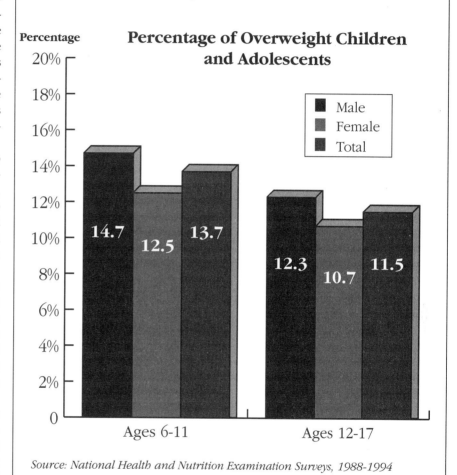

Many Children and Adolescents Are Overweight

Nearly 15 percent of American children and more than 10 percent of the adolescents are overweight, double the percentages since 1968. Studies show that up to 70 percent of overweight children ages 10-13 will be overweight or obese as adults.

Percentage of Overweight Children and Adolescents

Percentage

Legend: Male, Female, Total

Ages 6-11: 14.7 (Male), 12.5 (Female), 13.7 (Total)
Ages 12-17: 12.3 (Male), 10.7 (Female), 11.5 (Total)

Source: National Health and Nutrition Examination Surveys, 1988-1994

Some have suggested more drastic action. Kelly Brownell, a psychologist and epidemiologist at Yale University, believes the government should levy a tax on high-fat food with low nutritional value. Brownell says junk food is potentially as addictive as cigarettes and believes Americans should mount a public-health uprising similar to the one waged against the tobacco industry.

Others believe the problem needs a broader response. Moore of Shape Up America! says government should build more bike paths and create more recreational opportunities for children.

But she also says parents need to pay more attention to the basics when it comes to training, educating and rearing their children: "A tax on foods avoids the more serious challenge that simply must be faced if obesity is to be averted: People have to change the structure of their communities." ■

Notes

[1] For background, see Charles S. Clark, "Fast-Food Shake-Up," *The CQ Researcher*, Nov. 8, 1991, pp. 825-848.

[2] For background, see "Clinical Guidelines on the Identification, Evaluation and Treatment of Overweight and Obesity in Adults," National Heart, Lung and Blood Institute, 1998.

[3] For background, see "Obesity: Preventing and Managing the Global Epidemic," World Health Organization, 1998. An overview on obesity in America was presented at the American Dietetic Association annual meeting in Kansas City, Oct. 19-22, 1998. See *Journal of the American Dietetic Association*, September 1998, Supplement 1, Vol. 98, No. 9.

[4] See Mehmood Khan et al., "The Prevalence of Cardia Valvular Insufficiency Assessed by Transthoracic Echocardiography in Obese Patients Treated with Appetite-Suppressant Drugs," *New England Journal of Medicine*, Vol. 339, No. 11 (Sept. 10, 1998), pp. 713-718.

[5] For background, see Susan Phillips, "Dieting and Health," *The CQ Researcher*, April 14, 1995, pp. 321-344.

[6] For background, see Bruce Agnew, "Decisions, Decisions: NIH's Disease-By-Disease Allocations Draw New Fire," *The Scientist*, Vol. 12, No. 7 (March 30, 1998), p. 1.

[7] For background, see Richard L. Worsnop, "Dietary Supplements," *The CQ Researcher*, July 8, 1994, pp. 577-600, and Richard L. Worsnop, "Reforming the FDA," *The CQ Researcher*, June 6, 1997, pp. 481-504..

[8] Quoted in John Hendren, "Dieters Struggle With Weight Loss Without Diet Drugs," The Associated Press, Jan. 15, 1998.

[9] For background, see Justin Gillis, "Wave of Anti-Obesity Drugs in the Works," *The Washington Post*, Oct. 3, 1998, p. A1.

[10] For background, see Stephen Fried, *Bitter Pills* (1998), pp. 211-217.

[11] For background, see Yiying Zhang et al., "Positional Cloning of the Mouse Obese Gene and its Human Homologue," *Nature*, Dec. 1, 1994, pp. 425-31.

[12] For background, see Ricki Lewis, "Unraveling Leptin Pathways Identifies New Drug Targets," *The Scientist*, Vol. 12, No. 15 (July 20, 1998), page 1.

[13] See Anita Manning, "Hormone Appears to Fight Obesity," *USA Today*, June 15, 1998, page 1D.

[14] For background, see Christophe Fleury et al., "Uncoupling Protein-2: A Novel Gene Linked to Obesity and Hyperinsulinemia," *Nature Genetics*, March 1997, p. 269.

[15] For background, see Malcolm Gladwell, "The Pima Paradox," *The New Yorker*, Feb. 2, 1998, page 44.

[16] See Andrew Prentice and Susan Jebb, "Obesity in Britain: Gluttony or Sloth," *British Medical Journal*, 1995:311:437.

[17] For background, see Sally Squires, "Pound Foolish?" *The Washington Post*, June 9, 1998, p. Z6.

[18] For background, see Ross Anderson et al., "Encouraging Patients to Become More Physically Active: The Physician's Role," *Annals of Internal Medicine*, Vol. 127, pp. 395-400 (Sept. 1, 1997).

[19] See "Losing Weight — An Ill-Fated New Year's Resolution," *New England Journal of Medicine*, Vol. 338, p. 52 (Jan. 1, 1998).

[20] See William Chauncey Langdon, *Everyday Things in American Life, 1607-1776* (1943).

[21] For background, see Eleanor Mayfield, "A Consumer's Guide to Fats," *FDA Consumer*, May 1994, U.S. Food and Drug Administration.

[22] See *Diet and Health: Implications for Reducing Chronic Disease Risk* (1989).

[23] See William Grimes, "The Age of Indulgence," *The New York Times*, Nov. 26, 1997, page F1.

[24] See "Jenny Craig Agrees to Settle Ad Complaint," *Los Angeles Times*, May 30, 1997, page D1.

[25] For background, see David Brown, "FTC to Reaffirm Standards for Dietary Supplement Ads," *The Washington Post*, Nov. 18, 1998, p. A16.

[26] For background, see Nanci Hellmich, "Functional Foods, Supplement or Additive?" *USA Today*, Nov. 4, 1998, p. 1D.

[27] For background, see Sally Squires, "Obesity-Linked Diabetes Rising in Children," *The Washington Post*, Nov. 3, 1998, p. Z7.

[28] Address to U.S. Department of Agriculture Symposium on Childhood Obesity: Causes and Prevention, Oct. 27, 1998.

[29] For background, see Thomas Robinson, "Does TV Cause Childhood Obesity?" *Journal of the American Medical Association*, Vol. 279, pp. 959-960 (March 25, 1998).

FOR MORE INFORMATION

National Heart, Lung, and Blood Institute, 9000 Rockville Pike, Bldg. 31, #5A52, Rockville, Md. 20892; (301) 496-5166; www.nhlbi.nih.gov. This division of the National Institutes of Health oversees research on obesity and developed recent guidelines on what defines clinical obesity.

Food, Nutrition and Consumer Services, U.S. Department of Agriculture, 1400 Independence Ave., S.W., #240E, Washington D.C. 20250; (202) 720-7711; www.fns.usda.gov/fncs. This USDA branch administers domestic food-assistance programs and develops nutritional standards.

American Dietetic Association, 216 W. Jackson Blvd., Chicago, Ill. 60606; (312) 899-0040; www.eatright.org. This trade association for nutrition professionals promotes sound nutrition practices.

National Association to Advance Fat Acceptance, P.O. Box 188620, Sacramento, Calif. 95818; (916) 558-6880; www.naafa.org. The association fights discrimination against obese people.

Center for Science in the Public Interest, 1875 Connecticut Ave., N.W., Suite 300, Washington, D.C. 20009; (202) 332-9110; www.cspinet.org. The center conducts research on food and nutrition and focuses on better eating habits, food safety regulations and links between diet and disease.

American Obesity Association, 1250 24th St., N.W., Suite 300, Washington, D.C. 20037. 1-800-986-2373; www.obesity.org. This interest group lobbies Congress on obesity and health-related issues.

Bibliography

Selected Sources Used

Books

Fried, Stephen, *Bitter Pills*, Bantam, 1998.
An investigative journalist explores how Americans often incorrectly take medicines on faith, pointing to diet pills as one example of the dangers of self-medication.

Fumento, Michael, *The Fat of the Land*, Viking, 1997.
A controversial medical journalist, also a former obese person, traces the history of obesity in the United States and urges overweight people to accept responsibility for themselves. He also takes aim at larger and larger serving portions and foods that claim to be low-fat.

Stearns, Peter, *Fat History: Bodies and Beauty in the Modern West*, New York University Press, 1997.
A Carnegie Mellon University historian explores the focus on fat and dieting in the United States and France over the past century, concluding diets allow us to relish the consumer goods around us without feeling guilty about indulging in them.

Articles

Arnst, Catherine, and Amy Barrett, "The New Fracas Over Fat Pills," *Business Week*, Sept. 28, 1998, p. 72.
A year after the popular obesity drug combination fen-phen was pulled off the market, a Massachusetts Institute of Technology researcher ignites a new controversy by suggesting the drug combination Pro-phen, featuring the anti-depressant Prozac, could be just as dangerous.

Dortch, Shannon, "America Weighs In," *American Demographics*, June 1997.
The share of U.S. adults who are overweight is on the rise. Researchers know who is obese but don't have a proven treatment for what may be the nation's most threatening health problem after smoking.

Hill, James, "Environmental Contributions to the Obesity Epidemic," *Science*, Vol. 280 (May 29, 1998), p. 1371.
A University of Colorado researcher outlines what behaviors contribute to obesity, and how the environment fosters those behaviors.

Jacobs, Paul, "Heat Is On to Deliver Diet Drug," *Los Angeles Times*, Aug. 5, 1998, p. A1.
Drug and biotech companies are eagerly pursuing a new generation of anti-obesity treatments. But the safe, long-term use of such lucrative products is still in question.

Squires, Sally, "Obesity-Linked Diabetes Rising in Children," *The Washington Post*, Nov. 3, 1998, p. H7.
The incidence of obesity linked to diabetes has soared in U.S. children in the past few decades, illustrating how excess weight sets in motion a cascade of adverse long-term health effects.

"Sweets to Die For," *Nutrition Action*, Vol. 23, No. 5 (June 1996), pp. 1-7.
The Center for Science in the Public Interest details the calories and fat in some of the most popular sweets sold at malls, coffeehouses and sandwich shops. Part of a series of reports on the health merits of common foods.

Reports

***Clinical Guidelines on the Identification, Evaluation and Treatment of Overweight and Obesity in Adults*, National Heart, Lung, and Blood Institute, National Institutes of Health, June 1998.**
The first federal guidelines for physicians on identifying and treating overweight and obesity in adults. The guidelines estimate 97 million American adults — 55 percent of the adult population — are overweight or obese, and that total costs attributable to obesity-related disease approach $100 billion annually.

***National Health and Nutrition Examination Survey, 1988-1994* (NHANES III), National Center for Health Statistics, U.S. Department of Health and Human Services, 1997.**
The third and most recent installment of a nationwide sampling to assess the health and nutritional status of Americans through interviews and direct physical examinations. Topics investigated include obesity, diabetes, high blood pressure, cholesterol and dietary intake.

***Obesity: Preventing and Managing the Global Epidemic*, World Health Organization, 1998.**
This lengthy report of a 1997 WHO special meeting on obesity contrasts obesity trends around the world and outlines preventive and therapeutic strategies.

3 Childhood Depression

KATHY KOCH

Jessica was a happy toddler and preschooler. But the competitive environment of elementary school brought about a change.

She became listless and tearful, and her sense of self-worth took a nosedive. "She didn't have the energy to even try to cope with life," says her mother Sharon, a businesswoman in Terre Haute, Ind.* "She became a couch potato and started gaining weight."

Sharon, who takes medication for bipolar disorder (formerly called manic depression), recognized the classic signs of depression. So did her husband, also a depression sufferer.

A therapist who worked with Jessica put the 8-year-old on the antidepressant Prozac, saying that her depression was probably due to an inherited chemical imbalance.

"Now she's much more empowered to engage in life," says Sharon. She takes ballet, jazz and tap classes and even had the nerve to join a Little League team with only one other girl.

Jessica is among the estimated 1.5-3 million American children and adolescents who suffer from depression, a condition unrecognized in children until about 20 years ago. [1]

Some mental health specialists say childhood depression is on the rise and is appearing in younger and younger children. "I've even seen children as young as 3 years old with depression," says Lois Flaherty, a child and adolescent psychiatrist in Blue Bell, Pa.

Childhood depression can mimic adult depression, which is characterized by persistent listlessness, hopelessness and tearfulness, often ac-

---

* "Jessica" and "Sharon" are not their real names.

From *The CQ Researcher*, July 16, 1999.

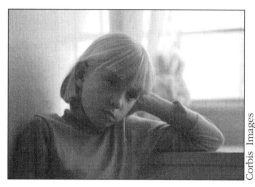

Corbis Images

companied by sleep disturbances and an inability to concentrate. [2] But depression in children and adolescents can also manifest itself as hostility, aggression and violence — especially in boys.

"A child who bullies his baby sister, picks fights at school or suddenly suffers frequent and unexplained aches and pains may be expressing his depression just as surely as the child who becomes tearful and withdrawn," writes Burlington, Vt., child psychiatrist David G. Fassler, co-author of a new book, *"Help Me, I'm Sad."* [3]

Teenagers' mental health problems have surged to the forefront of public consciousness in recent years after several incidents in which white, middle-class boys vented their frustration and anger — and some say their depression — by going on shooting rampages at their suburban schools.

Although such incidents are rare, many observers view them nonetheless as a wake-up call that the mental health needs of America's children are being ignored.

"The tragic school shootings in Littleton, Colo., demonstrated the potential consequences of unaddressed mental and emotional problems among our nation's children and youth," said Sen. Paul Wellstone, D-Minn., during Senate floor debate in May on the juvenile crime bill.

Left untreated, depression can take a devastating toll on a child, stunting the development of crucial social, emo-

tional and cognitive skills and damaging relationships with family and friends. Studies also show that the longer depression is left untreated the more likely a child will suffer recurrent depressive bouts throughout life. It can also lead to self-medication through drug and alcohol abuse, or to anorexia, bulimia, self-mutilation, school failure and trouble with the law.

Depression is also a major contributing factor in teen suicide, which is among the top causes of adolescent death. Researchers recently reported that adolescents diagnosed with depression as youngsters were 14 times more likely than their healthy peers to commit or attempt suicide during their lifetime. [4]

Childhood depression can be triggered by genetics, by an imbalance in brain chemistry or by a traumatic event, such as parents' divorce, prolonged exposure to violence, loss of a loved one, physical or emotional abuse or a romance gone sour.

While there are no statistics or studies showing definitively that depression among young children is increasing, many experts cite the teen suicide rate as proof that it is. The suicide rate for adolescents and young adults ages 15-24 tripled over the past four decades, while the rate for children under 15 quadrupled. [5]

"Suicide is the end stage of depression that hasn't been effectively treated," notes Martin Glasser, a Phoenix child and adolescent psychiatrist and spokesperson for the American Association of Child and Adolescent Psychiatrists (AACAP).

But others are more skeptical. David Shaffer, an authority on suicide, says it is cyclical and may be as much a function of substance abuse as of depression. In fact, he says, although adolescent suicide rates have tripled since the 1950s, they have been declining in recent years.

Non-Psychiatrists' Prescriptions Nearly Doubled

Primary-care physicians and pediatricians wrote nearly twice as many antidepressant prescriptions for children 18 and under in 1998 as in 1996. By contrast, the number of antidepressant prescriptions written by psychiatrists only increased 18 percent during the same period. Many psychiatrists worry that non-specialists may be administering the drugs without referring the children for psychotherapy, which they say should be an integral part of drug therapy.

Antidepressant Prescriptions for Children and Adolescents

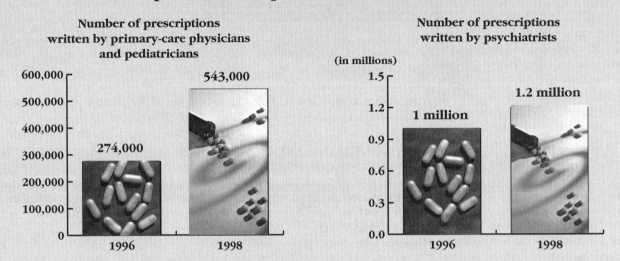

Number of prescriptions written by primary-care physicians and pediatricians

Number of prescriptions written by psychiatrists

(in millions)

1996: 274,000 — 1998: 543,000

1996: 1 million — 1998: 1.2 million

Note: Prescriptions were tallied for the six leading antidepressants: Prozac, Zoloff, Paxil, Serzone, Effexor and Luvox

Source: IMS Health

"Another reason we assume childhood depression is on the increase is because every generation since the 1920s has experienced an increase in adult depression. Presumably a lot of that started in childhood," says Flaherty.

"The increase may be real, and the disease may be spreading," says Glasser, "or we may just be more sensitive to identifying depressed children."

While no one knows for sure why childhood depression might be increasing and showing up in younger children, theories abound. Fassler, who is chairman of the American Psychiatric Association's Council on Children, Adolescents and their Families, blames a combination of factors. "Yes, it's more likely to be identified," he says, "but kids are under an awful lot more stress these days, and

they seem to have less stability in their lives."

Others cite such factors as the lack of adult and extended-family support systems — due to today's high divorce rate, greater family mobility and the preponderance of dual-career families — plus the increased exposure to death and violence in popular culture.

"If you do an environmental scan of society today, compared with society 10 or 20 years ago, it doesn't surprise me at all that youths have a higher rate of depression and suicide," says Glasser. "There aren't as many support systems for kids, and the rules for what is unacceptable behavior have been blown away. Kids function best with boundaries and there aren't any today."

In crime-ridden neighborhoods, the impact of living with the constant threat of violence can cause widespread trauma-induced depression, say other experts, especially if those children don't get adequate emotional support or counseling.

Some argue that depression may be showing up in younger kids because children today reach puberty earlier, and depressive symptoms often show up at adolescence.

Others argue that the apparent increase in depression may be the result of the availability of a whole new generation of safer antidepressants. "Perhaps people who once might not have married because they would have been too impaired to function are now able to have children thanks to the new drugs," says

Flaherty. "So there may be a genetic factor in the higher depression rates among this generation of kids."

While many may disagree about the causes, no one disagrees on one aspect of childhood depression: the number of American children taking antidepressants has increased dramatically in recent years. According to IMS Health, a pharmaceutical research company, children ages 2-18 received 1.9 million prescriptions for six of the new antidepressants in 1998 — an 86 percent increase in just four years. Prozac is even available now in child-friendly, peppermint-flavored liquid form, leading some to question whether such medications are being overprescribed for children. [6]

Some psychiatrists are particularly alarmed at the increase in drug use by children because about a third of the prescriptions are being written by non-psychiatrists, primarily pediatricians and family physicians. They fear that in at least some cases the drugs are being prescribed without referring the kids to a mental health professional for psychotherapy.

"Medication alone is never an appropriate treatment," says Fassler. "It should only be used as part of a comprehensive treatment plan, which includes individual therapy and perhaps family counseling."

Others claim doctors are being pressured by managed-care companies to cut costs by prescribing medication without doing an extensive evaluation and without prescribing the more expensive long-term psychotherapy, or "talk therapy." [7] Still others worry that, because none of the new antidepressants have been tested on children, doctors may actually be using them as guinea pigs. (*See story, p. 50.*)

But most doctors say the new antidepressants are rescuing thousands of children from lives of despair.

Yet only about a quarter of America's depressed children are receiving treatment, says the AACAP. "The majority of depressed kids really aren't getting the help they need," says Fassler, "which is a real tragedy because we have very good treatments for them."

Perhaps the most underserved populations are children in the inner cities and in juvenile-detention facilities, say mental health advocates. "Today, you have to have money or insurance to get medical help," says Glasser, noting that millions of Americans have no access to mental health services because they are uninsured but not poor enough to receive Medicaid.

Since the school shootings, many policy-makers have suggested hiring more school counselors or establishing more school-based mental health services. Even in many wealthier school districts few schools have full-time psychologists, and links between schools and community mental health services are weak or nonexistent, critics say.

Given the greater accessibility of guns in children's lives today, some experts predict that untreated childhood depression could mean ever-increasing juvenile homicide and suicide rates. When depressed kids use guns, it increases the chances that a suicide attempt will be successful.

To avoid such escalating juvenile violence, experts say, the country needs to make a more sustained and concerted effort to identify and help kids suffering from depression. As the issue is debated, here are some of the questions being asked:

Are antidepressants being overprescribed for children?

The 86 percent increase over four years in antidepressant prescriptions for children has led some to question whether doctors are overprescribing the new drugs. "Five years ago, one camper was taking Prozac and everyone remarked on it," said Regina Skyer of the Pennsylvania-based Summit Camp, the nation's largest summer camp for learning-disabled children. "Now, a quarter of the kids take it." [8]

Many doctors say the increase in prescription-writing only means physicians are doing a better job of recognizing childhood depression and are more willing to prescribe today's newer, presumably safer antidepressants. "We're just doing a much better job of identifying depression," says Carl Bell, a child psychiatrist in inner-city Chicago.

"I have no doubt that the use of these medications is increasing, but at the same time use of TCAs is decreasing," says Fassler. TCAs, or tricyclic antidepressants, the previous generation of antidepressants, had more dangerous side effects. "The increase may just reflect the fact that physicians are more comfortable using the new medications."

But while the newer medications, called selective serotonin reuptake inhibitors, or SSRIs, have been proven safe for adults they have not been widely tested on children as a treatment for depression.

"Antidepressants can be a very appropriate augmentation to psychotherapy, as long as the physician is properly trained and a complete, two-to-three-hour assessment has been done," says Glasser. "In the right hands, I don't think there is overprescribing. But when they are prescribed by physicians or nurse practitioners who don't have experience and training with children, there might be some overprescribing."

Sidney M. Wolfe, director of the Public Citizen Health Research Group in Washington, D.C., is more critical. He says the increase is due to "the somewhat casual and reckless prescribing of antidepressants" by non-psychotherapists, primarily pediatricians and family practitioners. "This is the group we are worried about."

IMS Health statistics show that between 1996 and 1998, pediatricians and primary-care physicians increased their antidepressant prescriptions for kids by 98 percent, while psychiatrists wrote only 18 percent more antidepressant prescriptions for children in the same time period.

Wolfe and others fear that such non-specialists may be prescribing antidepressants without also referring patients for psychotherapy. "If it's serious enough for antidepressants, it should be serious enough for psychotherapy," Wolfe says.

Some psychiatrists worry that pediatricians and primary-care physicians are being pressured by cost-conscious managed-care companies to prescribe antidepressants quickly, without an in-depth assessment or a trial of psychotherapy. "The average pediatrician spends less than 10 minutes with a child," says Glasser. "That's not enough time to go back and find out why they are depressed. Are they being battered, or are they the victim of incest?" You can't just give them a pill and send them back into a potentially toxic environment, he says.

Diane Schetky, a, child psychiatrist in Rockport, Maine, claims managed-care companies "have a real bias towards medication rather than therapy," because drugs are cheaper than psychotherapy. "And they think the family practitioner can handle these cases," she complains. "But they don't have four years of training in child psychiatry and aren't adequately trained in using psychotropic drugs."

"If you look at the pharmacy log of any managed-care plan, the majority of SSRIs are prescribed by primary-care doctors," Glasser says. "But most of those prescribing these medications don't have any special training in how to medicate a child."

Because the drugs have not been extensively tested for children, no clear age and dosage guidelines exist, and general practitioners can miss side effects that psychiatrists are trained to spot. Further, Glasser says, many kids are misdiagnosed with attention deficit hyperactivity disorder (ADHD) because the symptoms are often similar to depression. But the medications for the two disorders are very different — and a child's depressive symptoms may be masked if they are being medicated for ADHD. It takes skill to determine whether one problem is causing the other, and to find the appropriate treatment, he says.

According to a recent University of North Carolina survey, 72 percent of pediatricians and family practitioners polled said they prescribed antidepressants for children, but only 16 percent were comfortable with the practice, and only 8 percent said they had been trained to treat childhood depression. Many of the doctors had also prescribed antidepressants for conditions other than depression, including ADHD, aggressive-conduct disorder and bed-wetting.

Pediatric researcher Jerry Rushton, who conducted the study, said it did not examine whether antidepressants are being overprescribed. But it did show that, contrary to most perceptions, the drugs are not "replacing or supplanting" counseling therapies, he says. "Counseling is still being used. We were reassured by that finding."

Rushton said the 700 doctors he surveyed did not suggest that managed-care companies had influenced their prescription decisions. "But this is North Carolina," Rushton points out, "and managed care has not penetrated here to the degree it has on the coasts."

Ted Petti, a child and adolescent psychiatrist in Indianapolis, says managed-care companies put tremendous pressure on clinicians who work primarily with hospitalized youngsters. "Psychiatrists are being pushed to prescribe medication and get these kids out of the hospital within three or four days — before we've had enough time to do a good assessment," Petti says.

Some of the kids may even be suicidal, and the medication may not kick in for several weeks, he says, "but we are told to manage their care on an outpatient basis."

"Managed care is changing the way people with emotional or mental problems are treated," says Wolfe. "And although the short-term bottom-line figures of the HMO may look better, it's penny-wise and pound-foolish. In the long term it's not better for patients to be getting treatment that is demonstrably inferior," he says, citing a recent study showing more patients improve with a combination of therapy and drug treatment than with drugs alone. "The treatment should be a function of the problem, not of the payment system," he says.

But Glasser argues it is often the psychiatrists, not the managed-care companies, who are pushing drugs without therapy. As medical director for a managed-care company that serves military personnel, Glasser says he has trouble finding psychotherapists willing to do psychotherapy. "We want children to have psychotherapy, and we have no problem paying for it. But psychiatrists in this country today tend to do more medication management than psychotherapy. We really need a more balanced approach."

Others blame the increase in prescriptions on the fact that drug companies are now allowed to market directly to consumers. Harried parents having trouble with a rebellious teen may see the ads and ask their pediatrician for a prescription. "Much of the increase in prescriptions is due to more aggressive marketing by drug companies," says Wolfe, "It's a huge multibillion-dollar market, and the companies are eager to keep expanding it."

But drug company representatives point out that doctors are the gatekeepers for drugs. "You can't get a prescription without a doctor's approval," says Meredith Mayo, a spokesperson for the Pharmaceutical Research and Manufacturers of America. "The doctor knows what's best for his or her patients."

Some worry that children's social and emotional development may suffer if they learn to take pills to alleviate emotional upsets. If children learn to medicate sadness and anxiety away, how will they develop coping skills to weather psychic troubles on their own? they ask.

"Is the child seriously depressed or do they have a temporary sadness because somebody died, or they experienced some other loss?" Wolfe asks. "Many teenagers may have short-term sadness reacting to some situation that would make anyone sad, but now they may get put on antidepressants. Next we'll be giving teenagers antidepressants for shyness. Drugs have not yet been approved for every single mood disturbance, but that's the direction we are going."

Others bristle at the suggestion that antidepressants may be overprescribed. "You would never be asking me this question about insulin injections for diabetes," says Jenna Wallace, director of communications for the National Foundation for Depressive Illness. "Depression is a chemical imbalance in the brain. It is not a character weakness." Depression is probably being missed or misdiagnosed more often than it is accurately detected and properly treated, she insists.

Fassler agrees. "At the most, one in four children with a significant psychiatric problem is receiving appropriate treatment. If medications are used inappropriately, or if they are used as a substitute for other treatment or if they are used in the wrong dosages, I am concerned," he

Recognizing the Signs of Depression

Clinical depression goes beyond sadness or having a bad day. It is a form of mental illness that affects the way one feels, thinks and acts. Depression in children can lead to school failure, alcohol or other drug abuse and even suicide. The signs of depression are:

1 Persistent sadness and hopelessness.

2 Withdrawal from friends and activities once enjoyed.

3 Increased irritability or agitation.

4 Missed school or poor school performance.

5 Changes in eating and sleeping habits.

6 Indecision, lack of concentration or forgetfulness.

7 Poor self-esteem or guilt.

8 Frequent physical complaints, such as headaches/stomachaches.

9 Lack of enthusiasm, low energy or motivation.

10 Drug and/or alcohol abuse.

11 Recurring thoughts of death or suicide.

Source: National Mental Health Association

says. "But I am more concerned about all of the kids who really need treatment who aren't getting it."

Do we need more school-based child mental health services?

Since the rash of school shootings, more schools have been requesting assessments of apparently troubled students. "We're doing an awful lot of psychiatric evaluations in schools these days," Fassler says.

But evaluations aren't enough, he insists. "Many of these kids need ongoing monitoring and treatment," he says. "I strongly encourage expansion of early intervention and school-based mental health services."

Indeed, after the massacre in Littleton left 36 people dead or wounded, many mental health professionals argued that more counselors and mental health services in schools would help identify and treat troubled kids before they resort to violence.

"Historically in this country, we've really neglected children's mental health needs," argues Mark Weist, director of the Center for School and Mental Health Assistance in Baltimore, Md., and a proponent of an emerging national movement to establish mental health services in schools. Studies show 25 percent of kids will need some form of mental health services at some point in their lives, he says, "but less than one-third [of those] receive services, and far fewer receive effective services."

Community mental health services are grossly underdeveloped and

When Teen Depression Leads to Suicide

While much media attention has been focused on the fact that gun-wielding students killed 28 people in school shootings in the past three years, scant attention has been paid to the 2,000 teenagers who kill themselves every year. [1]

"Suicide is the end stage of depression that hasn't been effectively treated," notes Martin Glasser, a Phoenix child and adolescent psychiatrist and a spokesperson for the American Association of Child and Adolescent Psychiatrists (AACAP).

Indeed, some say many of the boys who went on the shooting rampages were acting out depression in suicidal ways. "I don't care if I live or die," shooter Eric Harris had written on his Web site before the April 20 shooting at Columbine High School in Littleton, Colo. [2]

A week later, T. J. Solomon, a 15-year-old at a suburban Atlanta high school, told a friend, "I have no reason to live anymore" after his girlfriend broke up with him. Three weeks later he opened fire on classmates,

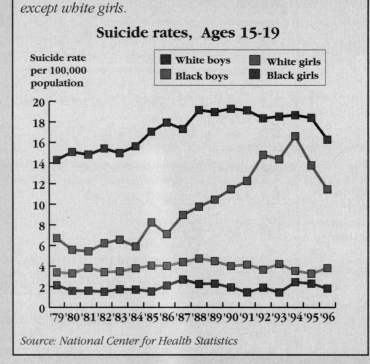

Suicide rates for boys are much higher than for girls. Rates began dropping in the mid-1990s for all groups except white girls.

Suicide rates, Ages 15-19

Suicide rate per 100,000 population

White boys   White girls
Black boys   Black girls

'79'80'81'82'83'84'85'86'87'88'89'90'91'92'93'94'95'96

Source: National Center for Health Statistics

injuring six students. Solomon was on the verge of suicide when he was disarmed.

"While depressed and suicidal kids and adults can engage in violent and destructive behavior," says David G. Fassler, author of *"Help Me I'm Sad,"* "homicidal behavior, thankfully, is relatively rare."

A recent study in the *Journal of the American Medical Association* found that adolescents diagnosed with depression as youths were 14 times more likely than their healthy peers to commit or attempt suicide during their lifetime. [3]

"One child in four thinks about suicide at least once a year," says Fassler. "By the end of high school, one child in 10 has actually made at least one suicide attempt, and usually the parents and teachers don't know about it." Some experts say for every child who commits suicide, up to 100 have tried and failed. [4]

According to federal health statistics:

• The rate at which Americans ages 15-24 commit suicide has tripled over the past four decades, from 4.5 per 100,000

underfunded, he says, so they have long waiting lists and concentrate only on critical cases. "In many communities the only kids who can access mental health services are the deeply disturbed," says Weist. Further, he says, kids and their families shun such centers because of fear, mistrust, transportation problems, family stress, insurance obstacles or other reasons.

Kids are more likely to talk to a school-based counselor they know, he says. "Community mental health

programs see three to four students a day," says Weist, who oversees a program providing comprehensive mental health services to 20 Baltimore schools. "In contrast, we see 15 a day."

"Schools are where students spend most of their waking hours," says Graeme Hanson, chairman of the AACAP's working group on schools. "Students would have a better chance of getting to their therapy hours if services were available there."

Because school-based services fo-

cus on prevention, they are also cheaper, says Weist. "If you don't bring these services to the kids where they are, many kids in dire need will not receive services," he says. If left untreated, their problems will likely worsen, become chronic and more costly to treat, perhaps eventually requiring hospitalization, he says. Or worse, he says, an untreated depressed child could turn to substance abuse or violence and end up in juvenile detention, where mental health services are notori-

in 1950 to 13.3 in 1995. Among children under 15, the rate quadrupled.

• In 1996, suicide was the third leading cause of death among Americans ages 15-24 and the fourth leading cause of death among those 10-14.

• Hispanic girls are twice as likely as non-Hispanics to commit suicide, and homosexual and bisexual adolescents also have much higher rates of suicide than heterosexuals.

• Up through age 14, boys and girls kill themselves at about the same rate, but after that boys are six times more likely than girls to commit suicide. [5]

Girls actually attempt suicide more than boys, but boys are more successful because they choose more violent means, Fassler points out. "Boys shoot themselves or crash their cars into trees," he says. Girls take overdoses or slit their wrists, he says, which are less-effective methods.

That may change, says child psychiatrist Diane Schetky, of Rockport, Maine. "Guns are becoming the favorite means of suicide for girls," she says.

Children apparently are starting to think about suicide at younger ages. "We've seen children who express thoughts of suicide as young as 4 and 5 years of age," says Glasser. In children that young, he says, the precipitating event is usually a divorce. "When you ask a child to choose between parent A or parent B, it can create tremendous feelings of desperation and hence depression, or acting out on self-destructive thoughts."

Others say suicide rates have escalated because kids today have greater access to effective methods of killing themselves — drugs, cars and weapons. "Historically, a suicidal person would have taken an overdose of pills, which is often unsuccessful. Now they have access to firearms," says Glasser.

Many argue that the escalating suicide rates prove that more kids are depressed today than at any time in history, and thus the skyrocketing rate of antidepressant prescriptions for kids is justified.

Others are not so sure. David Shaffer, a professor of

psychiatry at Columbia University School of Medicine and an expert in suicide, points out that suicide rates are cyclical and have recently begun to go down. They began declining for whites — more dramatically for boys than for girls — in 1988 and for blacks in 1994.

"The drug companies like to claim that these recent declines are due to the increases in the use of the new antidepressants among kids," he says. "But there's no evidence of that."

For one thing, he says, the decline is part of a worldwide pattern. Secondly, recent dramatic declines in suicide rates have been limited to boys. The suicide rate for females has been almost static for the past decade, he points out. "It never went up, and it never went down," Shaffer says. "If the declines were due to medication we should have seen a decline in the female suicide rate, especially since girls are more likely to seek help when they are depressed, and antidepressants are only available through prescription."

Instead, he suggests, variations in suicide rates across time are probably drug- and alcohol-related. Alcohol can cause depression, especially when taken intermittently and in large quantities, like the binge drinking done in high school and on some college campuses, he says. "Binge drinking plays havoc with your mood," says Shaffer.

[1] The number of suicides among children, teens and young adults up to and including age 24 has exceeded 5,000 since the late 1970s. The number peaked at 5,399 in 1985 and declined to 4,660 in 1996. About 60 percent of these deaths were among people ages 20-24.

[2] Nancy Gibbs, "Special Report: The Littleton Massacre," *Time*, May 3, 1999.

[3] Myrna Weissman, et al., "Depressed Adolescents Grown Up," *Journal of the American Medical Association*, May 12, 1999, pp. 1707-1713.

[4] For background, see Richard L. Worsnop, "Teenage Suicide," *The CQ Researcher*, June 14, 1991, p. 369.

[5] National Center for Health Statistics, Centers for Disease Control and Prevention and National Institutes of Mental Health.

ously lacking.

"But if you address depression in the beginning stages, we can treat it pretty quickly," Weist says.

School-based programs also give schools less expensive, more immediate options for dealing with disruptive kids, Weist says. Schools can send them to an on-site clinic for evaluation, rather than referring them to more expensive special-education classes or to a community program "20 minutes away that has a four-week waiting list," he says.

Such programs also increase students' ability to learn, say proponents, because kids can't learn if they are depressed, anxious or being abused. After only two years in existence, a new mental health program in Dallas schools showed reduced absenteeism and fewer disciplinary and special-ed referrals

Even if all schools don't establish comprehensive on-site mental health services, others argue that more school counselors are needed. The United States has about half the

number of guidance counselors, social workers and school psychologists recommended by a 1997 National Institute of Medicine study. And most high schools do not have a full-time psychologist on staff. [9]

"I think every high school in the United States should have a school psychologist," says Kevin Dwyer, president of the National Association of School Psychologists. School nurses have been cut back dramatically, and guidance counselors and school psychologists are stretched too thin with other duties to be available to troubled kids. As a result, when disturbed children "act out" their depression in school they often are expelled without a psychological evaluation or follow-up treatment because local mental health services have long waiting lists.

"What good is a waiting list for an acutely suicidal youth?" asks Schetky.

Yet during consideration of the juvenile crime bill on May 19, the Senate turned down a proposal offered by Wellstone to provide $340 million in matching funds for schools to hire 141,000 new school-based counselors and mental health providers.

"I am getting a little tired of hearing that the answer to everything around here is simply to throw more money at it," Sen. Orin G. Hatch, R-Utah, responded. "This is a Washington-knows-best, big-money answer to complicated questions that can best be addressed through local efforts." Wellstone's amendment was tabled on a 61-38 vote.

Others say school is not the place for delivering mental health services. "We don't think health care belongs in the schools," says Sheila Moloney, executive director of the conservative Eagle Forum. "Our kids can't read. They can't add. Yet there seems to be this massive emphasis on health care."

Most schools already have guidance counselors or school psychologists to help kids, she points out. Plus she doubts an on-site psychologist could have prevented tragedies like Littleton. The two shooters had attended anger-management classes, but it didn't stop them from shooting their classmates, she notes.

Taking care of a child's mental health is the family's job, insists Karen Holgate, president of the Parents National Network, a parental rights group based in Palm Desert, Calif. "Who is really responsible for the child — the taxpayer or the parent?"

she asks. "If a parent has a depressed child, it's the parent's responsibility to get treatment for him."

"That's fine if the family is handling the job," responds Weist. "But in many situations, the family is not doing the job." Many parents do not have the wherewithal to ensure that their kids get proper mental health care, Hanson notes.

Conservative family groups have grave misgivings about counseling being provided at school, just as they objected to medical clinics being established in schools a decade ago. Clinics, they complained then, were dispensing contraceptives to teenagers without parents' consent.

School-based counseling services threaten to similarly undermine parental authority and invade family and children's privacy, say critics. They particularly object to methods and questions used by health officials to discover whether a child is being sexually abused.

"Unless done properly, school health programs have a potential to go too far," says Dianna Lightfoot, director of the Physicians Resource Council of the Alabama Family Alliance. She and other opponents cite a Pennsylvania Head Start program in which preschoolers and kindergartners were required to undergo genital examinations along with their routine eye and hearing exams. The nurses who conducted the exams said they were looking for signs of sexual abuse.

"Although the parents had given their consent for a checkup, they had no idea the kids would be asked to drop their pants," says Moloney.

Holgate, Lightfoot and Moloney all complained that elementary school children have been sent to school psychologists — sometimes without their parents' consent — and have been asked intimate questions about the family. One father in St. Helena, Calif., permitted a school psycholo-

gist to test his twin daughters for educational aptitude. The psychologist asked one girl whether her parents were sexually abusing her. The child reportedly suffered nightmares and mental distress afterward, and the father is suing the school district.

Critics also object to the phrasing of some values-based questions on psychological tests given by schools, such as: Would your parents support you or condemn you if they found out you were having sex with your boyfriend/girlfriend?

"Such questions raise doubt in kids' minds about the validity of their parents' values," Lightfoot says.

Or a child may tell a therapist he is attracted to someone of the same sex. The counselor might tell the kid it's OK to feel that way. "We don't think a school counselor has any business giving that sort of approval to a child," says Lightfoot.

Some psychologists ask intimate questions about family life that imply parents are abusing children if they smoke in the same room as the child, drink more than two drinks a day or force the child to attend religious services, she says.

Lightfoot also complained about such vaguely worded questions as: "Do your parents ever hit you?" "Do they mean an open-handed slap on the buttocks of an 8-year-old who just spit in your face? Do they call that abuse?" she asks.

Conservatives want to know who will have access to such test results and if information from therapy sessions would become part of a child's permanent school file. "I would support mental health services being made available at the schools, but within certain parameters," says Lightfoot. Parents must be notified before any psychological tests are given and must be allowed to review the questions to be asked, she says.

Hanson admits that there are currently no guidelines for evaluating health and mental health needs of children in school settings but says a committee co-chaired by the American Academy of Pediatrics and the Association of School Nurses is currently drafting such guidelines.

He was surprised to hear that psychologists were giving written tests to determine parental abuse. "There are lots of [outward] indications that a child is in difficulty," he says. "You don't need to give them a written test to see that something has gone awry."

He also insists, "No responsible clinician would give a test or interview a child without obtaining a parent's permission." ■

BACKGROUND

Pioneering Research

Depression in adults has been recognized since biblical times. But it was not officially recognized in American children until 1980, when it was listed as a diagnosable psychiatric condition in the authoritative *Diagnostic and Statistical Manual on Mental Disorders (DSM-III)*.

However, as early as 1946, psychiatrist Rene Spitz had described what he called "anaclitic depression" in infants in orphanages, who failed to thrive when deprived of sufficient human contact.

And beginning in the 1950s, psychiatric researchers Leon Cytryn and Donald K. McKnew Jr. noted that chronically ill and hospitalized children often exhibited the same symptoms as classical adult depression.

In the 1960s and '70s, several pioneering psychiatric researchers attempted to differentiate between adult and childhood depression. Meanwhile, the first epidemiological study of a child population, done in England in the mid-1960s, identified depression in less than 1 percent of youngsters. A 1967 report by the U.S.-based Group for the Advancement of Psychiatry asserted that depression in children often presented itself differently than in adults. [10]

By the early 1970s, Cytryn and McKnew had suggested that there were three types of childhood depression: acute, chronic and masked. But the psychiatric community was not yet ready to recognize childhood depression as a separate pathology. "The absence of a name for this entity [in diagnostic manuals] forces many professionals to misdiagnose their depressive patients," they wrote in the 1979 *Basic Handbook of Child Psychiatry*. "This in turn perpetuates the misconception that the condition does not exist."

Throughout the 1970s, a handful of psychiatrists began diagnosing depression in children more frequently, and doctors began to realize that it had been underestimated in the past. But the diagnosis was still often contested, because most psychiatrists believed children lacked the emotional maturity to experience depression.

Then in 1980, psychiatrists Gabrielle Carlson and Dennis Cantwell wrote about childhood depression in kids with behavior problems. [11]

After the *DSM-III* identified the condition, it became a widely used diagnosis without a great deal of attention paid to how valid the diagnosis was, says Leon Eisenberg, a professor of social medicine at the Harvard School of Medicine. "When efforts were made to compare diagnoses for children across clinics, there were still much higher rates of disagreement [than in adult studies] as to whether childhood depression existed."

About that time, studies around the world showed that adult depression was increasing and appearing at younger ages than it had 50 years earlier. "It seemed more reasonable to think that we were missing depression in adolescents and in children," says Eisenberg.

Experts now know that more than half of depressive adults say they had their first bout with the disease before age 20, a fact that some say points to the urgency of catching and treating depression early in life. The NIMH estimates that up to 2.5 percent of children ages 5 to 12 and 8.3 percent of adolescents suffer from depression, although the AACAP puts the numbers at double that amount.

Some children are genetically predisposed to depression or have an imbalance in their brain chemistry. Often, one or both parents suffer from genetic depression. "Each of us has a certain vulnerability to depression that is inherited," says Glasser. "Children of mothers on Prozac often come in at 5 and 6 years old and are depressed."

If one parent is depressed, the child is 25 percent more likely to become biologically depressed, says Fassler. If two parents are depressed, the child has a 75 percent chance.

But it's not entirely genetic. "What happens to you in your life also affects whether depression occurs," says Fassler. "For instance, if you move five times before you are 5 years old, you are more likely to get depressed. If you are abused as a child, if you witness violence in your home, if you have a parent who has a substance abuse problem. All these experiences increase the risk of depression."

Symptoms and Causes

The symptoms of childhood depression vary with age. According to Fassler, a depressed infant or toddler may present a sad or emo-

Standing Up to School Bullies

Teenager Brian Head endured a never-ending series of bloody noses, broken eyeglasses and taunts about his weight from the bullies at his Marietta, Ga., high school. His father dismissed it as typical schoolyard teasing. Then one day in 1994, Brian walked into a classroom carrying a shotgun and shot himself to death.

As the recent spate of schoolyard killings has shown, however, some children seek payback for bullying. All of the teenage boys responsible for recent mass murders at schools complained that they had been picked on at school.

Parents, educators and mental health experts are increasingly realizing that ignoring chronic teasing and bullying — once considered an almost inevitable character-building rite of passage — can cause tragic consequences in an era of easy availability of guns. In recent years, bullying has become the subject of scholarly research, and many schools have adopted programs to teach kids how to deal with bullies or have tried to eradicate it from school campuses.

"It's really sort of a global phenomenon of growing interest," said Susan Limber, a developmental psychologist at the University of South Carolina who studied bullying among 6,300 fourth-, fifth- and sixth-graders in the rural South. [1]

Intense bullying can trigger depression in children and adolescents and cause lifelong emotional pain, according to psychiatrists. "Being bullied is a very powerful experience that can influence a person's self-esteem for a lifetime," says child psychiatrist David G. Fassler, co-author of *"Help Me, I'm Sad."* "If you ask adults who are struggling with depression when they first had problems, more than half will say it started in childhood, and many will relate stories about being bullied in school. When they tell those stories, they are almost as vivid today as they were when they were just happening."

Some experts suspect that today's teasing may be crueler and have more devastating effects than it did when today's parents were in school. For one thing, teenage pop culture, like the television show "South Park," glorifies vicious verbal assaults and disrespect of others.

In addition, 20 years ago children were more likely to have extended families, with brothers, sisters or cousins who could either intervene or at least support the child being bullied. "Back then, even if a kid was alienated from others in their school, they had a sizable number of kids in their extended family who wouldn't leave them out," said researcher Ahmed Motiar, a former teacher of kids with behavioral problems and author of *Defanging a Bully.* [2]

Many school anti-bullying programs teach kids to deal with bullies using humor and avoidance, but many also target the silent students who make up the bullies' audiences. For instance, in Aurora, Colo., next door to Littleton, where the most deadly school shooting occurred, Highline Community School's bully-intervention program is now a model for 300 schools nationwide. Officials there have declared it against the rules for a student to watch a fellow classmate being bullied without intervening or seeking help.

"Bullyproofing Your School," an anti-bullying program adopted by schools across the country, also focuses on those who stand by and watch. Without an audience, bullies fade into the background, says the program's developer, William Porter. "Kids who are bullies are obsessed with power," he said. "When they start to lose their power and their attention, they really do start to come around." [3]

Other schools are instituting a zero-tolerance policy toward bullying. In March, Georgia passed legislation, sought by the father of Brian Head, which makes bullying a crime and requires school officials to alert parents if it occurs.

"Bullying should not be tolerated in the schools," says Fassler. "It's detrimental and destructive, not just for the victim but for the bully as well. The victims are more likely to get depressed. The bullies are more likely to end up in jail" or as wife-beaters.

Martin Glasser, a child and adolescent psychiatrist in Phoenix, Ariz., said schools should not just expel bullies. "He may be bullying because his dad is beating him up or is beating up his mother," says Glasser. "The school needs the resources to figure out why he is bullying."

Fassler warns that schools should not try to create a school environment completely devoid of conflict. "Conflict is a real part of life," he says, "and kids need to learn how to deal with conflict, frustration and disappointment. But when it crosses the line into interactions that are dangerous either physically or emotionally, then the schools need to intervene to protect the kids."

---

[1] Quoted in Carol Masciola, "Experts say bullied kids' scars run deep," *The Orange County Register*, May 2, 1999.

[2] Quoted in Mike d'Amour and Nova Pierson, "Stopping Bullies, Slain Student's Father Calls for End to Taunting," *The Calgary Sun*, May 2, 1999.

[3] Quoted in Patricia Callahan and Karen Auge, "Schools seek way to defuse bullying," *The Denver Post*, April 23, 1999.

---

tionless face, minimal activity, withdrawal, excessive whining, too little or too much crying or verbal expressions of sadness. They may also fail to thrive, or may show speech and motor developmental delays.

Preschoolers may have frequent or unexplained stomachaches, headaches and fatigue, extreme restlessness, sadness, irritability, loss of pleasure in previously enjoyable activities and a tendency to portray the

Chronology

1940s-1950s
Early researchers describe depression in infants and children.

1946
Psychiatrist Rene Spitz describes a form of depression in institutionalized orphan infants, who fail to thrive when deprived of sufficient human contact.

1950s
Psychiatric researchers Leon Cytryn and Donald K. McKnew Jr. suggest that there are three types of childhood depression — acute, chronic and masked. They note that chronically ill and hospitalized children often exhibit the symptoms of classical adult depression.

1960s-1970s
Researchers attempt to differentiate between adult and childhood depression. A handful of psychiatrists begin diagnosing depression in children, and some doctors realize that it has been underestimated. But most of the psychiatric community is still reluctant to recognize childhood depression as a separate pathology.

1980s *Childhood depression becomes a more widely used diagnosis, but is still controversial among some doctors. Studies in the United States and abroad show that* adult depression worldwide is increasing and appearing at younger ages than 50 years ago. Mental health specialists begin to assume that the diagnosis has been missed in adolescents and in children.

1980
An article in the *American Journal of Psychiatry* identifies childhood depression in children with behavior problems. Childhood depression is officially recognized as a diagnosable psychiatric condition.

1990s *Diagnoses of childhood depression increase, as do pediatric prescriptions for new antidepressants. Three studies raise concerns that the new antidepressants may make a small population of patients exhibit manic tendencies.*

1994
The Food and Drug Administration addresses concerns that untested drugs are being given to children by proposing that pediatric data be required on all drug products that might be prescribed off-label for children.

1995
University of Pennsylvania research psychologist Martin E. P. Seligman writes in his book *The Optimistic Child* that American children are experiencing an "epidemic of depression" resulting partly from decades of misguided attempts to bestow unearned self-esteem on kids.

1996
The National Institute of Mental Health begins establishing a network of seven pediatric-pharmacology research units where clinical trials focus on the effects and safety of psychotropic medications on children.

1997
A University of Texas study shows that the new antidepressants are effective in treating childhood depression, but three of the treated children (6 percent) became manic. Congress encourages drug companies to conduct clinical tests on children by offering a six-month extension on their patents.

1998
After a string of schoolyard shootings by emotionally disturbed adolescent boys, Congress provides $180 million in block grants to help develop strong interagency collaboration between schools, local law enforcement and community mental health services so troubled kids can be identified and given treatment. Some schools begin providing mental health care.

1999
A month after the school shootings in Colorado and Georgia, the Senate refuses to provide money for additional school counselors and psychologists. The Senate adopts an amendment to the juvenile crime bill allowing states to use federal funds to assess detained youths and to put those with diagnosable mental conditions into treatment facilities. Another proposed amendment would allow states to use federal funds to train juvenile justice personnel in how to recognize and deal with mental disorders.

Many Drugs Prescribed for Children . . .

More and more children are being given Prozac and other new antidepressants, but no one really knows what their long-term effects will be on youngsters' developing brains.

None of the new drugs, known as selective serotonin reuptake inhibitors, or SSRIs, has been fully tested in children. No one knows what the appropriate dosages are for treating depression in children nor what the long-term effects are of manipulating serotonin, a brain chemical that affects mood.

"There's an awful lot we don't know about the long-term effects of using these medications," says child psychiatrist. David G. Fassler, co-author of "Help Me, I'm Sad."[1]

Designed for adults, SSRIs have been proven safer for adults than the previous generation of tricyclic antidepressants, or TCAs. Once the Food and Drug Administration (FDA) approves any drug for use in adults, doctors can legally prescribe them to children, a practice called "off-label" prescribing.

But off-labeling can be tricky. "Children are not just little adults," says Fassler. "Their dosages are different. Their metabolisms are different. The potential side effects are different."

Child psychiatrists are particularly worried because pediatricians and general practitioners, who are not trained to detect the subtle side effects of the new antidepressants, are increasingly prescribing psychiatric drugs for children. Many fear non-specialists are not able to monitor a child's behavior on the drugs as closely as a psychiatrist who is regularly seeing the patient for psychotherapy.

For instance, antidepressants that can cause agitation and nervousness in adults could trigger full-blown manic episodes in children. A 1997 University of Texas study showed that SSRIs were effective in treating childhood depression, but three of the treated children (6 percent) became manic.

"Until more sensitive studies of side effects occur, clinicians should be aware of a possible worsening of behavioral problems in children and adolescents treated with SSRIs, TCAs and other antidepressants," wrote the authors of a study reported recently in the Journal of the American Academy of Child and Adolescent Psychiatry.[2]

Fear about manic side effects prompted questions following the Columbine High School shooting, when it was learned that shooter Eric Harris was taking Luvox, an SSRI approved for treating obsessive-compulsive disorder in children but often prescribed off-label to treat depression. Further, of the nine boys involved in recent school shootings, five were depressed, and at least three were taking antidepressants or stimulant drugs, according to press reports.[3]

The fears prompted Solvay SA, the Belgian pharmaceuticals manufacturer that produces Luvox, to issue a prepared statement, saying, "'There is no evidence to suggest a causal relationship between the prescribed use of Luvox tablets and violent or suicidal behavior."[4]

Nonetheless, some say it is dangerous to give antidepressants to kids, particularly over the long term, until clinical, double-blind controlled trials show that they do not cause long-term problems. "There are significant gaps in what we know about the effects of these drugs on children," said Peter S. Jensen, a child and adolescent researcher at the National Institute of Mental Health (NIMH). "Especially in the area of depression, there is reason to be cautious about how these medications are being prescribed to children."[5]

But there could be "terribly unfortunate consequences" if doctors stop prescribing SSRIs for depressed youngsters, Jensen also said. "These medications might be safe and might be effective for children. We just don't really know."[6]

Indeed, only five of the 80 drugs most frequently prescribed in newborns and infants are actually labeled for pediatric use, and 80 percent of the drugs pediatricians routinely prescribe for children have never been tested on children.

"If it's unethical to give kids antidepressants, then it's

world as sad or bleak.

School-age children may develop school phobia, social isolation or antisocial behavior like stealing or lying, a poor self-image, poor grades, tearfulness, excessive worrying, changes in sleep patterns or frequent stomachaches, headaches or undue fatigue.

Older children and teenagers may have sad, hopeless or suicidal feelings, or they may experience extreme

mood swings, engage in dangerous activities, fail academically, run away from home, abuse drugs, steal or lie. Teenage girls may develop anorexia or bulimia or engage in self-mutilation — or cutting themselves — a phenomenon that is on the increase among teens. Males are less likely than females to seek help when they are depressed and more likely to use alcohol and drugs and to express their depression as uncontrolled rage.

Seventy percent of children with depression also have other problems, such as learning disabilities, ADHD and conduct and anxiety disorders. Depression is actually among the least prevalent of mental disorders affecting children.

Some mental health professionals say depression is increasing among children because modern life is more toxic and stressful. They also note that there are fewer adults in kids'

... Were Not Designed for Children — or Tested

unethical to give kids 80 percent of the medications they are given today, because they haven't been tested either," says Ted Petti, a child and adolescent psychiatrist in Indianapolis, Ind.

Concerned about untested drugs being given to children, the FDA in 1994 began requiring pediatric data on all drug products that might be prescribed off-label for children. The National Institutes of Health (NIH) also recently established a network of seven pediatric pharmacology research units where clinical trials will focus on the effects and safety of psychotropic medications on children.

In addition, in 1997 Congress encouraged pharmaceutical companies to conduct clinical tests on children by offering a six-month extension on their patents for those drugs being tested, thereby extending the time during which the drugs could not be copied by generic drug companies. Although generic drug companies tried to block the new rule, a federal judge in April turned down their request for an injunction.

Pharmaceutical companies have proposed studying the pediatric safety of more than 100 drugs, and have received FDA approval to begin research on nearly 50.

While awaiting the results of those studies, doctors are in a Catch-22 situation when deciding whether to give the untested remedies to depressed children. "If a child is depressed, without treatment they fall back in school, fall behind socially and are more likely to get depressed in the future," says Fassler. "So you have to weigh the risks and benefits, as with any course of treatment."

"If I've got a depressed and suicidal kid, do I put him on antidepressants for two months, which is not going to kill him or change his brain chemistry over the short term, but might stop him from killing himself?" asked Carl Bell, a Chicago child psychiatrist. "Me? I'm going to take the risk and save the life."

The difference is "night and day" for depressed patients when they take antidepressants, he says. "They tell me they feel so much better on the medication. I think it's criminal to withhold something that empirically works."

The real dilemma, says child psychiatrist Lois Flaherty of Blue Bell, Pa., is "when a 7- or 8-year-old comes in, and you're faced with prescribing an antidepressant over the long term."

Drug companies say finding child test subjects has been difficult for a variety of ethical, liability and logistical reasons. For one thing, says Marjorie Powell, assistant general counsel for the Pharmaceutical Research and Manufacturers of America, parents usually don't want to subject a sick child to additional burdens.

"Is it ethical to give a child a placebo for a double-blind, controlled study, thereby withholding treatment that could reduce the child's suffering?" she asks. Plus, a 3-year-old can't give informed consent, notes Powell. "Is it right for a parent to make this decision for a kid that cannot comprehend what is happening to him?" Some state courts have held that a parental consent form is no longer valid once the child reaches 21 years of age, she said.

Testers must also determine what the long-term effects might be on a child's brain or physical development. "Following kids for 5-10 years is more difficult than following adults," she says. "And it's more difficult to test on pubescent kids, whose hormones are fluctuating wildly. And how do you get young kids to take medicine if it can't be made into a liquid form or the taste can't be camouflaged?"

---

[1] David G. Fassler and Lynne S. Dumas, *"Help Me, I'm Sad"* (1997).

[2] Graham J. Emslie, et al. "Nontricyclic Antidepressants: Current Trends in Children and Adolescents," *Journal of the American Academy of Child and Adolescent Psychiatry*, May 1999.

[3] "Patterns of Violence," *Time*, May 3, 1999.

[4] "Belgian drugs manufacturer denies link to violence after school shooting," The Associated Press, May 5, 1999.

[5] Quoted in Marc Kaufman, "Are Psychiatric Drugs Safe for Children?" *The Washington Post*, May 4, 1999.

[6] *Ibid.*

---

lives and that they lack a sense of connectedness to their communities. "Kids today are more likely to have moved many times, to have experienced multiple separations from important people," says Fassler. "In addition, they are less likely to have consistent and stable relationships with role models. Isolation increases chances of depression. Kids today are less likely to be connected to their neighborhood, their community

or an extended family."

Further, in the AIDS era, adolescents exploring intimacy and sexuality must deal with the fear of death. "All these factors increase the difficulty adolescents face in trying to separate from the family and find comfort in the outside world," says Glasser.

Children today also see more violence inside and outside the home, experts say. Studies show that expo-

sure to violence and severe stress at an early age can cause permanent physical and chemical changes in the brain that predispose one to depression. "Experiencing very severe stress over a long enough period of time changes the brain chemistry," says Flaherty. "These changes can be irreversible for the immature brain."

"Family violence is a significant contributing factor in child and adolescent depression," says Glasser.

"Some of the conditions that are thought to be depression come from a phenomenon of demoralization, such as when a child is caught in a family setting with tremendous domestic violence. These children become extremely distraught and sometimes commit suicide."

Glasser says today's lack of values and boundaries contribute to teen depression. "Over the last five years, the bar for what is appropriate human behavior in our culture has totally disappeared," he says. "The removal of any type of censorship or reasonable judgment in music, movies and sensational TV news reports is likely to affect the most vulnerable youths.

"Since KISS, every new shock-rock group has tried to out-gross each other: Marilyn Manson feigns killing cats on stage, claims he has a cat eyeball in his head, spits blood and every other human secretion out onto the audience. At what point do we say there is a limit to what kids can be exposed to?" Glasser asked. "I had a 16-year-old psychotic patient who really believed that he was absolutely communicating with the anti-Christ by listening to Manson's music.

"Adolescents function best when they know they can't go beyond certain limits," Glasser continues. "It makes an adolescent much less secure when there are no clear boundaries. But it seems that society has totally removed some of the parameters of what is acceptable behavior. I'm appalled that there's no lid on the kind of terribly bizarre, obscene things that are packaged, marketed and sold to kids as entertainment."

Experts say childhood depression is treatable

Research psychologist Martin E. P. Seligman of the University of Pennsylvania, past president of the American Psychological Association, says in his book *The Optimistic Child* that American children are experiencing an "epidemic of depression" resulting partly from decades of misguided attempts to bestow unearned self-esteem on kids.

"America has seen 30 years of a concerted effort to bolster the self-esteem of its kids," Seligman writes. "But they have never been more depressed." [12]

Constantly telling children they are "special" and that they can "be anything they want to be" without making them work hard to master skills sets them up for depression, he says.

"By emphasizing how a child feels, at the expense of what the child does, parents and teachers are making this generation of children more vulnerable to depression," he wrote.

The good news is that childhood depression is highly treatable, usually with antidepressants combined with counseling. Although depression typically lifts within about nine months, even without treatment, Fassler emphasizes that it should not be left to run its course.

Untreated depression could result in "severe emotional and developmental setbacks," he says. Moreover, within three years up to 50 percent of depressed kids will have a recurrence, he says. "The longer the initial episode goes ignored, the sooner the next will occur," he says, and the more likely it will persist into adulthood.

In light of the new research showing dramatically higher suicide rates among adults whose depression began in childhood, some say it is more imperative than ever that all doctors be on the alert for depression in kids, and that treatment be started as soon as possible.

"Our findings argue for the early identification of depressed adolescents," the authors of the *JAMA* study wrote. "Any debate about whether society can afford the cost of their psychiatric treatment needs to take the consequences of adolescent [depression] into consideration." [13] ∎

CURRENT SITUATION

Focus on Schools

Some professionals hope that the outrage over this year's school shootings will focus public attention beyond installing more metal detectors to the deeper problems of how America is neglecting the mental health needs of its children.

Critics complain that the current system for providing mental health services for youths at community mental health centers is fragmented, uncoordinated and underfunded. Links between schools, community mental health services and the juvenile justice system are often nonexistent or haphazard. As a result, only the most critical cases receive attention from public mental health services.

And in most schools, mental health professionals concentrate on children in special-education programs. So unless a troubled child's parents can afford private therapy, he is not likely to get treatment until his situation erupts into a crisis. Hanson notes that about 25 percent of children are not covered by insurance but are not poor enough to receive Medicaid.

"No one takes responsibility for adolescents until they get into trouble," says Glasser. "If an adolescent is depressed but doesn't make trouble in school, he is ignored. If he acts out, he is expelled, but that just puts society at an even greater risk.

At Issue:

Do we need more school-based mental health services?

HOWARD S. ADELMAN, PH.D.

Professor of Psychology and Co-director, School Mental Health Project/Center for Mental Health in Schools, University of California at Los Angeles

WRITTEN FOR *THE CQ RESEARCHER*, JUNE 1999.

*e*very day too many youngsters encounter barriers that interfere with their healthy development. From an educational perspective, such barriers encompass any factor that interferes with children's academic performance — including factors that make it difficult for teachers to teach effectively.

Among those living in poverty, major inequities of opportunity exist that interfere with school readiness, and this contributes to the large proportion of learning, behavior and emotional problems found in urban and rural schools serving economically impoverished families.

How many youngsters are affected? Estimates vary, but the number is large and growing. With specific respect to mental health concerns, between 12 percent and 22 percent of all children are described as suffering from a diagnosable mental, emotional or behavioral disorder, with relatively few receiving mental health services anywhere. If one adds the many others experiencing significant psychosocial problems, the numbers grow dramatically. The reality for many large urban and poor rural schools is that over half of their students manifest learning, behavior and emotional problems.

Clearly, young people are facing multiple barriers to their successful development and learning. It is critical to deal with these barriers in ways that enable more youth to achieve successfully in school. However, as is widely acknowledged, schools are not in the mental health business. Their primary mission is to educate. At the same time, educators, policy-makers, families and communities have long recognized that schools must play an expanding role in addressing barriers to learning so that all students can learn and perform effectively. Thus, the question before policy-makers isn't whether schools should be involved in such matters. The real question is how to address the many barriers and promote healthy development most effectively.

Although mistakes have and will be made in finding better ways to do all this, such errors are not reasons for backing away from major efforts to ensure that schools address psychosocial and mental health concerns. If we back away from these responsibilities, we will surely jeopardize the futures of too many young people and ensure the failure of current policy initiatives for school reform and renewal. Schools can and must strive to do a better job in meeting their responsibilities to protect everyone's rights, and this especially includes ensuring that no young person is deprived of interventions that are essential to enabling them to benefit appropriately from the school's instructional program.

KAREN HOLGATE

President, Parents National Network, Palm Desert, Calif.

WRITTEN FOR *THE CQ RESEARCHER*, JUNE 1999.

*c*ongress and state legislators should look carefully at the facts before endorsing mental health services at public schools. Before engaging in feel-good "knee-jerk" reactions to the Littleton tragedy, or before authorizing massive expansion of school-based mental health services, issues of privacy, confidentiality, parental rights, funding and the proper role of government (and public schools) in the lives of citizens must be addressed.

Psychological evaluations are already being conducted on children in classrooms across America — often without parental notification or permission. Teachers often administer surveys that ask children whether their parents treat "other children" in the family better than they treat them, whether their parents are headed for a divorce and other personal questions.

In Minnesota, Dr. Karen Effrem, says that school-based clinics allow mental health screening, tracking and referrals without parental knowledge or consent and that parents and/or the parents' insurance is often billed for these services — again without parental permission or even review of records. She points out that the guidelines for diagnosing mental health are extremely broad and vague.

The opportunity for wide-scale abuse is staggering. Parents are already complaining about the abuse of current school practices. For example:

• Twelve third-graders were sent to the school psychologist. After being asked numerous personal questions about their families, the children were told not to talk to anyone outside the classroom about the "counseling group."

• Parents who gave permission for an educational aptitude test for their fourth-grade twin daughters were shocked when the girls told them they were grilled about possible sexual abuse and whether their parents yelled at them.

• A single mom learned her seventh-grade son was labeled at-risk and had been seeing a school psychologist for six weeks. He told her he hadn't realized he was such a "burden" until the counselor told him.

Parental rights are at risk. In California, parents are notified at the beginning of each year that their child may be removed from campus for "confidential medical services" without their consent.

There are already procedures and agencies in place to aid children and parents — whether the problem is mental or physical. Let's not compound the problem by increasing government intrusion into the private lives of families.

Yet if the school principal calls the mental health services, they are often told their hands are full with more critical cases. And the juvenile justice agencies don't want to hear from him until the child commits a crime.

"There is absolutely no coordination between social services, probation and education, the three agencies — all federally supported — that are supposed to support youth in America," he continues. "The question Congress needs to ask is, 'What are the preventive services for youth in America today, and how can we make them work better?' Here we have crisis every two weeks telling us that the system we have isn't working."

While some want more school counselors in the schools, others want comprehensive, full-service mental health centers on school grounds. Such programs would be based on school-based health centers that have been established around the country since the 1980s. Although some were shut down by conservatives complaining they were nothing more than "conduits for condoms," at least 1,200 such health centers still operate at schools today.

School-based health providers consistently report that mental health services are an "overwhelming" unmet need in these centers. As a result, dozens of schools are expanding the services offered at school health centers to include mental health care. Some offer just counseling and referrals, while others offer a full-range of services, including assessment, treatment, case management, prevention and individual therapy. Most are partnerships between school systems and community mental health services and sometimes medical schools.

"The notion of school-based mental health services is expanding around the country," says Weist. "Five states now have funding to enhance infrastructure for such centers." There

is also increasing interest among professional organizations, including the AACAP, the American Psychological Association, the National Association of School Psychologists and the American School Health Association, he says.

The federally funded center that Weist runs in Baltimore — another operates in Los Angeles — offers technical assistance to any community wishing to set up such a program. School administrators often resist the concept until they realize that the programs "are really in-kind contributions to the school and in the long run will improve tests scores," he says.

If the community mental health program cannot take a troubled kid, the school often has no option but to put the child into its special-education program, which can cost up to $8,000 a year per child, much more than the usual per-child education cost.

"Right now, school systems get saddled with the cost and liability for youths with emotional and behavior issues," says Weist. "And sometimes the student ends up needing expensive out-of-state residential treatment at $120,000 a year. Is it appropriate for the school system to be saddled with that cost, while the mental health community sits back and lets that happen? The agencies need to come together and share costs and responsibility for children."

Who Pays the Bill?

Perhaps the biggest obstacle to providing mental health services to troubled children is figuring out who will pay. School administrators aren't keen about having to provide mental health services unless more money is provided. "Principals and teachers

are often prohibited from mentioning the "M" word (mental health problems of students), because their superintendents fear the school district will be asked to pay for it," says Glasser. "I've heard it 20 times."

School-based services are usually funded through a variety of state, local and federal public and private sources, and various payment options are offered to students based on need.

If students are eligible, Medicaid pays the bill. But the Medicaid stream could dry up soon, as managed-care companies aggressively solicit clients among Medicaid recipients, says Weist. Managed-care companies have resisted funding school-based mental health services.

Some funding relief may be coming from Washington. The federal government last fall passed a law providing $180 million in block grants for the states to develop "school and community mental health prevention and treatment intervention services" for kids. Applications for these Safe Schools, Healthy Kids block grants were due June 1.

"To be eligible for this program, communities must develop a plan that includes school-based mental health services," says Sandra McElhaney, special assistant to the president of the National Mental Health Association (NMHA). "This is really innovative stuff. It is a real strong federal investment in prevention and mental health services. It's unprecedented. In the past, there hasn't been any funding for preventive services in mental health."

Last year's school shootings were the impetus behind the law. "The shootings really brought these problems to the attention of Congress as well as the general public," she says.

The program's primary goal is to urge strong interagency collaboration between schools, local law enforcement and community mental health services so that troubled kids can be identified sooner and given treatment before the situation reaches a crisis.

In the wake of the school shootings, many communities are scrambling to strengthen the safety net for troubled kids by improving the lines of communication between schools, parents, law enforcement and the mental health community. A proposed bill to reauthorize the Substance Abuse and Mental Health Services Administration, expected to be debated later this month, would also provide funds for communities to establish comprehensive, interagency, collaborative programs linking schools with mental health service providers.

Communities that do not receive the new block grant funds can pursue a variety of other ways to ensure that troubled kids get services, says Fassler. If students cannot afford private treatment and aren't eligible for Medicaid, schools can ask university clinics to offer services on a sliding scale. Or the school may ask local clinicians to provide services.

"There are clinicians in the community who are interested in and available to provide services," he says. "It's up to the schools to be creative about reaching into the community to work with a wide variety of clinicians to make sure there are services. It's not enough for the schools to say that our backup is the community mental health program. You need access and availability of appropriate services."

Glasser contends that mental health services can be provided to schools without sending psychotherapists into the schools to do on-site therapy. "You don't have to have a shrink in the schools," he insists. "It would never be accepted in some areas."

He suggests making child welfare agencies more responsive to school administrators, having mental health professionals consult with teachers about particular cases that concern them and training student peer counselors to work with troubled classmates.

Problems in detention centers for juveniles

Depressed children — especially adolescent boys — often express their pain in inappropriate ways, which lands them in juvenile detention. The NMHA estimates that as many as 60 percent of kids in the juvenile justice system have some kind of diagnosable mental health problem.

Yet Justice Department investigations show that screening and treatment for children's mental illness is grossly inadequate in juvenile facilities. The department is suing several states for failing to provide institutionalized children with mental health care.

The National Association for the Mentally Ill recently released a study showing that many mentally ill children in juvenile facilities are being abused instead of treated. Some are left in isolation for weeks, others are kept in restraints. Often kids are punished for asking for their medications or for exhibiting the symptoms of their mental disorder.

"If kids have mental health problems, they need treatment, not incarceration," says Fassler. "And the earlier we can identify and treat these mental health problems, the less likely the child is to have long-term, ongoing difficulties."

Besides seeking proper treatment for youths in detention, mental health advocates want juvenile justice employees, judges and law enforcement officials to be trained in how to recognize depression and mental illness in kids.

During debate in May on the juvenile crime bill, the Senate adopted two Wellstone amendments allowing states to use federal juvenile justice funds to assess and treat mentally ill youths and to pull those with diagnosable conditions out of detention and put them into treatment facilities. One amendment would allow states to use the funds to train juvenile justice personnel in how to recognize and deal with mental disorders. ■

OUTLOOK

Fighting Back

In Baltimore, Weist predicts that some schools will reach out more to the religious community to help provide for children's mental health needs. For instance, he is negotiating with local churches that he wants to provide parishioners who would act as youth mentors in the schools.

"We are working hard to break down the barriers between the mental health and religious communities," he says. "There's been a lot of reticence on both sides, but when you bring the two groups together, you'd be amazed at the level of communication and the lightbulbs going off in people's heads. We don't have enough resources for kids, but folks from the religious community typically are invested in kids. Rather than bashing each other, we need to build bridges."

Meanwhile, at the Food and Drug Administration's urging, drug companies are doing more research on the impact of antidepressants on children. If they prove safe, many companies are expected to expand their marketing campaigns, targeting even more pediatricians and parents.

"In a year or so, one or more of the SSRIs will be approved for kids," Wolfe noted. "Will this increase the use of them by non-psychotherapists? Probably yes. It is already out of control."

Several mental health professionals predict that within five to 10 years brain imaging will be so sophisticated that doctors will be able to pinpoint the cause of a patient's distress, and eventually medicines will be developed to specifically address a patient's unique problems.

"Treatments will become more specific," says Fassler. "We will be better able to identify which kids are most likely to respond to which treatments. And with regard to prevention, we will have a better handle on which kids are at highest risk, and, hopefully, we will have progressed to the point where we will be better able to prevent the first episode of depression in kids."

Some schools and mental health professionals say the best hope is to prevent depression through "resilience training," teaching kids to be better able to handle disappointments and frustration.

In *The Optimistic Child* Seligman outlines a program for immunizing kids against depression by teaching them optimism. Parents and teachers can help cure children's helplessness by teaching them how to:

• Recognize the thoughts that automatically cross their minds when they feel low.

• Evaluate these automatic thoughts and acknowledge that they may not accurately reflect reality.

• Generate more-accurate explanations to replace the less-accurate thoughts.

• "Decatastrophize" things that go wrong by disputing their own negative interpretations of them.

• Master new skills, so their self-esteem will be boosted legitimately.

But, of course, the biggest challenges are still figuring out how all kids can get access to mental health care and who will pay for it. "We have ample mental health professionals for children, adolescents and their families, but we have a disconnect

FOR MORE INFORMATION

American Academy of Child and Adolescent Psychiatry, 3615 Wisconsin Ave. N.W., Washington D.C. 20016; (800) 333-7636; www.aacap.org. An organization of child and adolescent psychiatrists that monitors research and legislation concerning mentally ill children and provides information on child abuse, youth suicide and drug abuse.

National Assembly on School-Based Health Care, 666 11th St. NW, Suite 735, Washington, D.C. 20001; (888) 286-8727; www.nasbhc.org. A nonprofit association representing school-based health-care providers and supporters that promotes school-based mental health care for children.

National Institute of Mental Health, 6001 Executive Blvd., Room 8184, MSC 9663, Bethesda, Md. 20852; (301) 443-4513; www.nimh.nih.gov. A branch of the National Institutes of Health that researches the causes, diagnosis, treatment and prevention of mental disorders.

National Mental Health Association, 1021 Prince St., Alexandria, Va. 22314-2971; (800) 969-6642; www.nmha.org. The NMHA encourages research on mental illness, helps establish community mental health centers, participates in litigation supporting patients' rights and serves as a clearinghouse for information on mental health issues.

with access," says Glasser. "The problem is not in having enough trained professionals, it's who should pay for them."

Meanwhile, having thousands of kids walking around suffering from untreated depression is a tragedy, says Fassler. "We can help almost all kids with major psychiatric problems," he says. "We can't cure them all. But we can significantly reduce their symptoms, pain and suffering." ∎

Notes

[1] The lower estimate is from the National Institute of Mental Health; the higher estimate is from the American Academy of Child and Adolescent Psychiatry.
[2] For background, see Richard L. Worsnop, "Depression," *The CQ Researcher*, Oct. 9, 1992, pp. 857-880.
[3] David G. Fassler, and Lynne S. Dumas, *"Help Me, I'm Sad,"* 1997.
[4] Myrna Weissman, et al., "Depressed Adolescents Grown Up," *Journal of the American Medical Association*, May 12, 1999, pp. 1707-1713. For background, see Richard L.

Worsnop, "Teenage Suicide," *The CQ Researcher*, June 14, 1991, pp. 369-392.
[5] The suicide rate for adolescents and young adults ages 15-24 rose from 4.5 deaths per 100,000 in 1950 to 13.3 deaths in 1995, according to the National Center for Health Statistics; 60 percent of the suicides were among the young adults.
[6] For background, see Mary H. Cooper, "Prozac Controversy," *The CQ Researcher*, Aug. 19, 1994, pp. 721-744.
[7] For background, see Adriel Bettelheim, "Managing Managed Care," *The CQ Researcher*, April 16, 1999, pp. 305-328.
[8] Quoted in Mary Crowley, "Do kids need Prozac?" *Newsweek*, Oct. 20, 1997, p. 73.
[9] For background, see Kathy Koch, "School Violence," *The CQ Researcher*, Oct. 9, 1998, pp. 881-904.
[10] "Psychopathological Disorders in Childhood: Theoretical Considerations and a Proposed Classification," Report No. 62, Group for the Advancement of Psychiatry, New York, 1967.
[11] Gabrielle Carlson and Dennis Cantwell, "Unmasking Masked Depression," *American Journal of Psychiatry*, 1980.
[12] Martin E. P. Seligman, *The Optimistic Child*, (1995), pp. 27-36.
[13] Weissman, et al, *op. cit.*

Bibliography
Selected Sources Used

Books

Cytryn, Leon, and Donald H. McKnew Jr., *Growing Up Sad, Childhood Depression and Its Treatment*, W. W. Norton, 1996.
Two psychiatric researchers discuss the causes, symptoms and treatment of childhood depression.

Fassler, David G., and Lynne S. Dumas, *Help Me, I'm Sad*, Penguin, 1997.
A child psychiatrist advises parents how to recognize, treat and prevent childhood depression.

Seligman, Martin E. P., *The Optimistic Child*, HarperPerennial, 1995.
A University of Pennsylvania experimental psychologist and former president of the American Psychological Association explains how parents and teachers can teach children optimism skills that will help immunize them against depression.

Articles

"Belgian drugs manufacturer denies link to violence after school shooting," AP, May 5, 1999.
After it was learned that Eric Harris, one of the shooters in the Littleton, Colo., school massacre, was taking the antidepressant Luvox, the Belgian pharmaceuticals manufacturer that produces it insisted there is no evidence of a causal relationship between the prescribed use of Luvox and violent or suicidal behavior.

Callahan, Patricia, and Karen Auge, "Schools seek way to defuse bullying," *The Denver Post*, April 23, 1999.
An anti-bullying program adopted by schools across the country focuses on those who stand by and watch. Without an audience, bullies fade into the background, says the program's developer, William Porter.

Crowley, Mary, "Do kids need Prozac?" *Newsweek*, Oct. 20, 1997, p. 73.
A dramatic increase in antidepressant prescriptions for children has led some to question whether doctors are overprescribing the new drugs, many of which have not been proven safe for kids through clinical trials.

d'Amour, Mike, and Nova Pierson, "Stopping Bullies: Slain Student's Father Calls for End to Taunting," *The Calgary Sun*, May 2, 1999.
The father of a student shot by a classmate who complained he had been picked on in school called for an end to bullying.

Gibbs, Nancy, "Special Report: The Littleton Massacre," *Time*, May 3, 1999.
The Jefferson County sheriff in Littleton, Colo., said the boys who raged through Columbine High School shooting classmates on April 20 were actually on a suicide mission.

Kaufman, Marc, "Are Psychiatric Drugs Safe for Children?" *The Washington Post*, May 4, 1999.
Peter S. Jensen, a child and adolescent researcher at the National Institute of Mental Health, says there are significant gaps in what is known about the effects of the new antidepressants on children.

Masciola, Carol, "Experts say bullied kids' scars run deep," *The Orange County Register*, May 2, 1999.
Researchers are taking a new interest in the long-term impact and the emotional scars left by excessive bullying.

Weissman, Myrna, et al., "Depressed Adolescents Grown Up," *Journal of the American Medical Association*, May 12, 1999, pp. 1707-1713.
Researchers report that adolescents diagnosed with depression as youngsters in the early 1980s were 14 times more likely than their healthy peers to commit or attempt suicide during their lifetime.

Reports and Studies

Emslie, Graham J., et al. "Nontricyclic Antidepressants: Current Trends in Children and Adolescents," *Journal of the American Academy of Child and Adolescent Psychiatry*, May 1999.
The authors review the current data on the safety and efficacy of using the newest antidepressant drugs on children. They recommend that double-blind, placebo-controlled trials be conducted.

Jensen, Peter S., et al., "Psychoactive Medication Prescribing Practices for U.S. Children: Gaps Between Research and Clinical Practice," *Journal of the American Academy of Child and Adolescent Psychiatry*, May 1999.
Many psychotropic drugs are given to children without evidence of safety and efficacy, says a group of NIMH and FDA researchers.

Psychopathological Disorders in Childhood: Theoretical Considerations and a Proposed Classification, Report No. 62, Group for the Advancement of Psychiatry, New York, 1967.
This early report asserted that depression in children often presented itself differently than in adults.

4 Asthma Epidemic

KENNETH JOST

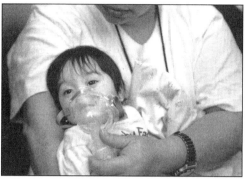

Nadine Anderson's son Aaron was not yet 1 year old when she heard the telltale cough. "It was not like a regular cough," she recalls. It was "dry" and "dull" — "like he was choking."

Aaron's doctor recognized his wheezing and coughing as classic symptoms of asthma and treated him with albuterol — one of many strangely named medicines that Anderson now talks about with familiarity. The medicine, converted into a fine mist by a device known as a nebulizer and inhaled through a mask, opened Aaron's clogged airways enough for him to go home and breathe easily, at least until his next asthma attack.

On that day four years ago, Aaron joined the rapidly growing number of children who have been diagnosed with asthma, a chronic and debilitating breathing disorder that affects more than 5.3 million youngsters under age 18 in the United States and 17.3 million people overall.

While doctors and public health officials have been making progress against other chronic diseases, asthma has been increasing in numbers and in severity over the past two decades — for reasons that are not completely understood.

"We have an alarming increase in the prevalence of asthma, which may be considered of epidemic proportions," says Virginia Taggart, director of the division of lung diseases at the National Heart, Lung, and Blood Institute, part of the National Institutes of Health (NIH) in Bethesda, Md. "The increase has been large. It's not clear why it has happened. And it's certainly had a profound impact on our lives."

Technically, the increased incidence of asthma that is being noted

From *The CQ Researcher*, December 24, 1999.

in the United States and other industrialized countries does not qualify as an epidemic, a term normally used for infectious diseases spread by viruses or bacteria. Asthma, instead, appears to be a disease born from some genetic predisposition or early disorder of the immune system.

The condition, misleadingly dormant much of the time, can be triggered by the body's allergic response to indoor air contaminants, outdoor air pollution or, in some individuals, to cold, exercise or stress. [1] An attack leaves the asthma sufferer gasping for breath. A severe attack can require hospitalization or — in a small but disturbing number of extreme cases — can be fatal.

Whether an epidemic or not, doctors and public health officials are seeing more and more asthma cases, especially in inner-city neighborhoods and especially among blacks. "It's going up at a very rapid rate in the inner city and at a rapid rate elsewhere," says Lawrence Lichtenstein, director of the Asthma and Allergy Center at Johns Hopkins University Medical Center in Baltimore. In the South Bronx, researchers estimate that 9-14 percent of youngsters have asthma. A study by the Children's Health Fund earlier this year found that among children in New York City shelters the rate was alarmingly high: 38 percent. [2]

Treating homeless children with asthma poses particularly difficult

problems, according to Shawn Bowen, an asthma pediatrician with the asthma initiative being conducted jointly by the Children's Health Fund and Montefiore Medical Center.

"Children in the homeless shelter don't have a medical home," says Bowen, who is also an assistant professor in the division of community pediatrics at Montefiore Medical Center/Albert Einstein College of Medicine. "They get most of their care in an emergency room or clinic. As a result, there's very little continuity. And since asthma is a chronic disease, the only way to treat it is to have continuity of care." [3]

Aaron, who until recently lived in a shelter with his mother, has improved greatly, thanks in no small part to her efforts to learn how to deal with the disease. Anderson, a single parent in her 30s who came to the United States from Jamaica as a teenager, knows how to listen to Aaron's chest to gauge his breathing. "When he's wheezing, it sounds like the wind blowing through the trees," she says.

Initially, Aaron's asthma was classified as persistent and severe, the most serious of the four diagnostic gradations. (The others: intermittent/mild, persistent/mild and persistent/moderate.) Aaron needed two types of medications: bronchodilators — so-called rescue medicines — that relieve the immediate symptoms of an asthma attack by relaxing the bronchial tubes and allowing normal breathing to resume; and corticosteroids — so-called controller medicines — that reduce the chronic inflammation of the airways and thus help reduce the long-term severity of the disease.

Today, Aaron is only taking albuterol, one of the most common bronchodilators. He was once taking controller medicines up to four times a day but is no longer on daily

Childhood Asthma on the Increase

The rate of asthma among children under age 18 almost doubled from 1982 to 1998, while the rate among all ages increased by almost two-thirds. An estimated 17.3 million Americans had asthma in 1998, including 5.3 million children under 18.

Estimated Number of Asthma Cases

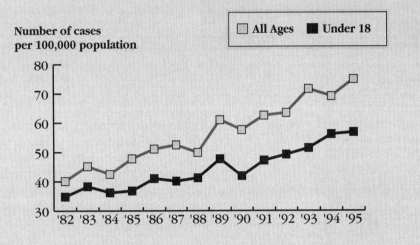

Number of cases per 100,000 population

☐ All Ages ■ Under 18

Source: National Center for Health Statistics, "National Health Interview Survey," 1982-1995

medication at all. Anderson, who now has her own apartment and works as a security guard at the shelter where she once lived, is clearly pleased. But she still keeps a close eye on Aaron. "I don't let him run too much," she says. "I don't let him cry too much."

Anderson's crash course in asthma parallels the experience of millions of other parents around the country, in well-to-do suburbs as well as inner cities. "Every day, we pull down about 50 or 60 requests for information, and the vast majority of those are from parents of children under age 6," says Nancy Sander, president of the Fairfax, Va.-based support network known as Allergy and Asthma Network/Mothers of Asthmatics.

"Many of the families are just newly diagnosed, so they don't know what they don't know," says Sander, who has asthma herself and has a daughter with the disease. "They're searching for help, understanding, information."

Oddly, many better-off families resist the diagnosis. "Parents are often reluctant to have their kids labeled as asthmatic," says John Carl, a pediatric pulmonologist at Rainbow Babies and Children's Hospital in Cleveland. "The label is not a negative thing. It may be a defining thing that may help other health-care providers provide appropriate treatment."

One reason for families' reluctance to acknowledge asthma in their children may be the widespread misunderstanding about the disease. Ancient Greek physicians recognized asthma, but its exact causes remain a mystery today. As recently as 50 years ago, many doctors believed — mistakenly — that the disease was largely psychosomatic. Still today, asthma is widely thought of as a not especially severe disease — even by some people who have asthma.

The asthma "epidemic" is helping to correct some of those mispercep-

tions, as more people deal with the disease in their families or encounter other people who have it. Meanwhile, public health officials are working to improve the care and treatment of people with asthma, while researchers look for more effective medicines to control the disease or — in the longer-term future — prevent it.

As the efforts continue, here are some of the questions being debated:

Are environmental factors causing the increase in asthma?

When the 12th-century rabbi and physician Maimonides treated an Egyptian prince for asthma, he prescribed, among other things, escape from the urban pollution of the time. With the advent of the Industrial Revolution in the 19th century, outdoor air pollution again became a leading suspect in either causing or aggravating asthma — and remained a major focus of asthma investigators into the 1980s.

Since that time, however, doctors and researchers have devoted greater attention to other possible "triggers" for asthma, especially allergens found in the air inside homes and offices. Today, tobacco smoke, cockroach infestation and dust mites rank as the leading suspects for aggravating the condition.

Indoor air problems are "a much more likely explanation of why asthma is increasing," says Carlos Camargo, an epidemiologist at Massachusetts General Hospital in Boston. "There's all kind of evidence that inhalation of things like dust mites, [decaying] cockroaches and other allergens worsen asthma. And they're also associated with a higher risk of developing asthma."

Researchers hypothesize that modern living conditions, including enclosed homes and offices and reduced outdoor time in particular for children, exacerbate the effect of indoor air problems and thus the potential for either causing or aggravating asthma. By contrast, outdoor air pollution has been reduced in the United States in recent years as the incidence of asthma was increasing.

"Twenty years ago, people did suspect that outdoor pollution was high on the list of either causing or aggravating asthma, or both," says Taggart at NIH. "Today, it's highly unlikely that outdoor pollution is on the list of causing asthma, though it does aggravate the disease."

One study often cited for discounting the role of air pollution in causing asthma compared the rates of the disease in east and west Germany after unification. Surprisingly, east Germany had a lower incidence of hay fever, bronchial asthma and other respiratory diseases than west Germany despite markedly worse outdoor air pollution in the former communist state. The researchers described the results as "paradoxical," though they nonetheless concluded, "environmental factors . . . do influence the development" of the disease. [4]

Some researchers disagree with the de-emphasis on the role of outdoor air pollution in asthma research. Patrick L. Kinney, an associate professor and environmental health expert at the Joseph L. Mailman School of Public Health at Columbia University in New York City, says some studies provide evidence of a relationship between living near busy streets and having respiratory problems. In addition, other studies also suggest that diesel fuel particles — a contributor to outdoor air pollution — can "enhance" people's response to allergens.

"We know that air pollution exacerbates asthma," Kinney adds, "but we don't know that that's the only thing it does."

In recent years, another suspect has been added to the list of possible causes of asthma: changes in human immunology. Some researchers believe that public health improvements — such as reduced incidence of respiratory infections among children,

Deaths Among Blacks Increased the Most

Deaths from asthma among blacks increased by more than 150 percent from 1979 to 1997, compared with a 91 percent rise among whites. Among all Americans, deaths increased by 92 percent during the same period. Nearly 90 percent of the 5,434 asthma deaths in 1997 were among adults age 35 and older.

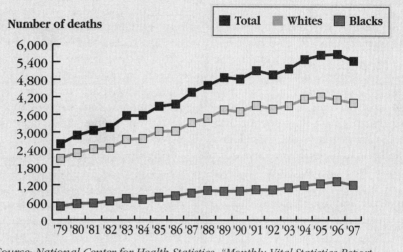

Estimated Number of Asthma Deaths

Source: National Center for Health Statistics, "Monthly Vital Statistics Report, 1979-1997"

increased use of antibiotics and improvements in diet — may be stunting the development of immunological protections against allergens.

"By modifying the normal immune mechanisms in people, we've allowed for an increase in the incidence of asthma," says William Busse, president-elect of the American Academy of Allergy, Asthma and Immunology and a professor of medicine at the University of Wisconsin. "We're getting a changed immune response."

The variety of hypotheses leaves researchers and health-care professionals frustrated.

"We don't know what causes asthma," Taggart says. "We are increasingly convinced that it's some interplay between the environment, the genetic predisposition to having allergies and the developing immune systems and lungs. Which thing is the most important, or which comes first to start the

chain of events, we really don't know."

Are health services adequate for people with asthma?

When he was struggling with asthma as a youngster in the 1930s, Lichtenstein of Johns Hopkins University was advised to spend every winter in Florida to take advantage of its warm, sunny climate. Today, as one of the country's leading asthma researchers, Lichtenstein says his doctor's advice was flat wrong.

"For asthmatics, some of the most common irritants are dust mites, mold and other substances you'll find in a wet climate, like Florida," Lichtenstein writes. His doctor "didn't know enough about asthma to realize that I would wheeze and cough as much — if not more — during our winter vacation at the beach." [5]

Health care for people with asthma has improved dramatically since that time. Doctors and other medical professionals are better informed. Some misconceptions — like the idea that asthma was primarily psychosomatic — have been dispelled. New medications and new devices have been introduced to control and prevent asthma attacks.

Still, the asthma epidemic has focused attention on shortcomings in the care and treatment of asthmatics. Public health experts say that youngsters in medically underserved areas — inner-city neighborhoods in particular — often go undiagnosed until their asthma reaches an advanced state and may get inadequate care after that because they do not have a regular primary-care provider. [6] Children in families that do have good medical care also may not be properly diagnosed or treated because some general practitioners fail to recognize the symptoms or fail to prescribe the right course of treatment after making the diagnosis.

In addition, Lichtenstein and others say that the present treatment options are still short of a cure. "What we're doing is treating the symptoms rather than the underlying disease," he says.

For many patients, however, even symptomatic treatment is far from ideal. In the inner cities — where asthma is increasing most rapidly — too many people see doctors only at times of acute attacks. "They have episodic contact with the health-care system, usually in the emergency room," says Irwin Redlener, president of the Children's Health Fund, a New York City-based organization working to improve health services for children in medically underserved areas.

"The ER ends up being both the receiving and monitoring point for people whose asthma is out of control," says Michael McDermott, an emergency room physician at Cook County Hospital in Chicago. "It's theoretically possible that asthmatics should never come to an emergency room once they're properly trained."

Redlener, who is also president of the Children's Hospital at Montefiore Medical Center in the Bronx, says that inadequately trained physicians are also a problem. "Many kids go to doctors that aren't even close to up-to-speed with respect to the latest treatments that are available to children."

Too many general practitioners tend to be late in diagnosing asthma, according to Bruce Bender, a doctor at the National Jewish Medical and Research Center in Denver, a leading asthma research and treatment facility. "Treating asthma earlier can prevent it from being worse later on," Bender explains.

Meanwhile, researchers are trying to develop more effective medications. NIH's Taggart calls the research "very exciting and very promising." "We'll get more therapies that will target the earlier parts of the inflammatory process so that we can stop this chain reaction earlier in the cycle," she says.

Some asthma experts, however, say they want to see more attention paid to improving existing services without waiting for therapies that are years away from being introduced. "We have excellent tools right now to achieve reasonable disease control, but the system is providing for inadequate application of those controls," says Carl, at Rainbow Babies and Children's Hospital. "We can do much better nationally than we are doing." ■

BACKGROUND

Gasping for Breath

Ancient Greek physicians as early as Hippocrates in the fifth century B.C.E. used the word "asthma" (meaning panting) to refer generally to conditions of gasping or breathlessness. [7] Only in the 17th century did the English physician Sir John Floyer and others develop the modern view of asthma as a condition distinct from other breathing disorders.

Diagnosis of asthma advanced in the 18th and 19th centuries with the development of new medical techniques and tools. The 18th-century Viennese physician Leopold Auenbrugger introduced the now standard technique of chest examination in a 1761 treatise, "On Percussion of the Chest," that explained how tapping on a fluid-filled chest cavity produces a different sound than tapping on a clear one. In the early 19th century, the French physician Rene Laënnec invented the stethoscope for listening to the heart and lungs.

Treatment of asthma also improved, but remained fairly primitive through the 19th century. In the United States, asthma was widely recognized as a common ailment, and medical hucksters advanced a variety of cures and treatments for the disease. Opium, cocaine and tobacco were often prescribed: As stimulants, they help open airways, but they also have adverse side effects. A variety of powders and inhalants were also advertised as cures.

By the turn of the century, some experimenters were working on ways to deliver medications into the lungs with devices that used air or steam instead of smoke — forerunners of today's inhalers.

Doctors remained divided about the causes of asthma through the 19th century. As early as the 17th century, the German physician Konrad Schneider had identified dust as an irritant of the disease. In the mid-19th century, the English physician Henry Slater identified animal dander as an asthma trigger. By then,

Chronology

several researchers had concluded that the underlying cause of bronchial asthma was a spasm of the bronchial musculature. But the dominant theory linked asthma to a nervous disorder.

Early Breakthroughs

In 1910, though, American scientist Samuel Meltzer put forth the theory — close to the modern understanding — that asthma is caused by a spasm of the bronchioles triggered by some specific substance to which a person with the disease is hypersensitive. [8]

The great medical breakthrough in treating asthma came with the introduction of corticosteroids to control asthma attacks in the 1950s. [9] Biochemists had identified the importance of the natural hormones produced by the cortex of the adrenal gland as early as the mid-19th century. Extracts of the adrenal cortex were purified during the 1930s, and the individual steroids were identified, including the most important: cortisone. After the U.S. physician Philip Hench demonstrated that cortisone could be used to treat acute arthritis, doctors tried it on other diseases, including asthma.

"It was very quickly evident," the English physician Donald Lane writes, "that steroids would combat severe life-threatening attacks of asthma." But "disappointing relapses" occurred when the steroids were withdrawn. So doctors turned to prescribing steroids as long-term maintenance for some asthmatics. The results were generally positive, but a rash of side effects produced a reaction against the use of steroids in the 1960s. Concerns about side effects were alleviated, however, by the development of manufactured corticosteroids — more powerful than the natural sub-

Before 1900
Asthma is recognized, but causes are not completely understood and treatments are primitive.

1600s
German physician identifies dust as asthma trigger.

1820s
Invention of the stethoscope helps doctors better diagnose asthma.

Mid-1800s
English physician Henry Slater systematically documents asthma cases, identifies animal dander as trigger.

Late 1800s
Opium, cocaine, tobacco and other inhalants are widely prescribed for treating asthma in the United States.

1900s-1960s
Biochemists make progress in understanding the body's response to allergens.

1920s
Adrenaline is used to relieve asthma symptoms despite potential side effects.

1940s
Cortisone — a hormone produced by the adrenal gland — is isolated and used to treat arthritis.

1950s-1960s
Manufactured corticosteroids are introduced to treat asthma; bronchodilators are developed to relieve symptoms with fewer side effects.

1980s *Asthma rates increase in United States and other industrialized countries; outdoor air pollution is thought to be major factor in causing disease.*

1990s *Public health agencies and support groups mount campaigns to increase public awareness of asthma "epidemic"; indoor air contaminants viewed as major factor in causing or triggering disease.*

1991
National Heart, Lung, and Blood Institute prescribes guidelines for diagnosing and treating asthma; updated in 1997.

1997
Researchers suggest exposure to tuberculosis virus may reduce susceptibility to asthma.

1999
Clinical trials continue on anti-IgE therapy; companies plan to seek government approval for use of the drug in 2000.

A Guide to Asthma Medications

Asthma patients and their families can easily feel bewildered by the array of medications and devices used to manage the disease and the instructions on how to use them. Moreover, many specialists and asthma advocates believe that doctors often fail to educate patients adequately and tend to underprescribe the anti-inflammatory medications that decrease swelling in the airways and thus provide long-term protection against severe attacks.

Many asthma patients, however, believe doctors are insensitive to complaints about side effects of asthma medications, such as jitteriness and rapid heartbeat and growth reduction in youngsters who take anti-inflammatory corticosteroids on a regular basis. But asthma specialists believe the side effects are minimal — most youngsters reach their anticipated height anyway, they say — and in any event are outweighed by the benefits of the medications.

People with "persistent" asthma — symptoms more than twice a week — are typically given two types of medications: anti-inflammatory ("control") medicines and so-called bronchodilators ("rescue" medicines) for symptomatic relief. Here's a brief guide:

Anti-inflammatory medicines — Corticosteroids, not to be confused with the anabolic steroids used and abused by athletes and body-builders, are most commonly prescribed to reduce the asthmatic's chronic inflammation of the airways. Typically, they are inhaled so that more of the medicine reaches the lungs instead of other parts of the body — thus allowing lower doses and minimizing side effects. Some brand names: Vanceril, Pulmicort, Flovent and Azmacort.

Cromolyn and nedocromil are non-steroid, anti-inflammatory drugs that block allergens from attaching to and triggering certain inflammatory cells that line the airways. Both are inhaled. Brand names: Intal and Tilade. Anti-leukotrienes are another non-steroid drug that target one type of inflammatory cells, leukotrienes. Two pills are being aggressively marketed since winning approval two years ago: Accolate and Singulair.

Bronchodilators — These drugs provide short-term relief of coughing, wheezing and shortness of breath by relaxing the constriction of the bronchial muscles that causes breathing difficulties in an asthma attack. The most widely used is albuterol, also sold as Ventolin and Proventil. It comes in metered-dose inhalers or in a solution for use in a nebulizer, a mist-creating machine used by infants or other people who have difficulty operating an inhaler. Another bronchodilator, salmetrol, acts for up to 12 hours but takes longer to start working.

Alternative-medicine advocates list a variety of non-pharmacological methods of treating asthma, including reducing air pollutants, taking vitamins or dietary supplements and decreasing stress.[1] Some of the approaches are "quite mainstream," says Virginia Taggart, director of the division of lung diseases at the National Heart, Lung and Blood Institute, part of the National Institutes of Health. But she says the use of herbal teas, acupuncture and meditation "have not been adequately studied" to assess their effectiveness.

---

[1] For background, see Richard L. Worsnop, "Alternative Medicine's Next Phase," *The CQ Researcher*, Feb. 14, 1997, pp. 121-144, and Charles S. Clark, "Alternative Medicine," Jan. 31, 1992, pp. 73-96.

---

stances — and by physicians' greater familiarity with their use.

The second medical breakthrough came with the development of bronchodilators — chemicals that open up the narrow airways by relaxing the bronchial muscle.[10] The natural hormone adrenaline was first used for treating asthma at the end of the 19th century and introduced into commercial use in the 1920s. But, as Lane explains, adrenaline is a general stimulant that causes higher blood pressure and a number of other adverse physical changes.

Biochemists worked to produce more selective agents that would operate only on the bronchial muscles and by the 1960s had created what Lane calls "a daunting array" of bronchodilators with fewer side effects. In addition, the development of the metered-dose inhaler made it easier for patients to administer bronchodilators themselves, getting a small, measured dose directly into the clogged airways.

Unexplained Epidemic

Doctors and asthma researchers were encouraged by their progress in treating the disease in the 1960s and '70s. They took further encouragement from the gradual decline in the number of asthma deaths among young people reported in the United States beginning in 1968 and continuing through the next decade.

In the 1980s, however, asthma-related deaths began a steady rise that has continued up to the present. By the beginning of the 1990s, two experts writing in the *Journal of the American Medical Association* labeled the trend "an alarming reversal" in the progress against the disease.[11]

Now, at the end of the decade, experts still profess bafflement at the increased incidence of asthma and asthma-related deaths. "There are a lot of thoughts," says Thomas Casale, an asthma researcher at the Nebraska Medical Research Institute in Papillion. "I don't think we have a clear-cut answer." Lichtenstein at Johns Hopkins agrees: "Basically, we don't know the reason why, which is a little discouraging."

Focus on Education

Through the decade, asthma advocates worked to increase public awareness of the disease. "There remains a pervasive attitude, among physicians as well as patients, that asthma is not all that serious," medical writer Robin Marantz Henig observed in a 1993 article. [12] Educating patients and physicians remains a major concern today.

"We think a lot of people have adjusted to a lower quality of life than they need to," the NIH's Taggart says. "It's a matter of changing ways that people look at the disease. It's a chronic disease that needs daily therapy for most people who have asthma."

Among physicians, asthma specialists have long complained that primary-care providers are not aggressive enough in treating asthma. General practitioners rely too much on bronchodilators for symptomatic relief rather than turning to steroids to relieve the chronic inflammation of the airways, specialists say.

"Half of the people with asthma are being undertreated," Busse says. He blames the cost of medication in part but places primary responsibility on what he calls "lack of aggressiveness on the part of the physician."

With asthma rates continuing to climb in the United States, researchers continued to look for explanations for the increase. A new hypoth-

esis emerged toward the end of the decade that, paradoxically, suggested improved childhood health might be partly responsible for the increased incidence of asthma. In January 1997, a team of English and Japanese physicians reported that they found a higher rate of asthma among children in a Japanese village who had been exposed to the tuberculosis virus than those who had not. [13] In effect, the researchers hypothesized, the immune system's response to exposure to the tuberculosis virus served to inhibit the development of asthma.

Other researchers have broadened the idea into a so-called "hygiene hypothesis" that suggests children's immune systems get stronger by fighting off viruses and allergens but have less opportunity to develop fully today because of improved sanitation, greater use of antibiotics and more widespread immunizations.

"Some people think that immunizations have been so effective that kids' immune systems are shifted in a way that they might be more prone to having allergies," Casale explains. He stresses that the hypothesis is "not proven."

By the end of the decade, public awareness of the asthma "epidemic" was increasing with greater media coverage of the issue. The National Heart, Lung, and Blood Institute issued updated guidelines for doctors, stressing early diagnosis and aggressive treatment. Asthma organizations were putting out concrete checklists for patients on how to manage the disease and reduce exposure to asthma "triggers." Still, researchers had no agreed-upon explanation for the cause of the epidemic.

"Ten allergists will give you 10 different answers — maybe 15 or 20," James Wedner of the Washington University School of Medicine in St. Louis said in a *Newsweek* cover story in May 1997. "No one really knows." [14] ■

CURRENT SITUATION

Helping the Poor

The key to improving health care for people with asthma is better education for both patients and doctors, according to asthma specialists and advocacy groups. But people in inner-city neighborhoods where the asthma epidemic is most severe face a variety of obstacles in coping with the disease. And asthma specialists say that the rise of managed care hampers the ability of primary-care providers to educate patients and families regardless of their economic status. [15]

For the asthma patient without a regular primary-care provider, medical care is too often hit and miss. Families are "whisked in and out of the emergency room," says Bowen of the New York City asthma initiative. "A patient's history has to be taken over a month really to be treated adequately. The people in the ER don't get that because too much is going on."

Families in homeless shelters or public housing may also have difficulty controlling the environmental factors that can trigger asthma attacks. "If you live in public housing, you may not have good control over such things as cockroach infestation, or it may not be as easy to go outdoors and smoke," says Floyd Malveaux an asthma expert and acting dean of the Howard University medical school. "It also may not be as easy to get good ventilation or to control individual heating and cooling."

In addition, poor families may be less able — either because of limited education or preoccupation with other day-to-day problems — to make sure children are taking asthma medications regularly. "Non-compliance is a bigger problem with inner-city kids," says Bender at National Jewish Hospital. "Even if they have inhaled corticosteroids, they're taking them very erratically."

Families that do have a regular, primary-care physician and health insurance coverage may still not receive the kind of education and treatment needed to manage asthma effectively. One problem, specialists say, is that many primary-care providers do not understand the importance of daily medication for most people with asthma. "Too many people — more poor than rich, but both poor and rich — are being undertreated," says Lichtenstein at Johns Hopkins Medical Center.

"Everybody but the 'intermittent' [sufferer] should be treated with an anti-inflammatory on a daily basis," says Carl, the Cleveland physician. "Our goal is to enable someone to have a fully active life without the intrusion of acute symptoms."

Carl also says primary-care physicians and health-plan administrators do not refer as many patients to specialists as they should. "We don't need to see three-quarters of the patients with asthma," Carl says. "But for the sickest quarter, specialty care needs to be viewed not as the enemy but as a partner with the primary-care community."

Seeing specialists is "not happening across the country," agrees Sander of the asthma-support network. "That has less to do with the individual doctor than with the way managed care and HMOs are set up."

Even specialists may fail to do a good job in patient education, however. Cook County Hospital's McDermot says a recent survey found that only about one-tenth of the asthma specialists in Chicago had any educational program for patients other than informal consultation in the office. "It is unlikely that ad-equate education could be done under those circumstances," he says.

New Treatments

Ever since Maimonides prescribed chicken soup as part of an anti-asthma regimen, doctors have been looking for medications to cure, or at least control, the disease. Today, researchers are optimistic about a new drug that might rid the body of the chemical that touches off an allergic asthma attack. Some doctors are skeptical, however, saying the search for new treatments diverts attention from making better use of the anti-asthma drugs already available.

The new drug — known as anti-IgE — is aimed at blocking the anti-body Immunoglobulin E that is released in the body when someone susceptible to allergic asthma or hay fever comes into contact with an allergen.[16] The IgE binds to cells in the bronchial or nasal passages — known as mast cells — which then release the substances — histamines and leukotrines — that cause runny noses and sneezing among hay-fever sufferers and gasping and wheezing among asthmatics.

Once scientists discovered exactly how IgE binds to the mast cells, they set about trying to manufacture an antibody that would block the process and interrupt the so-called allergic cascade. Scientists at the California-based biotech company Genentech genetically engineered anti-IgE from mouse cells.[17] Genentech is now partnering with the Swiss-based pharmaceutical company Novartis in conducting clinical trials of the drug in the United States and Europe.

Casale, the Nebraska asthma specialist and one of the people supervising the trials, says the results are encouraging. "This anti-IgE has been shown to improve the quality of life of people with asthma, to decrease the need for their rescue inhaler, to decrease their symptom scores and to enable patients to reduce the dose of oral or inhaled steroids they are using to treat their asthma," he says.

The drug appears to have caused few side effects, Casale adds, aside from the discomfort of regular injections every two to four weeks. Genentech says it hopes to seek Food and Drug Administration approval for the anti-IgE therapy in May.

One new type of drug already on the market treats asthma in a different way from bronchodilators and inhaled steroids by inhibiting the release of leukotrines, one of the inflammatory agents produced in an allergic attack. Two so-called leukotrine modifiers are being marketed in the United States under the brand names Accolate and Singulair. These drugs are taken once a day but are useful only in mild cases.

McDermott, the Chicago physician, is strongly skeptical of the new drugs. The leukotrine modifiers, he says, are "not very good" and are "very expensive." As for the anti-IgE therapy, he feels it is being oversold. "Rather than use inhaled steroids, we're going to introduce a new product which is not nearly as good and claim that it is salvation," he says. ∎

OUTLOOK

Research vs. Prevention

Researchers at National Jewish Hospital in Denver are halfway through a five-year research project aimed at finding out whether intensive assistance to at-risk families can reduce the incidence of asthma

At Issue:

What changes are needed to improve the treatment of asthma?

Educate Patients

NANCY SANDER
President, Allergy and Asthma Network/Mothers of Asthmatics, Fairfax, Va.

*m*ost people view asthma as little more than a nuisance, but each day it drowns 15 people in their own mucus and fluids escaping from inflammatory cells that line their airways. Talk to the families of loved ones that have died. They'll tell you they didn't know asthma could kill. They'll ask why their doctors didn't tell them. It's what they didn't know that hurts.

If you don't have the facts about asthma, you'll believe the myths and suffer the consequences. Education is important whether you are the patient, the family, the physician or a legislator. What you know affects how you breathe. It's that simple.

Education, learning and applied knowledge begin in a skilled physician's office and should continue for the patient and family over a lifetime. It's asthma's nature to play hide and seek with symptoms. Those unaware will suffer more than those in the know. That's why our organization — the Allergy and Asthma Network/Mothers of Asthmatics — dedicates every dollar to patient education and outreach.

Across-the-Board Improvements

IRWIN REDLENER, M.D.
President, Children's Health Fund

*m*odern medicines for asthma can keep patients essentially symptom-free, with no missed school days and no limitation of activity — not even the dreaded chronic nighttime cough. Yet countless hospitalizations, emergency room visits and missed school days are the reality for too many asthma sufferers. The costs are staggering — and almost totally avoidable.

What's needed are "medical homes" where children get competent care from concerned, informed providers; great follow-up; education for themselves and their parents; and proper medications.

But with more than 11 million uninsured children in the United States, and millions more facing other barriers to appropriate and timely care, true control of the asthma epidemic is not possible. Furthermore, many children who are getting some care do not receive state-of-the-art information from their doctors.

My prescription: (1) More money for research on the underlying causes of asthma; (2) universal access to health insurance and comprehensive health services; (3) community education and awareness programs; (4) improving awareness of providers, parents and patients; and (5) unencumbered availability of needed medications.

Better Physician Training

MICHAEL McDERMOTT, M.D.
Department of Emergency Medicine, Cook County Hospital, Chicago

*a*lmost 10 years have passed since the first edition of the National Institute of Health's asthma guidelines. Nonetheless, a recent survey in one large city shows that only 50 percent of one class of specialists gave out peakflow meters to patients to measure asthma problems at home, and only 60 percent of asthmatics received written plans for how to deal with attacks. These are basic steps agreed upon for all serious asthmatics.

Many physicians have neither the training, skills nor interest to work with the crucial educational and behavioral parts of asthma. Even if the correct medications are prescribed, the feedback and questioning to develop proper medication habits are not done. The predictable result is more attacks, and blaming the patient as non-compliant.

There's no crying need for a new asthma magic bullet. There is a crying need for physicians who can work with patients to help them take meds regularly, to watch their asthma closely, to change their meds early in an attack. And our health-care system needs to help doctors get the training and take the time to do the job right.

Find New Treatments

WILLIAM BUSSE, M.D.
President-elect, American Academy of Allergy, Asthma and Immunology

*e*ach year, we are learning more and more about the mechanisms of asthma, and this information is giving us insight into how we might best treat this disease.

The experimental anti-IgE therapy — which controls the antibody that causes all allergic reactions — has been shown to be safe and potentially effective in treating allergic asthma. Anti-IgE may make it possible to remove one of the most important keys to allergic reactions and thus lessen the severity of asthma.

Genetics may play an important role in our attempts to control asthma. Once the genes responsible for asthma are discovered, it will be possible to establish their functions and the products they regulate and to develop medications to block these products. In addition, it should be possible to more accurately diagnose the disease early in its course.

With further advances in knowledge, it may be possible in the next decade to use compounds that have greater specificity to treat asthma or even prevent it. That is the hope — and there is promise for its fulfillment.

among infants. After identifying 180 low-income families in Denver with infants who had visited doctors at least three times for wheezing problems, the project sent nurses to visit the homes more than a dozen times a year. The nurses tried to help the families reduce indoor allergens, improve communication with physicians and deal with other problems.

The results so far? "We know that we've reduced allergens in some of the homes, and we've reduced cigarette smoke in some of the homes," says Mary Klinnert, who is supervising the study. "We can say that we have had some positive effects in the process part of it. But nobody knows whether that will translate into less asthma or less severe asthma."

The $1.8-million, NIH-funded project epitomizes one approach — prevention — to trying to stem the asthma epidemic. Research into new treatments represents a second. The two approaches need not conflict, but they do compete for the time and attention of health-care policy-makers and for financial support from government and health-care institutions.

Public health advocates are eager to see more time and money invested in prevention. "If we can make resources available, especially in our impoverished communities and in our underserved population, we can dramatically improve the statistics," says Howard University's Malveaux. "If you put resources into prevention and wellness, you will reduce the numbers of hospitalization use, of emergency room visits."

Other experts voice greater enthusiasm about the potential payoff of research into new therapies. "The new treatments may be helpful, and they may also tell us something more about the disease," says the University of Wisconsin's Busse. "We still don't know the basic mechanisms of the disease. These treatments become

very informative for investigators."

"Five years down the road, we're going to be able to recognize some of the genes that are characteristic of asthma," Busse adds. "By understanding the disease better, we're going to get a very different therapeutic approach, not five years from now but 10 years."

For the moment, though, experts expect the incidence of asthma to continue rising in the United States. "It's going to get worse in the sense that more people will have it," says Camargo at Massachusetts General Hospital. But he sees doctors making progress in managing the disease.

Others are less optimistic. Carl says he is "frustrated at the way the system is structuring care, the way that specialists are [not used enough] in the current system." At National Jewish Hospital, Bender worries about the quality of patient education. "That's where we're getting stuck," Bender says.

For her part, Sander of the asthma-support network hopes that prevention efforts and research will combine to help give people with asthma the power to cope with the disease without letting it dominate their lives. "The more we know as consumers about ourselves and what medical research has to offer us," she says, "the more likely we are to put asthma in its place and get on with our lives."

"I don't want my son or daughter to wake up every morning and say, 'I have asthma,' and identify themselves with this disease," Sander adds. "Taking care of my airways is just as important as taking care of the rest of my life, and that is the place I want to help other people to reach. Taking care of asthma is just part of what they do." ■

Notes

[1] For background, see Richard L. Worsnop, "Indoor Air Pollution," The CQ Researcher,
Oct. 27, 1995, pp. 945-968.

[2] See The New York Times, May 5, 1999. Further details can be found on Children's Health Fund Web site: www.childrenshealthfund.org.

[3] For background, see Charles S. Clark, "Emergency Medicine," The CQ Researcher, Jan. 5, 1996, pp. 1-23.

[4] Ring et al., "Environmental Risk Factors for Respiratory and Skin Atopy: Results from Epidemiological Studies in Former East and West Germany," International Archives of Allergy and Immunology, Vol. 118, pp. 403-407 (1999).

[5] Lawrence M. Lichtenstein, Conversations About Asthma (1998), p. vii.

[6] For background, see Bob Adams, "Primary Care," The CQ Researcher, March 17, 1995, pp. 217-240.

[7] Some background drawn from National Library of Medicine/National Institutes of Health, "A Breath of Life," exhibit on display March 23, 1999-June 30, 2000.

[8] See E. L. Becker, "Elements of the History of Our Present Concepts of Anaphylaxis, Hay Fever and Asthma," Clinical and Experimental Allergy, Vol. 29, p. 880 (1999).

[9] Background drawn from Donald J. Lane, Asthma: The Facts (1st ed.) (1979), pp. 123-126. The 1996 edition includes a somewhat shorter version of the history, pp. 148-149.

[10] See ibid. (1st ed.), pp. 109-111; (3d ed.), pp. 138-139.

[11] Journal of the American Medical Association, Oct. 3, 1990, pp. 1683-1687. (asthma mortality); pp. 1688-1692 (asthma hospitalization among children).

[12] Robin Marantz Henig, "Asthma Kills," The New York Times Magazine, March 28, 1993.

[13] Shirakawa et al., "The Inverse Association Between Tuberculin Responses and Atopic Disorders," Science, Vol. 275 (1997), p. 77.

[14] Quoted in Geoffrey Cowley and Anne Underwood, "Why Ebonie Can't Breathe," Newsweek, May 26, 1997, p. 60.

[15] For background, see Adriel Bettelheim, "Managed Care," The CQ Researcher, April 16, 1999, pp. 305-328.

[16] Some background drawn from Arthur Allen, "Breath of Life," The Washington Post Magazine, Oct. 31, 1999, p. 21.

[17] For background, see Craig Donegan, "Gene Therapy's Future," The CQ Researcher, Dec. 8, 1995, pp. 1089-1112.

Bibliography

Selected Sources Used

Books

American Lung Association, *Family Guide to Asthma and Allergies: How You and Your Children Can Breathe Easier*, **Little Brown, 1997.**

A practical guide to dealing with asthma including a glossary, references, a list of lung association state chapters and other asthma organizations and state-by-state listings of asthma camps for children.

American Medical Association, *Essential Guide to Asthma*, **Pocket Books, 1998.**

A comprehensive guide to understanding what causes asthma, how to diagnose and treat the disease and how to control asthma attacks, with resources, short bibliography and glossary.

Casler, Kristin, *Asthma: Questions You Have ... Answers You Need*, *People's Medical Society*, **1998.**

A question-and-answer format provides straightforward explanations of the causes of asthma and medical procedures for diagnosing and treating the disease, with a list of organizations and glossary.

Chaitow, Leon, *Asthma and Hayfever: Safe Alternatives Without Drugs* **[rev. ed.], Thorsons, 1998.**

The book discusses consequences of conventional pharmacological treatment of asthma and details alternative treatments, including nutritional regimens.

Lane, Donald J., *Asthma: The Facts* **(3d ed.), Oxford University Press, 1996.**

Lane, a physician, gives a detailed but accessible medical account of the causes of asthma and methods of treating the disease.

Lichtenstein, Lawrence M., with Kathryn S. Brown, *Conversations About Asthma*, **Williams & Wilkins, 1998.**

Lichtenstein, director of the Johns Hopkins Asthma and Allergy Center, gives a very practical guide to living with asthma, including steps to "asthma-proof your world" and work with health-care providers to better manage the disease, with a list of organizations with addresses, telephone numbers and Web addresses.

FOR MORE INFORMATION

Allergy and Asthma Network/Mothers of Asthmatics Inc., 2751 Prosperity Ave., Suite 150, Fairfax, Va. 22031-4397; (703) 641-9595; www.aanma.org. The organization maintains an informative Web site and also publishes a quarterly magazine.

American Academy of Allergy, Asthma and Immunology, 611 East Wells St., Milwaukee, Wis. 53202; (414) 272-6071; www.aaaai.org. The academy has about 6,000 members, including allergists, asthma specialists and immunologists.

American Lung Association, 1740 Broadway, New York, N.Y. 10019; (212) 315-8700; www.lungusa.org. The association's Web site offers a variety of information, including current statistics on asthma rates.

Children's Health Fund, 317 E. 64th St., New York, N.Y. 10021; (212) 535-9400; www.childrenshealthfund.org. The fund seeks to improve health services for children in underserved medical areas, it cosponsors the Childhood Asthma Initiative with Montefiore Medical Center and Schering-Plough Corp.

National Heart, Lung, and Blood Institute, 6701 Rockledge Drive, Suite 10138, Bethesda, Md. 20892; (301) 435-0233; www.nhlbi.nih.gov/nhlbi/nhlbi.htm. The institute maintains a detailed Web site with information for laypersons and medical professionals.

National Jewish Medical and Research Center, 1400 Jackson St., Denver, Colo. 80206; (303) 388-4461; www.njc.org. The center is a leading asthma hospital and research facility with an informative Web site.

Articles

Allen, Arthur, "Breath of Life," *The Washington Post Magazine*, **Oct. 31, 1999, pp. 8-13, 20-22.**

Allen discusses the current asthma "epidemic" by focusing on the experiences of two Washington-area children of differing socioeconomic backgrounds.

Stolberg, Sheryl Gay, "Poor People Are Fighting a Baffling Surge in Asthma," *The New York Times*, **Oct. 18, 1999, p. A1.**

Stolberg gives a comprehensive overview of the current asthma "epidemic," with interviews with a wide variety of national experts.

Reports and Studies

National Heart, Lung, and Blood Institute, National Asthma Education and Prevention Program, Expert Panel Report 2: Guidelines for the Diagnosis and Management of Asthma, 1997.

The 153-page report — an update of a 1991 report — sets out guidelines for diagnosis and treatment of asthma and education of asthma patients.

5 Vaccine Controversies

KATHY KOCH

I t's school immunization season, and parents like Suzy Richards, of Friendsville, Tenn., give public health officials nightmares.

Richards* recently decided to discontinue vaccinations for her boys, ages 10 and 6, even though they haven't reacted negatively to earlier vaccines. "There's no way to know for sure whether they will have a negative reaction to the next one," she says.

Her fears were raised by reports about adverse vaccine reactions in *Parents* magazine and on ABC's "Nightline" — sources she trusts. "I've just heard and read too many things about how kids can be harmed or develop autism," she says. "I think they're just cramming these kids full of too many shots too early in life."

Richards worries because the number of vaccines recommended for children has been dramatically increasing. In 1960, children received 19 doses of four different vaccines before they reached school age. Today, an American child receives up to 39 doses of 12 different vaccines, most given during the first two years of life. And, unlike in previous decades, today's youngsters often are given multiple inoculations on the same day.

But immunization experts like Samuel L. Katz, a pediatrics professor emeritus at Duke University, say that parents like Richards threaten the nation's health. "Unless we continue to achieve high levels of immunization," he says, "terrible diseases will return — some in epidemic form."

That's what happened in the former Soviet Union, when vaccination rates dropped in the early 1990s,

*Suzy Richards is not her real name.

From *The CQ Researcher,*
August 25, 2000.

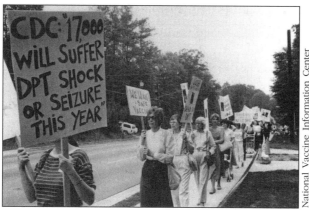

In the first demonstration of its kind, scores of parents who say their children suffered adverse effects from the DPT vaccine protest outside the Centers for Disease Control and Prevention in Atlanta in May 1986.

public health officials say. A diphtheria epidemic broke out, and diphtheria cases skyrocketed from 839 in 1989 to nearly 50,000 cases in 1994 (including 1,700 deaths), the U.S. Centers for Disease Control and Prevention (CDC) reports. [1]

The CDC is quick to point out that most parents do not share Richards' fears. "Vaccination rates are as high as they've ever been," says Benjamin Schwartz, acting director of epidemiology and surveillance for the CDC's National Immunization Program (NIP). "The vast majority of Americans support vaccinations."

But for a growing number of parents, getting their children vaccinated — once a no-brainer — has become an agonizing and confusing decision. It pits parents against their child's pediatrician and school, other parents and local health officials.

A mother in South Carolina recently found out just how hard it is to buck the system. The federal government had compensated her after her first daughter was left with severe brain injuries following a DPT (diphtheria-pertussis-tetanus) vaccine. But when local health authorities found out she was not planning to let her youngest daughter get the same vaccine, they threatened to charge her

with child abuse and take her child away.

"We see cases like this all the time," says Barbara Loe Fisher, president of the National Vaccine Information Center (NVIC), in Vienna, Va. "She finally told them she had a gun and would leave the state to protect her child from vaccine damage if they did not leave her alone."

Fisher helped found the NVIC in 1982 after her own son suffered brain damage after his fourth DPT shot. She later co-authored a book, *A Shot in the Dark*, about the dangers of the pertussis shot and the politics surrounding its continued use in the United States, 15 years after a safer version was available in Japan (*see p. 89*).

Other parents around the country — including lawyers, scientists and even public officials — who say their children have been injured or killed by vaccines have followed in her footsteps, organizing lobbying groups and Web sites advocating safer vaccines, more informed consent about potential risks and more freedom to choose which vaccines their children receive.

"I'm not anti-vaccine," Richards insists. "I just think the government needs to do a better job of making sure they are as safe as possible."

Vaccine reformers were somewhat vindicated in recent years after the CDC agreed to replace the DPT and oral polio vaccines with safer versions, eliminate mercury from childhood vaccines and recall the new, genetically engineered rotavirus vaccine (for severe diarrhea) after it caused potentially life-threatening illnesses in some children. [2]

But those actions just fueled the controversy and catapulted the debate from Internet chat rooms to congressional hearing rooms. In the past year,

Today's Children Get Many More Shots

Children today typically receive 39 doses of 12 different vaccines by the age of 6. By comparison, children in 1940 only received 9 doses in three vaccinations to prevent diphtheria, tetanus and pertussis (whooping cough).

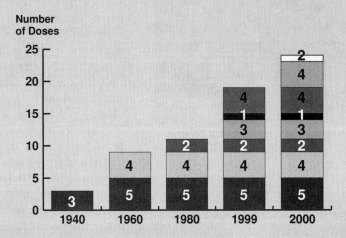

Vaccine Doses in the First Six Years of Life

Number of Doses	Type of Vaccine	Disease Prevented
2	Hepatitis A	Mild form of hepatitis
4	Pneumococcal	Pneumonia, meningitis, sinus infection and sepsis
4	Hib	Meningitis and pneumonia
1	Varicella	Chickenpox
3	Hepatitis B	Severe hepatitis, cirrhosis, liver cancer
2	MMR	Measles, mumps, rubella/German measles
4	Polio	Poliomyelitis
5	DPT	Diphtheria, pertussis/whooping cough and tetanus

Source: Advisory Committee on Immunization Practices

House committees have held hearings on the safety of a new hepatitis B vaccine, conflicts of interest among federal vaccine policy-makers, possible links between vaccines and autism, the safety of mercury in vaccines and whether the federal program that compensates people injured by vaccines is working.

And it's not just childhood vaccines that have come under fire.

Hundreds of men and women in the military have chosen early retirement or court-martial rather than be vaccinated with a controversial anthrax vaccine. Other soldiers claim multiple vaccines they received against biological weapons are partly to blame for the mysterious Gulf War Syndrome afflicting many veterans — a claim the Defense Department has denied.

Ironically, the vaccine debate is partly the result of the success of mass immunizations. Childhood immunization rates are at an all-time high, except for pockets in some inner cities. And once-dreaded childhood diseases, such as measles, diphtheria, mumps and whooping cough, are at or near record lows. Smallpox has been wiped off the Earth, and polio has been eradicated from the Western Hemisphere.

"Vaccines have prevented thousands of deaths," says the CDC's Schwartz.

But as vaccination rates climb, chronic diseases and conditions, like asthma, allergies, diabetes, autism and learning disorders, are increasing nationwide among children, often at alarming rates. Some parents and doctors are questioning whether the rise in chronic disease may be a long-term effect of childhood vaccinations.

"Are we living in a different society where people have fewer infections because of immunizations and we have somehow changed our immune systems?" asked Edward Bailey, medical director of the Springfield, Mass., school system. [3]

Critics say much of their concern stems from the fact that today's new vaccines are not for diseases that occur in epidemic proportions, at least not in the industrialized world. In the 1990s, for instance, the four new vaccines added to state mandatory-immunization schedules were for hepatitis B, rotavirus, *Haemophilus influenzae* (Hib) and pneumococcal disease — infections that don't sweep through populations, wiping out victims by the thousands.

Today's vaccines are different in another way. With the advent of new technologies and years of heavy investment and research in DNA-based vaccines, dozens of biotech companies are now competing with traditional manufacturers to produce genetically engineered vaccines for all kinds of conditions. Parents who think their kids are already getting too many vaccines might be shocked to learn that more than 200 new vaccines are in the pipeline, to treat everything from cocaine addiction to herpes.

Just because a new childhood vaccine is available, critics say, it shouldn't automatically be included on the mandatory-immunization schedule. That question was raised after the CDC recommended a vaccine for the relatively innocuous chickenpox and one for hepatitis B — a disease primarily found among prostitutes, gay men and drug abusers. (*See sidebar, p. 74.*)

"We are not discriminating as to which are the appropriate vaccines for the appropriate populations, taking into account what the reasonable risk for that population is," says Ronald Kennedy, professor of microbiology and immunology at the University of Oklahoma.

Vaccine-policy critics also note that once a new vaccine is added to the federal childhood immunization schedule, manufacturers have a guaranteed market because every child in America is generally required to receive it before entering school. The recommendations are also taken into consideration when the World Health Organization (WHO) recommends vaccines for use in Third World countries.

Yet those same manufacturers, as well as pediatricians who administer the shots, are largely exempt from lawsuits by parents of injured children, thanks to a 1986 law that made the government, not the vaccine producers, liable for damages caused by mandatory vaccinations. The fund is financed with taxes on vaccines. As a result, activists argue, both the government and the billion-dollar vaccine industry have powerful stakes in downplaying vaccine problems.

As the debate over vaccines continues, here are some of the key questions being asked:

Are vaccines safe?

Vaccines are among the "safest pharmacological interventions for disease prevention available," says epidemiologist Roger Bernier, associate director for science at the CDC's National Immunization Program.

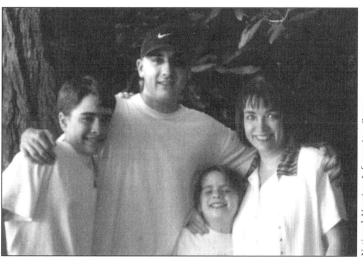

Barbara Loe Fisher helped found the National Vaccine Information Center, an advocacy group for children damaged by vaccines, after her eldest son, Chris (center), suffered brain damage following his fourth DPT shot.

National Vaccine Information Center

Health officials are quick to point out that the odds a child will die or become disabled from the diseases targeted by vaccines are far greater than being harmed by the vaccine. Without the diphtheria vaccine, Bernier says, 6 million people would have died during the 20th century.

"The real question," says Paul Offit, chief of infectious diseases at Children's Hospital of Philadelphia, is, "Do the benefits of vaccines definitively outweigh the risks? For all children's vaccines, that is clearly the case."

That was even true for the rotavirus vaccine, he contends. "A million children got the vaccine, and 100 got sick and one died. Yet now that it's off the market, if a million children don't get the vaccine, 16,000 will be hospitalized and 10 will die. It's still safer to get the vaccine."

Still, Offit adds, vaccines are not completely harmless. Of the 3 million children who receive vaccines each year, "a small percentage will have a severe allergic reaction, such as hives, difficulty breathing and low blood pressure," he says.

Such statements enrage parents like Michelle Helms, whose son Zachary died 33 hours after receiving his childhood vaccinations.

"Why aren't parents told about the real dangers these vaccines pose?" she asks on the Web site for the Global Vaccine Awareness League, the advocacy group she co-founded after Zachary's death. "Knowing that, I could have seen the tell-tale signs of a vaccine reaction and done something to save his life." [4]

Public trust in official reassurances about vaccine safety began eroding in 1976, when many people reportedly contracted Guillain-Barré Syndrome after being vaccinated against the swine flu, an epidemic that never materialized. In the 1980s, a television documentary about the dangers of the DPT shot spurred a flurry of lawsuits against DPT manufacturers. Then in the early 1990s, Persian Gulf War veterans began questioning the safety of the many vaccinations they received before shipping out.

Other incidents and revelations have spurred skepticism about vaccine safety, including:

Critics Blame Hepatitis Vaccine for Injuries ...

Bonnie S. Dunbar is not your typical anti-vaccine activist. A professor of molecular and cell biology at Baylor College of Medicine in Houston, she has been honored by the National Institutes of Health for her pioneering vaccine work.

But she began challenging federal vaccine policy six years ago, after her brother and a medical student who worked for her developed severe complications following a series of hepatitis B shots.

Her brother developed severe joint and muscle pain, fatigue, vision impairment and multiple sclerosis-like symptoms. "He hasn't been out of bed since," she says.

The lab worker lost vision in one eye three weeks after her second injection and ended up in the hospital for two months after her third booster.

Alarmed, Dunbar scoured the medical literature on adverse reactions to the shot, the nation's first genetically engineered vaccine made with recombinant DNA. She found 121 articles in medical journals from around the world listing a variety of adverse reactions, including multiple sclerosis, rheumatoid arthritis, optic neuritis, Bell's Palsy, Guillain-Barré Syndrome and diabetes. In addition, Dunbar insists, a dozen specialists confirmed that her brother had suffered a classic adverse reaction to the vaccine.

Eventually, Dunbar filed a Freedom of Information (FOI) request for all reports from the Food and Drug Administration's (FDA) Vaccine Adverse Event Reporting System (VAERS). "I was overwhelmed by the thousands of reports I received, hundreds of which were identical to the reports I had filed," she told the House Government Reform Subcommittee on May 18, 1999.

Dunbar is now in the vanguard of an increasingly vocal group of parents, health workers and scientists who claim that, for a small segment of the Caucasian population, the hepatitis B vaccine may be worse than the disease. They want the government to study whether some people may be genetically predisposed to react negatively to the shot. And they want it to be voluntary, especially for newborns, which are at minimal risk of contracting the disease.

Public health officials and representatives of health-provider organizations insist that any connection between the vaccine and chronic or autoimmune diseases is purely coincidental.

"Hepatitis B vaccines are among the safest vaccines we have," Harold S. Margolis, chief of the Hepatitis Branch at the Centers for Disease Control and Prevention's (CDC) National Center for Infectious Diseases, told the congressional panel. "Several reviews have not shown a scientific association between hepatitis B vaccination and severe neurological adverse events such as optic neuritis and Guillain-Barré Syndrome. In addition, preliminary data from French and British studies have shown no significant association between hepatitis B vaccination and multiple sclerosis."

Dunbar and other critics say they have repeatedly asked the CDC for copies of those studies, but so far have not received them. "We are still waiting for the data they keep quoting," says Dunbar.

Susan S. Ellenberg, director of biostatistics and epidemiology at the FDA's Center for Biologics Evaluation and Research, echoed Margolis' comments. "At present, we have ... little in the way of verified serious risks" from the hepatitis B vaccine, she said.

Benjamin Schwartz, acting director of epidemiology and surveillance for the CDC's National Immunization Program, points out that while more than 24,000 adverse reactions have been reported to VAERS, more than 30 million people have been vaccinated safely since the early 1990s.

Necessity of Hepatitis B Questioned

Observers say the fate of the hepatitis B vaccine is being closely watched because it is the first genetically engineered vaccine. Hundreds more are in the pipeline. The so-called Hep B vaccine has been controversial ever since 1991, when the CDC recommended that all newborns receive it before leaving the hospital. States officials then added the vaccine to their mandatory-immunization schedules for public school entrance eligibility, and immunizing newborns became standard pediatric practice.

Hepatitis B is rampant in some Asian and African countries, but in the United States it is primarily spread through infected blood or sex, and those at greatest risk of the disease are intravenous drug addicts, gay men and prostitutes, or babies of infected mothers. Why not just immunize babies whose mothers were carriers of the disease, critics ask.

"The idea of giving this vaccine to a 1-day-old baby, a newborn, is preposterous," Mayer Eisenstein, chairman of the Department of Medicine at St. Mary of Nazareth Hospital in Chicago, told a 1997 Illinois Board of Health hearing. [1]

"There is no raging hepatitis B epidemic among babies in this country," says Michael Belkin, whose 5-week-old daughter Lyla Rose died in 1998 with a swollen brain 15 hours after receiving her second hepatitis B booster shot.

Critics say a baby is more likely to have an adverse reaction than it is to contract the disease. Subcommittee Chairman John L. Mica, R-Fla., cited a recent New Hampshire study he "found shocking," showing that serious reactions to the vaccine — including 11 deaths — "were 16 times greater" than incidents of the disease. [2]

In the early 1990s, federal immunization officials decided to immunize newborns because they felt that not enough adults in the high-risk groups were being immunized. Even though incidence of the disease had been declining for five years, "it wasn't declining fast enough for some of us," says Louis Cooper, vice president-elect of the American

... But Health Officials Say It's Safe

Academy of Pediatrics (AAP). "It appeared we had the potential to wipe this disease out, because we had a vaccine that was safe and effective."

But some critics see a more sinister motive for vaccinating hours-old newborns. "It's a perfect way to disguise any adverse reaction," says Clifford Shoemaker, a Vienna, Va.-based attorney who has represented vaccine-injured children for 30 years. "Then the parent can't say, 'Before the vaccination, my child was like this.'"

Vaccinating infants is the most effective way to combat the disease, which is a serious public health threat, health officials say. "Hepatitis B kills 4,000 to 5,000 Americans each year," Margolis told the House panel. He said national studies carried out by the CDC have shown that 5 percent of Americans — 12.5 million people — have been infected with hepatitis B, and that about 300,000 were infected with the disease every year between 1970 and 1990, including 25,000 children.

Critics say such estimates are way overblown in an effort to frighten parents. They cite the CDC's own annual report on communicable diseases, which says only about 1,000 Americans die each year from hepatitis B, and only 10,416 new cases were reported in 1997. Only 26,611 cases were reported in 1985, when the disease reached its peak, and cases have been declining ever since, according to the report.[3]

Health officials say the estimates seem high because only about one-tenth of actual cases get reported to the CDC, and three times as many people are asymptomatic carriers of the disease as those who actually get it.

In 1998 a group representing 15,000 French parents and others sued SmithKline Beecham, alleging, among other things, that vaccine companies and health officials had exaggerated the risks associated with hepatitis B. The manufacturer was fined about $20,000 for causing at least one case of multiple sclerosis, and French health authorities later discontinued their mandatory hepatitis B vaccination program for adolescents.

Safety Studies Described as Inadequate

Critics contend that safety studies conducted for the vaccine were too small, too short and too limited to detect long-term adverse reactions. For instance, when he asked a manufacturer's representative to show him the evidence that the vaccine is safe for 1-day-old infants, Eisenstein said the representative told him, "We have none. Our studies were done on 5- and 10-year-olds."[4]

The drug companies' own product inserts state that the vaccines were tested on fewer than 2,000 persons, who were monitored for only five days after receiving them. And critics told the House panel that several often-cited long-term safety studies for the vaccine were conducted

on Alaskan natives or Asians — not Caucasians, who have been reporting the most adverse reactions.

In fact, the long-term studies in Asia and Alaska were done for an earlier plasma-derived conventional hepatitis B vaccine, not for the genetically engineered version. The FDA allowed the manufacturers to do "abbreviated studies" on the genetically engineered version of the vaccine "to assure they were comparably effective," says William Shaffner, chairman of the Department of Preventive Medicine at Vanderbilt University and an expert on the hepatitis B vaccine. Most mainstream scientists believe genetically engineered vaccines are safer than older versions, but others say more study is needed on their long-term impact.

"The manufacturers and public health officials keep saying there's no study proving that the vaccine is causing these adverse reactions," Belkin says. "I say back to them: 'Show us the proof that these vaccines are safe for all genetic populations.' They don't have any."

A 1994 Institute of Medicine (IOM) study also complained that no large, controlled, observational studies or clinical trials investigated the kinds of long-term adverse reactions described in the medical journals. "The lack of adequate data regarding many of the adverse events was of major concern to the committee [which] ... encountered many gaps and limitations in knowledge bearing directly or indirectly on the safety of vaccines," the report said.[5]

Marcel Kinsbourne, a pediatric neurologist who often testifies in vaccine-injury cases, suggests that there are no long-term studies because "the best defense in a product-liability case is no research. Then the plaintiffs cannot prevail."

Margolis said several ongoing studies are investigating whether adverse events are associated with the vaccine. But he warned that case reports rarely provide a convincing link between the adverse event and vaccination.

Dunbar says she and other critics will withhold judgment on the studies until they are allowed to see actual data and all of the scientific controls used, with long-term follow-up information. But, she says, "If the studies only concentrate on ethnic, inner-city populations, they still will not prove that the vaccine is safe for all populations, especially Caucasians."

---

[1] Quoted in "Hepatitis B Vaccine: The Untold Story, The Vaccine Reaction," National Vaccine Information Center, September 1998.

[2] Quoted in John Hanchette, Gannett News Service, May 19, 1999.

[3] "Summary of Notifiable Diseases, United States, 1997," *Morbidity and Mortality Weekly Report*, Centers for Disease Control and Prevention, Nov. 20, 1998.

[4] "Hepatitis B Vaccine," *op. cit.*

[5] "Adverse Events Associated with Childhood Vaccines," Institute of Medicine, National Academy of Sciences, 1994.

Adverse Effects of Childhood Vaccines

Scientists believe that some vaccines can cause certain diseases and adverse reactions in rare instances. In other cases, they have noted varying indications of causal links but no conclusive evidence.

VACCINES	◄◄◄ STRONGER EVIDENCE		WEAKER EVIDENCE ►►►	
	EVIDENCE ESTABLISHES A CAUSAL RELATION	EVIDENCE INDICATES A CAUSAL RELATION	EVIDENCE IS CONSISTANT WITH A CAUSAL RELATION	EVIDENCE FAVORS A CAUSAL RELATION
Diphtheria and Tetanus Toxoids	Anaphylaxis (shock)			Guillain-Barré Syndrome Brachial neuritis
DPT Vaccine		Anaphylaxis; protracted, high-pitched screaming	Acute encephalopathy shock; unusual "shock-like state"	
H. Influenzae Type B				Early-onset H. Influenzae B disease
Measles Vaccine	Death from measles-strain viral infection			Anaphylaxis
MMR Vaccine	Thrombocytopenia; Anaphylaxis			
Oral Polio Vaccine	Polio in recipient or contact; death from polio vaccine-strain viral infection			
OPU/IPUb Vaccine				Guillain-Barré Syndrome
Rubella Vaccine		Acute arthritis	Chronic arthritis	
Hepatitis B Vaccine	Anaphylaxis			

Sources: Institute of Medicine, "Adverse Effects of Pertussis and Rubella Vaccines: A Report of the Committee to Review the Adverse Consequences of Pertussis and Rubella Vaccines," *(1991);* "Adverse Events Associated With Childhood Vaccines: Evidence Bearing on Causality" *(1994)*

• Studies linking the DPT vaccine to seizures and brain damage in rare cases. The U.S. government finally licensed a safer, but less profitable, version of the vaccine (DTaP) in 1996 — 15 years after the Japanese had begun using it. [5]

• In another series of studies, the Institute of Medicine (IOM) concluded that the diphtheria-tetanus vaccine could cause Guillain-Barré Syndrome and death, the rubella vaccine could cause acute and chronic arthritis and the live measles and oral polio vaccines could cause viral infection and death. [6]

• A French court ruled in 1998 that SmithKline Beecham's hepatitis B vaccine had caused a child to get multiple sclerosis, prompting France to suspend compulsory hepatitis B vaccinations for schoolchildren. U.S. public health officials say there is no proof that the vaccine, the first genetically engineered vaccine to be mandated, causes multiple sclerosis or any other chronic or autoimmune disease.

• Mandatory inoculations with the new rotavirus vaccine, genetically engineered from a monkey-human hybrid virus and widely hailed as a breakthrough in the prevention of dehydrating diarrhea, were suspended in 1999 after a significant number of inoculated infants suffered from life-threatening bowel blockages.

How Parents Can Prevent Vaccine Reactions

Parents can help to prevent vaccine deaths and injuries by asking themselves these eight questions before having their children vaccinated, according to the National Vaccine Information Center. The NVIC is a nonprofit educational organization founded in 1982 to prevent vaccine reactions by improving information about vaccines available to the public.

- Is my child sick right now?

- Has my child had a bad reaction to a vaccination before?

- Does my child have a personal or family history of vaccine reactions; convulsions or neurological disorders; severe allergies; immune system disorders.

- Do I know if my child is at high risk of reacting?

- Do I have full information on the vaccine's side effects?

- Do I know how to identify a vaccine reaction?

- Do I know how to report a vaccine reaction?

- Do I know the manufacturer's name and lot number?

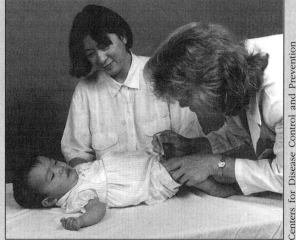

Centers for Disease Control and Prevention

• The Food and Drug Administration (FDA) acknowledged in 1999 that vaccines expose infants in the first six months of life to levels of the neurotoxin mercury considered unsafe by the Environmental Protection Agency (EPA). The CDC recommended a voluntary transition to mercury-free vaccines by next spring, despite urgings from some scientists and parent groups that it should be phased out faster.

• The CDC recommended in January that live, oral polio vaccines be replaced by the inactivated, injectable version because the live vaccine caused up to 10 cases of polio a year among children and their caretakers.

• Scientists are studying whether vaccines produced from animal tissue, like monkey and bovine cells, can transfer previously undetected viruses that can cause cancer or other diseases in humans.

In addition, vaccine-safety advocates cite the warning flags sent up by the government's own Vaccine Adverse Event Reporting System (VAERS). It receives more than 10,000 reports annually, but the FDA says

that only about one-tenth of actual cases are reported for all health conditions. (*See table, p. 76.*) The NVIC's own survey found that only 2.5 percent of New York doctors report death or disabilities that occur after a vaccination.

But the CDC's Schwartz says VAERS is not a reliable indicator. "Just because someone reports something doesn't mean that the condition was caused by the vaccine," he says. "It only means that it could possibly be caused by the vaccine."

Moreover, vaccine supporters point out, only 15 percent of VAERS reports describe events considered serious. Even for the more serious reactions, there is often only a "temporal, or time-based" association between the illness and a recent vaccination, said Surgeon General David Satcher.

Critics of vaccine policy also cite the government's National Vaccine Injury Compensation Program, which has paid more than $1 billion to patients who claimed injury from a vaccine. But health officials say the program's standard of proof is very low, and that just

because someone is compensated does not necessarily mean a vaccine caused their condition.

Vaccine-reform advocates worry that the government's accelerated childhood-immunization schedule may put some children at risk for serious adverse reactions. They say that in a dramatic departure from previously established protocols, children now get more vaccines at earlier ages, receive multiple vaccines on the same day and are vaccinated even when they are sick.

"This whole thing about hitting the newborns with all these shots before they get out of the hospital is really kind of frightening," said Arizona physician Jane Orient, executive director of the Association of American Physicians and Surgeons (AAPS).[7]

The University of Oklahoma's Kennedy says giving babies inoculations for up to nine diseases at once is "just asking for trouble," because the infant immune system is different than an adult's. "I don't even give the monkeys in my lab nine vaccines in one day."

But the CDC's Schwartz disputes

Court Links MMR, DPT Vaccines ...

Anna had been a bright, healthy baby and had started walking at 13 months. When she had her first MMR shot (for measles, mumps and rubella) at 15 months, the pediatrician told her mother to expect a mild reaction 10 days to two weeks after the shot that might include cold symptoms or a rash.

Nine days later, Anna had a runny nose and a low-grade fever. Although her cold symptoms eventually disappeared, Anna did not return to the happy, playful toddler she had been; instead, she constantly cried and wanted to be held.

Then Anna started tripping and falling down. When her mother called the pediatrician, he told her to put ice on the leg he had injected and give her Tylenol.

Over the next six weeks, Anna lost the ability to sit or walk. One doctor suggested that Anna be seen by a psychologist to determine why she was refusing to walk. A neurologist her mother consulted immediately hospitalized Anna with a suspected tumor on her spinal cord. The MRI scan of her brain showed there were lesions in the white matter of her brain; the other tests came back negative.

Anna continued to deteriorate. When she tried to sit up, she would flop over like a rag doll. Nearly every week

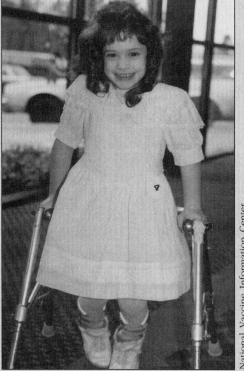

Anna was a healthy baby until she received an MMR (measles, mumps and rubella) vaccination at 13 months that eventually left her paralyzed from the waist down.

National Vaccine Information Center

she would run a fever for several days. Lab tests turned up nothing. In a four-week period, she endured seven spinal taps.

Eventually Anna was put on steroid therapy, which helped her to regain her personality and stopped her brain from further deteriorating. However, her lower body remained paralyzed.

Today, 8-year-old Anna attends third grade in a wheelchair. As she becomes taller and heavier, it is hard for her to sit upright. Anna loves to swim underwater because she says it makes her feel free.

In 1993, the U.S. Court of Claims in Washington, D.C., ruled that Anna had suffered post-vaccination encephalopathy following her MMR vaccination and paid a claim to her parents under the Vaccine Injury Compensation Program.

Richie's Death Followed His First DPT Shot

Richie was a thriving 2-month-old, the second son of a family in upstate New York, when he got his first DPT shot. Richie's brother had had severe reactions to his DPT shots, including high fever, uncontrollable screaming, diarrhea and vomiting, but the pediatrician had reassured Richie's mother, a nurse, that these were "normal" reactions.

the notion that multiple vaccinations overload an infant's immune system. "When a baby is born, it has a repertoire of white blood cells that can respond to more than 100,000 foreign substances," he says.

"It's unfortunate that people believe that [multiple vaccines harm children]," he adds, "because when a new vaccine comes along it provides a wonderful opportunity for us to prevent additional diseases. It would be horrible if some unfounded fears led to underutilization of these important products."

According to a CDC fact sheet on

vaccine safety, a multiple vaccination gives the child maximum protection with the least trauma while saving parents both time and money. In fact, researchers want to combine even more antigens into single injections — such as adding chickenpox to the MMR vaccine.

Critics bristle at such plans, arguing that safety considerations often take a back seat to economic concerns and the federal push for higher immunization rates. Rick Rollens, a parent in Granite Bay, Calif., whose son became autistic, says that at fed-

eral advisory committee discussions on accelerating the immunization schedule, "the discussions have nothing to do with safety and everything to do with maximizing as many medical services as possible when you have the child at the hospital or in the doctor's office."

Schwartz says that if a child has had an allergic reaction to a vaccine, it should not get a booster injection of that vaccine.

Public health authorities are constantly concerned about vaccine safety, Duke University's Katz says.

... in Children's Paralysis, Death

By the evening of the day Richie got his shot, the area around the injection began to swell, but Richie's mother remembered how his brother's leg had swelled. Then Richie's hip turned red and purple. Still, Richie didn't have a fever and continued to drink from his bottle so Richie's mother didn't worry.

In the morning Richie woke up screaming "like a cat in pain." After a nap, Richie woke up crying again, but his cry was weaker. He had a bottle and fell back to sleep. An hour later, he had severe diarrhea with mucous in his diapers. Then he fell asleep again until he again woke up crying.

When his mother picked him up, he had soaked through two receiving blankets and gave off a musty, pungent odor. While she washed him, she noticed he was limp and staring at her with "dark eyes."

Richie slowly drank eight ounces of water from his bottle and later that day had three more diapers with diarrhea in them. His leg still seemed to be sore. When he slept, his fingers twitched

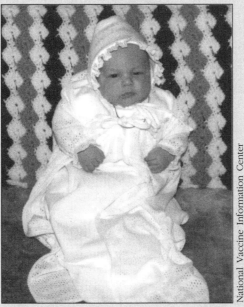

Two-month-old Richie died 33 hours after receiving his first DPT vaccination. The coroner attributed death to "irreversible shock" from the vaccine.

slightly. Later he gagged on his bottle and vomited a little. Richie's Mom remembered how Richie's brother had had diarrhea and vomiting after his shots, so she didn't worry.

That evening, while Richie was having a bottle, he suddenly stopped sucking and his breathing became shallow and irregular. Alarmed, his mother described the

symptoms to the doctor and asked him to meet them at the emergency room. The doctor said it wasn't necessary, but within minutes Richie had died in his mother's arms as his father and 6-year-old brother watched. It had been 33 hours since a doctor had injected him with his first DPT shot.

Fourteen weeks after his death, Richie's parents received the autopsy report describing an enlarged thymus gland (the gland that helps regulate the immune response in the body) as well as congestion and edema in the lungs and brain.

Not satisfied with the autopsy findings, Richie's parents talked with the coroner, who suggested the death had been caused by sudden infant death syndrome (SIDS). But they knew it wasn't SIDS. Armed with the *Physician's Desk Reference* and studies on DPT vaccine, his mother described in detail exactly what had happened. The coroner listened to her and noted on the death certificate that death had been caused by "Irreversible shock due to a probable reaction to DPT."

Richie's family filed a claim with the Vaccine Injury Compensation Program and, as in Anna's case, the U.S. Court of Claims awarded them compensation, ruling that the vaccine had caused his death.[1]

[1] See Harris Coulter and Barbara Loe Fisher, *A Shot in the Dark* (1991).

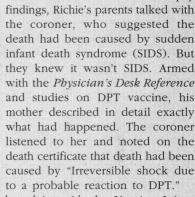

The move to eliminate mercury from vaccines "didn't come from the anti-vaccine people," he says. "It came from the vaccine establishment. They made that decision even though there was no evidence at all that the trace amounts in vaccines are harmful. It was just a theoretical risk."

But James Turner, a Washington consumer lawyer, says the vaccine establishment has known about mercury in vaccines for nearly three decades. "I remember attending hearings in 1973 at which the danger from mercury in vaccines was discussed."

Is the government doing sufficient research on vaccine safety?

Parents of vaccine-injured children say that because neither the government nor the manufacturers study the potential long-term or chronic adverse effects of vaccines, they are not recognizing the true scope of the damage done by vaccines.

"Rates of asthma and attention-deficit disorder have doubled; diabetes and learning disabilities have tripled; and most states have experienced a 300 percent or more increase in autism," says Fisher, who has

served on the National Academy of Science and Food and Drug Administration vaccine advisory panels.

"The whole problem with vaccine-adverse effects is that there are too many hypotheses without scientific support," Oklahoma's Kennedy says. "We need to support careful scientific investigations in this area, but unfortunately the federal government and the pharmaceutical companies don't agree and don't support such efforts."

"They are not doing the studies they need to do to put some of these fears to rest," says AAPS's Orient.

Is Your Child Getting the Right Vaccine?

L ast year the Centers for Disease Control and Prevention (CDC) recommended an unprecedented number of new vaccine formulas. But this doesn't guarantee that your doctor is using the safest medicine available. According to the National Vaccine Information Center, here's what parents should ask before their children get shots:

Which polio vaccine do you use? Between 1996 and 1999, children usually received two kinds of polio vaccines: two doses of inactive injected vaccine and then two doses of an oral version containing the live virus. Live polio cells can pass through the baby's stool, and in rare cases they cause polio in the child or his caretaker. In January, the CDC recommended that children get all four doses of the inactive vaccine. Most doctors made the switch, but it's still prudent to double-check.

Are you using the new DTaP vaccine? Although sales of the older, cheaper DPT vaccine are dropping, it has not been taken off the U.S. market. Your doctor may still be ordering the older version. So far, the new vaccine really does seem to have fewer side effects. In one study, only 3 to 5 percent of DTaP recipients developed a fever, compared with 16 percent of the patients who received the old formula. Be sure to ask for DTaP when you schedule your appointment. Then, when you're in the office, ask to see the actual vial the vaccine comes in.

Can I get mercury-free vaccines? At least one brand of every vaccine is now made without thimerosol, a mercury-based preservative. Make sure your doctor is using those brands. If he or she isn't, ask the doctor to order them for you. (For a complete list, call the CDC at (800) 232-2522.)

What are the symptoms of a vaccine reaction? After vaccination, you should know how to monitor your child for signs and symptoms that a vaccine reaction is taking place so that you can call your doctor. Depending on the vaccine or combination of vaccines given, signs and symptoms of a vaccine reaction can vary from minutes to several weeks or months. Most adverse reactions to DPT or DTaP vaccine occur within the first 72 hours to seven days and include high-pitched screaming or uncontrollable crying; excessive sleepiness; high fever; unusual twitching, shaking or stiffening of the body; limpness and inability to react normally to stimulation that may signal seizures or brain inflammation. With other vaccines, such as MMR, it can take several weeks for those signs to develop.

What about revaccinating? If your child's health has deteriorated severely following vaccination and you believe a vaccine reaction has taken place, you should consult several health professionals before revaccinating. A previous vaccine reaction can increase a person's risk of having a more severe reaction when more vaccine is given. You have the right to defer vaccination if you believe your child is at increased risk of having a vaccine reaction until you are confident about the medical advice you are being given.

How do I report a vaccine reaction? You should keep your own records of vaccinations your child has received and whether any adverse symptoms occurred. No detail is too small to record. If your child had a severe health problem after vaccination, you have the right to report it to the Vaccine Adverse Event Reporting System (VAERS) — even if your doctor denies it is because of the vaccination and refuses to file such a report. Contact VAERS at (800) 822-7967. The National Vaccine Information Center (NVIC) also accepts vaccine reaction reports and serves as a consumer watchdog on the VAERS system. You can report adverse vaccine events to NVIC at www.909shot.com.

What about compensation for vaccine-related injuries? If your child has been injured by vaccination, you can seek compensation under the National Childhood Vaccine Injury Compenstion Act of 1986. Call (202) 219-9657 for information.

"There are so many unknowns that the children receiving these immunizations really are experimental subjects."[8]

"A genuine and vigorous effort to identify risk factors would help dissipate the impression that some citizens have formed that vaccine safety is not a high priority," Marcel Kinsbourne, an expert on vaccine injury, told the House Government Reform Committee last year.

Microbiologist Howard Urnovitz, founder of the Chronic Illness Research Foundation, in Berkeley, Calif., says the government's compensation figures are understated and its cost-benefit analyses skewed because they don't take into account the cost of treating chronic diseases that may be triggered by vaccines. The government "must study whether chronic illnesses, such as learning and behavior disorders, autism, arthritis, cancer, diabetes, chronic-fatigue syndrome and multiple sclerosis, are triggered by vaccines," he says, "and then calculate the cost of treating those diseases when it makes its cost-benefit analyses."

"They say there's no scientific evidence to prove that vaccines cause chronic diseases, but they won't fund any research in that area either," Urnovitz says. "If you don't look for something, you won't find it."

The government is also not looking for evidence that some children may be genetically predisposed to react negatively to a particular vaccine, Fisher says. "We've seen cases in which three or four children in one family will have already been injured by a particular vaccine, but the health officials still insist that other children in the family be vaccinated or that the already-injured children receive boosters," she says.

"The government has no business forcing vaccinations on these people, or adding more vaccines to the schedule while refusing to do research to discover the genetic markers that would identify who is susceptible to adverse reactions," she says. "It's unconscionable."

The University of Oklahoma's Kennedy says certain vaccines should not be given to individuals with a family history or predisposition to autoimmune diseases, such as lupus, rheumatoid arthritis or multiple sclerosis.

But the CDC's Schwartz says, "There is no good data to support the concept of a familial risk of adverse events. In contrast, we know that vaccines protect against real and significant diseases. In the absence of scientific data, we believe vaccination is the best policy in such a case."

However, the CDC is in the process of setting up a better way to check on adverse events reported to the VAERS, Schwartz says. "We will be following up on people who report certain conditions to VAERS," he says, including neurological conditions or multiple sclerosis. "We know that there are concerns that this is one of the conditions where a genetic predisposition might be involved."

Meanwhile, Schwartz insists, the CDC *is* looking at possible connections between vaccines and chronic diseases. "The implication that we are ignoring things is not true," he says.

Schwartz warns, however, that just because an allegation is made about a vaccine does not mean that a full-blown study will be done to determine a connection. The first step is to look at whether a certain condition is more prevalent in a vaccinated population, compared to an unvaccinated population, he says. To do that, the agency established the "Vaccine Safety Datalink," which allows officials to check the health records from four large West Coast managed-care companies.

The CDC is also entering into a contract with the IOM and the National Institutes of Health (NIH) to work with an independent panel being set up to look at emerging issues in vaccine safety, including possible links between vaccines and autism. (*See sidebar, p. 88.*)

Rollens, the California father of an autistic child, will be watching to see if that panel investigates the possible connection between vaccine ingredients and autism.

"Vaccines contain numerous active agents, such as live viruses, bacterial agents, preservatives, and toxic chemicals, including formaldehyde and mercury, as well as human, animal and plant [genetic material]," Rollens told the House Government Reform Committee in July. "[Yet] not a single safety study has ever been done on the short-term or long-term effects of the interaction of this potent cocktail on the developing brain and immune systems of our children."[9]

He called manufacturers' safety studies, which range from a few days of surveillance to a couple of weeks, "woefully inadequate," and said, "I must ask the public health community: Where is the science?"

Oklahoma's Kennedy also complains that manufacturers sometimes do not do sufficient research before vaccines are licensed. Vaccines have gone "directly from rodent studies into human clinical trials," bypassing the monkey phase of testing, he told the committee. Or when problems cropped up during the monkey phase, "these were ignored and the product went into human clinical trials anyway," he said.

Unfortunately, says Neal A. Halsey, director of the Institute for Vaccine Safety at Johns Hopkins University School of Hygiene and Public Health, just when the FDA needs highly qualified scientists and resources to address increasingly complex vaccine-safety issues, the research budget for the agency's Center for Biologics and Evaluation Research has been drastically reduced.[10]

"Safe, effective vaccines save lives," Rep. Dan Burton, R-Ind., chairman of the committee, responded. "Vaccines that have not been thoroughly tested and reviewed can be dangerous." He cited the rotavirus vaccine as a good example: "The government and manufacturers ignored the warning signs. A lot of babies were injured and required surgery. One baby died before the vaccine was pulled from the market."

Do vaccine manufacturers have too much influence over government immunization policymakers?

Federal immunization policy emanates from two advisory committees. The FDA's Vaccines and Related Biological Products Advisory Committee (VRBPAC), recommends whether new vaccines are safe and effective. The CDC's Advisory Committee on Immunization Practices (ACIP) recommends which vaccines should be included on the national Childhood Immunization Schedule, which is usually automatically adopted by most states. They then require all children to have the specified vaccinations before entering school.

Critics have long claimed that certain members of those committees have incestuous ties with agencies that stand to gain power or manufacturers that stand to reap enormous profits from federal vaccine policy. And even when members recuse themselves from specific votes, they are permitted to participate in discussions, and thus influence the decisions, critics say.

"Vaccines are the only substances that a government agency mandates a United States citizen receive," said Burton during a hearing of his committee on June 15. "Families need to have confidence that the vaccines that their children take are safe, effective and truly necessary. Doctors need to feel confident that when the FDA licenses a drug, that it is really safe and that the pharmaceutical industry has not influenced the decision-making process. Has that trust been violated?"

Burton's committee staff investigated how the two advisory panels had approved the ill-fated rotavirus vaccine.

The investigation found that in clinical trials five children out of 10,000 developed bowel obstructions after taking the vaccine, Burton said. "There were also concerns about children failing to thrive and developing high fevers, which, as we know, can lead to brain injury," he added. Despite these concerns, and others, both advisory committees unanimously approved the vaccine, he said.

Burton's staff also examined the finances of advisory committee members and found that:

• The chairmen and members of both advisory committees own stock in vaccine-manufacturing companies, and some members of both advisory committees own patents for vaccines affected by decisions of the committee.

• Three out of five of the members of the FDA's advisory committee who voted for the rotavirus vaccine had conflicts of interest that were waived.

Burton also noted several specific examples of potential conflicts of interest, including:

• John Modlin, chairman of the rotavirus working group of the CDC ad-

visory group, owned $26,000 worth of stock in Merck, one of the largest manufacturers of vaccines, and serves on Merck's Immunization Advisory Board.

• Children's Hospital's Offit, a member of the CDC advisory committee who voted to recommend adding the rotavirus vaccine to the Vaccines for Children program, holds a patent on a rotavirus vaccine and receives grant money from Merck to develop it.

• Harry Greenberg, chairman of the FDA committee, owns $120,000 worth of stock in Aviron, a vaccine manufacturer. He is also a paid member of the board of advisers of another vaccine manufacturer and owns $40,000 worth of its stock. This stock ownership was deemed not to be a conflict and a waiver was granted. To the FDA's credit, Burton noted, Greenberg was excluded from the rotavirus discussion because he holds the patent on the rotashield vaccine.

If panel decisions on all vaccines on the national immunization schedule had as many conflicts as those discovered for the rotavirus vaccine, Burton said, "then the entire process has been polluted and the public trust has been violated."

Linda A. Suydam, senior associate commissioner for the FDA, responded that the agency has given high priority to selecting the most qualified clinical and scientific experts for its advisory committees and to "rigorously complying with the statutes and regulations governing these advisory committees." They are often pre-eminent scientists in their field, she said, and since academic biomedical research in the United States today is increasingly financed by industry, "most active researchers in the private sector have some ongoing or past relationship with regulated industry."

If the FDA were to exclude any scientist with a relationship with industry from its advisory committees, "We would not get the top scientists

in the field, and the recommendations of the advisory committees would not be of the highest scientific nature, with a likely impact on public health," she said.

Dixie Snider, the CDC's associate director for science, said each committee member is required to report stock ownership, honoraria, employment, general partnership interests, contracts and receipt of grant funds that they — or their spouse or minor children — have had within the past 12 months. If members do have a potential or actual financial conflict, she says, they may be granted a limited waiver to participate in committee discussions but must publicly disclose relevant interests at the beginning of each meeting and abstain from votes involving those interests.

Offit says his relationships with pharmaceutical companies don't cloud his judgment. "When pharmaceutical companies pay me to speak about vaccines, they do it via unrestricted educational grants," he says. "They have no input in what I say, nor would I ever allow that to happen. If I think a vaccine has certain weaknesses, I say it. Never have they said, 'Wait a minute, this is not what we want people to hear.'"

Duke University pediatrics Professor Katz, who has served on immunization committees of the CDC, WHO, IOM and FDA, says, "Government doesn't fund clinical studies of vaccines. Industry does. And nearly everyone who has ever been involved in developing a vaccine has been involved in a clinical study funded by industry."

Nevertheless, he says, "People are much more sensitive to this issue now than they were 10 years ago. In the past, a lot of us did take consultation fees."

But Katz says now he does not take any honoraria, "and I make sure neither I nor any members of my family have financial interests in vaccine companies."

Should vaccines be mandatory for all?

As questions about vaccine safety persist, the debate over whether some parents should be allowed to exempt their children from mandatory vaccines has intensified. It's a debate that pits personal freedom of choice on one side and public health and safety on the other.

All states require children to get all mandated shots — based on the federal immunization schedule — before they can attend school, or day care, in some states. Each state also allows medical exemptions for those with immune system problems, who have allergic reactions to vaccine constituents or who are moderately or severely ill. Fifteen states allow philosophical exemptions, and all states except two allow religious exemptions.

A small but increasing number of parents are seeking exemptions from some or all vaccines. They argue that until there is more convincing scientific evidence that vaccines are safe, they prefer to decide for themselves which, if any, vaccines their children will receive.

Hundreds of military men and women are also caught up in the debate. They have chosen retirement or court-martial rather than be vaccinated with a controversial anthrax vaccine.

But with a new push for higher vaccination rates, some say local health departments and managed-care firms have increased the pressure on non-complying parents.[11] Un-inoculated children are being kicked out of school. Doctors are balking at treating patients who refuse to have their kids vaccinated; others report

non-compliant parents to social service agencies, which then try to charge the parent with neglect.

Politicians have gotten into the picture as well. States have begun withholding portions of welfare checks from mothers who do not inoculate their children. Members of Congress have suggested disallowing federal income tax exemptions for unvaccinated children.

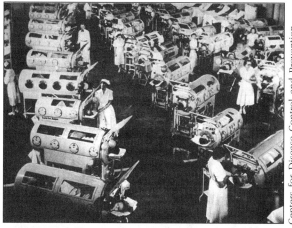

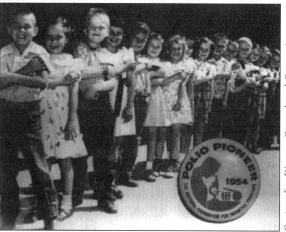

Parents' fear of polio in the 1940s and '50s was fed by news stories and pictures of children encased in iron lungs, which helped them breathe (top). After a massive nationwide immunization effort, polio cases fell by 90 percent.

The debate has grown even testier as the CDC has mandated vaccines for chickenpox and hepatitis B, which many parents consider non-essential. After all, they say, chickenpox is only a mild discomfort for most children,

and hepatitis B is transmitted through contaminated blood, dirty needles or risky sexual activity. Yet hundreds of recipients say they have suffered serious, sometimes permanent, adverse reactions from the hepatitis vaccine, a claim public health officials say is unproven.

"With hepatitis B vaccine, the case for mandatory immunization with few exemptions is far less persuasive than with smallpox or polio vaccines, which protected against highly lethal or disabling, easily transmissible diseases," the AAPS's Orient says. (*See sidebar, p. 74.*)

Absent a public health emergency, "People should have the right to choose whether to get all these new vaccines," says consumer lawyer Turner, who is helping to organize a new group, Parents and Professionals for Vaccine Choice.

Orient complains that mandating vaccines profoundly changes the relationship between the patient and doctor. "The [vaccine] manufacturer and the physician administering [it] are substantially relieved of liability for adverse effects," she says, and the physician "becomes an agent of the state."

"I have heard reports of physicians threatening to call Child Protective Services to remove the child from parental custody if a parent refused a vaccine," even after the child had reacted negatively to an earlier dose of the vaccine, Orient says.

She contends that mandating vaccines marks a fundamental change in the concept of public health. Traditionally, individuals were quarantined only when they had contagious diseases that posed "a clear and present danger to public health," she says. "Today, a child may be deprived of his liberty to associate with others or his right to a public education simply because of being unimmunized."

And that's just as it should be, says Offit of Children's Hospital. "It is no more your right to catch and transmit a potentially fatal illness than it is your right to run a red light," he says.

"Parents should not be able to get their kids exempted from vaccines," he says. "The notion that one creates a risk-free situation by not vaccinating is incorrect. It is not a medically neutral thing. You are just creating a different risk." He cites a 1991 outbreak of measles in Philadelphia, which centered on a fundamentalist church where most children weren't immunized. Some of the children from the church died, he says, but so did two other children who lived nearby, who were too young to be immunized.

"As long as the great majority of children receive their vaccines, we will be able to maintain our current level of disease control," Duke University's Katz says. But if the level of community protection drops significantly, "we instantly return to a past era when epidemics were an accepted part of life."

The nation experienced that during 1989-91, when immunization rates dropped and there was a measles outbreak, he said. There were 55,622 cases of measles, mainly in children younger than 5, more than 11,000 hospitalizations and 125 deaths. ■

BACKGROUND

Early Breakthroughs

The first vaccine breakthrough in modern times came in 1796, when Edward Jenner, an English country physician, noticed that dairymaids exposed to the milder disease cow-

pox were immune to smallpox. He took some fluid from a patient's cowpox sore and later introduced it into a scratch in the arm of an 8-year-old boy. Forty-eight days later, when Jenner exposed him to smallpox, he resisted the infection. Jenner named his substance "vaccine" after the Latin word for cow.

Another breakthrough came in the late 19th century, when Louis Pasteur, a French chemist, developed chemical techniques to isolate viruses and weaken their effects so they could be used as vaccines.

Yet vaccination continued to provoke controversy. Pasteur's first administration of rabies vaccines to humans was strongly protested by physicians and the public, and efforts to immunize British troops against typhoid at the turn of the century were bitterly opposed despite the serious risk of typhoid faced by troops serving in the Boer War in South Africa.[12]

By the turn of the century, other scientists had developed "killed" vaccines against typhoid, plague, rabies and cholera. By the mid-1920s, vaccines had been developed against diphtheria — an often-deadly childhood disease characterized by a severe inflammation of the throat — and pertussis, or whooping cough, another often-fatal childhood disease characterized by a loud "whooping" sound as the victim struggles to get air into the lungs after violent fits of coughing.

Children and parents of the 1940s and '50s especially dreaded paralytic polio, which could paralyze arms, legs or respiratory muscles. News stories showed children with metal braces on their legs or encased in the so-called iron lungs that helped them to breathe.

Two teams of scientists led by Jonas Salk and Albert Sabin each developed a polio vaccine. The Salk vaccine, using killed viruses, was licensed in 1954 and used in mass-immunization campaigns. Within six years, polio cases dropped 90 percent.

But the Salk vaccine did not provide complete immunity against all three polio viruses. By 1961, Sabin had developed an oral vaccine that did, using a live, attenuated virus. It all but replaced the injectible Salk version in the United States. But because it used a live virus, about a dozen persons a year contracted polio from the vaccine or from being exposed to a recently vaccinated child. Consequently, public health officials decided last January to phase out the live, oral vaccine.

By the 1960s, routine vaccination was no longer controversial among the public and the medical community, and live-virus vaccines had been developed for measles (1963), rubella/German measles (1966) and mumps (1968).

Mandatory Vaccinations

To be effective, vaccination depends on universal immunization. Otherwise, anyone who is not immunized can contract a disease and spread it to others. State laws requiring immunization date from the early 1800s, when Massachusetts required smallpox vaccinations. Britain established the principle of universal free vaccination for smallpox three years later. In recent times in the United States, local immunization laws aimed at schools and licensed day-care began with efforts to eliminate measles in the 1960s and '70s.

Opposition to mandatory vaccinations — largely based on religious, legal, medical or safety grounds — emerged almost as soon as they were implemented. In 1905, the U.S. Supreme Court upheld compulsory-vaccination laws, but anti-vaccination sentiment prevailed in some states.[13]

Nonetheless, the incidence of smallpox continued to decline. The United States reported its last natu-

STD Vaccines for Children May Be Next

The Institute of Medicine and the National Academy of Sciences last year released a report on new vaccines being developed for sexually transmitted diseases and other infectious diseases that may be recommended for adults or children of various ages within the next 20 years. The following vaccines are among those in the works:

- **Cytomegalovirus vaccine.** Cytomegalovirus, a member of the herpes virus group, is spread through blood transmission or sexual activity. May be recommended for all 12-year-olds.

- **Influenza vaccine.** Guards against certain strains of the flu virus. May be recommended for all children and adults.

- **Streptococcus pneumoniae vaccine.** This type of pneumonia is caused by bacteria. May be recommended for all infants.

- **Chlamydia vaccine.** Chlamydia, a sexually transmitted disease, is a type of bacteria that causes genital infections. May be recommended for all 12-year-olds.

- **Hepatitis C virus vaccine.** Hepatitis C is transmitted primarily through infected blood. The U.S. blood supply was contaminated with hepatitis C virus before routine screening was performed. May be recommended for all infants.

- **Herpes simplex virus vaccine.** This virus, transmitted sexually, causes genital, oral and other lesions on the body. May be recommended for all 12-year-olds.

- **Human papillomavirus vaccine.** This virus, transmitted sexually, causes genital warts. May be recommended for all 12-year-olds.

- **Neisseria gonorrhoeae vaccine.** Gonorrhea, another sexually transmitted disease, is a genital-tract infection caused by a bacteria. May be recommended for all 12-year-olds.

- **Respiratory syncytial virus vaccine.** This virus causes the common cold as well as more serious respiratory infections. May be recommended for all infants and 12-year-olds.

Source: National Vaccine Information Center

---

rally occurring case in 1949. In 1971, routine vaccination for smallpox was discontinued.

By contrast, the polio vaccine resulted in an immediate push for federal action to make the vaccine widely available. After Salk reported positive results from his vaccine in 1955, members of Congress from both parties urged the government to distribute the vaccine itself or help the states.

The Republican administration of Dwight D. Eisenhower branded a Democratic-sponsored bill for universal free vaccines as a form of socialized medicine. By August, Congress had drafted a compromise measure, the Poliomyelitis Vaccination Act, which provided $28 million to the states for free universal polio vaccines.

Over the next 45 years, the nation would experience a cyclical pattern: Disease risk would appear to diminish thanks to immunization; then politicians would cut back on immunization funds; vaccination rates would drop, followed by disease outbreaks; then there would be an outcry for more funding for immunizations. [14] For example, polio aid was curtailed in 1957, only to be revived in 1960 after outbreaks of the disease in several cities. To provide broader assistance, President John F. Kennedy asked Congress in 1962 to authorize aid to states to buy vaccines against diphtheria, whooping cough and tetanus, as well as polio.

DPT Under Attack

By the early 1980s, infectious epidemics that killed hundreds of children a year had drifted into distant memory, and some parents were beginning to start questioning the need for massive inoculations. [15] A small number of those parents felt that their children had been damaged by vaccines that were not as safe as they could be — particularly the DPT shot.

Among them was the NVIC's Fisher. In 1980 her toddler Chris suffered a severe reaction after his fourth dose of DPT and an oral polio vaccine. After studying the medical literature on vaccine reactions, she learned that he had suffered convulsions and collapsed shock, a rare, adverse reaction to a DPT shot.

After that, Chris was different — physically, mentally and emotionally. "He no longer knew his numbers or the alphabet, he had poor concentration levels, constant ear infections and diarrhea that would not stop,"

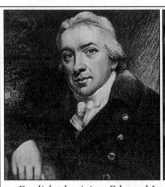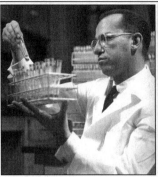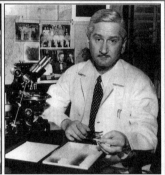

English physician Edward Jenner (left) coined the term "vaccine" after discovering how to protect against smallpox. Jonas Salk (center) led the team that developed the first polio vaccine in 1954 in Pittsburgh. Albert Sabin (right) developed an improved oral polio vaccine in 1961 at his University of Cincinnati lab.

Sources: Centers for Disease Control and Prevention, Archive Photos and Corbis-Bettmann Photos.

Fisher says. "He became emaciated and stopped growing."

Fisher learned that similar adverse events related to the DPT shot in Japan, Sweden and the United Kingdom had led to drops in immunization rates in those countries, and subsequent epidemics of pertussis.

In 1982, Fisher and other mothers founded the advocacy group that evolved into the NVIC. Their goal: get Congress to demand safer DPT vaccines.

By then Japan was already using a safer version of the vaccine, produced, ironically, with technology developed by the NIH. In fact, a U.S. company, Eli Lilly, had marketed the safer version in the 1960s and '70s, but when Wyeth bought Lily in 1976, it discontinued the product. A 1977 Wyeth internal document said producing the safer DPT shot would result in "a very large increase in the cost of manufacture." [16]

"Sure, you can produce a much less toxic product in very low yields, and anyone who has worked on pertussis knows this," Dennis Stainer, an assistant director of production and development at Connaught Medical Research Laboratories in Canada, told a 1982 symposium sponsored by U.S. health officials. "What we are faced with is going from a vaccine that costs literally cents to produce to one that I believe is going to cost dollars to produce." [17]

By the mid-1980s, at least 300 lawsuits had been filed against U.S. DPT manufacturers. "They knew that the older pertussis vaccine was making kids sick," recalls Ted Warchafsky, a Milwaukee attorney who represented parents seeking damages.

In 1991, Fisher documented the development of the DPT vaccine in *A Shot in the Dark*, explaining how the more toxic whole-cell pertussis portion of the shot was causing so many problems, and why a safer, acellular version had not been widely marketed in the United States.

"When word went out that I was writing that book, people started leaving packages of documents, with transcripts from government meetings, on my doorstep in the middle of the night," Fisher says. "One physician told me, 'You are on the right track, but I will never stand up beside you publicly and say that.'"

Fisher says "it was all about money," but, in fact, health officials and drug firms also wanted to keep the price of vaccines low enough for impoverished Third World governments.

"It's the same for every . . . vaccine," said Stanley Plotkin, medical and scientific director for Pasteur-Merieux-Connaught, a Paris-based pharmaceutical company. "Research costs are recouped in North America and Europe, and the vaccines are sold in the developing world at much, much lower margins." [18]

Stainer went on to ask at the 1982 meeting whether it was right to switch to the safe DPT vaccine: "Are we . . . going to have two vaccines, one for the wealthy and one for the rest? I don't think any of us want that."

But that is exactly what has happened. The U.S. government stopped purchasing the whole-cell DPT vaccine in 1996 and recommended that doctors switch to the acellular DTaP version. Only about 6-7 percent of the pertussis vaccines in the U.S. still contain the whole-cell DPT. But it is widely used in the Third World.

But back in the mid-1980s, faced with increasing lawsuits, one of the three DPT producers stopped producing it, and the remaining manufacturers found it was increasingly difficult to obtain liability insurance. "Shortages of the vaccine occurred in some areas of the country, and prices escalated dramatically," Duke University's Katz recalled. [19]

But instead of selling the safer Japanese vaccine, Warchafsky says, U.S. manufacturers asked Congress to limit their liability for adverse reactions to any vaccine mandated by the government, hinting they might stop producing children's vaccines without it.

"And then the industry started buying up the experts," he contends, citing the example of James Cherry, a widely recognized pertussis expert who has served on both the ACIP and the AAP's vaccine advisory committee.

Cherry was a principal author in a

Chronology

1900-1940s
Large-scale immunization programs launched in U.S.

1905
U.S. Supreme Court upholds state law mandating smallpox vaccinations.

1906
Vaccine against pertussis (whooping cough) is developed.

1921-1928
Effective vaccine against diphtheria is developed.

———— • ————

1950s-1960s
Vaccines against polio and other diseases are developed. Congress approves aid to ensure free polio vaccinations.

1954
Jonas Salk develops first polio vaccine in United States. An oral vaccine later developed by Albert Sabin is approved in 1961.

1955
Poliomyelitis Vaccination Assistance Act funds free distribution of polio vaccine.

1962
Vaccination Assistance Act authorizes government purchase of vaccines at negotiated prices and provides grants to states for mass vaccinations.

1963
Measles vaccine is licensed; incidence of the disease drops by 95 percent in U.S. within five years.

1970s-1980s
Decrease in government support for immunizations leads to new outbreaks of some diseases. U.N. begins worldwide immunization program.

1981
Japan licenses safer DPT shot, the acellular DTaP shot, partially developed at the National Institutes of Health.

1982
Vaccine against hepatitis B becomes available. Parents of vaccine-injured children establish Dissatisfied Parents Together to push for safer DPT vaccines. It eventually becomes the National Vaccine Information Center.

1986
Vaccine Injury Compensation Act establishes a no-fault compensation system for persons who suffer serious side effects from legally required vaccination.

1987
Vaccine against *Haemophilus influenzae* type B (Hib), the leading cause of bacterial meningitis, is licensed.

1989-1991
U.S. measles epidemic causes 132 deaths.

———— • ————

1990s-2000s
President George Bush increases funding for immunizations but is faulted for not doing more. President Clinton proposes plan to assure universal access to vaccines for poor and underinsured children.

February 1991
Federal Centers for Disease Control and Prevention (CDC) recommends universal infant immunization with the first genetically engineered vaccine — for hepatitis B.

June 1991
President Bush refuses request for extra funds to boost lagging immunizations.

April 1, 1993
Clinton administration introduces plan to increase immunization rates but later modifies provisions for universal government purchase of vaccines.

1996
CDC's Advisory Committee on Immunization Policy recommends that doctors use the safer DTaP shot instead of the whole-cell pertussis shot.

1998
French court rules that SmithKline Beecham's hepatitis B vaccine had caused a child's multiple sclerosis. France suspends compulsory hepatitis B vaccinations for teens.

1999
New genetically engineered rotavirus vaccine is pulled off market after significant numbers of inoculated infants become seriously ill. FDA acknowledges that vaccines expose infants to unsafe levels of mercury. Congress begins hearings on vaccine safety.

2000
CDC recommends replacing "live" oral polio vaccine with inactivated injectable version because live vaccine caused up to 10 cases of polio a year.

Parents of Autistic Children...

An audible gasp erupted from the audience at a congressional hearing in July after a presentation by a group of parents of autistic children from New Jersey.

Their 85-page report on their exhaustive search of medical literature included a chart listing 75 symptoms characteristic of autism — such as social withdrawal, obsessive-compulsive traits, arm flapping, head banging and toe walking. Alongside those traits, they had listed 75 symptoms attributable to mercury poisoning. As they read the chart, members of the audience gasped. The two lists of symptoms were nearly identical — for all 75 symptoms.

"As a trained scientist, my reading of the mercury literature indicates that every trait that defines autism can be induced by organic mercury [poisoning]," said Albert Enayati, a chemist and president of the New Jersey chapter of the Cure Autism Now Foundation (CAN), which did the study. His son Payam developed normally until he received his DPT and MMR shots, after which he stopped talking and interacting with people and began toe walking, head banging and arm flapping.

Enayati and other parents at the hearing claimed that excessive amounts of mercury from multiple vaccines may have triggered their children's late-onset autism, a new type of autism in which a normally developing child suddenly loses speech and social and cognitive skills. Classic autism is considered a genetic condition that exists from birth.

Theories about autism have been tested and discarded for decades. Medical associations and public health officials insist there is no scientific evidence that vaccines cause autism. However, in recent years — with rates of the disorder skyrocketing across the country — frantic parents are increasingly questioning the vaccine-autism connection.

And mercury in vaccines is not the only concern. Doctors and researchers are examining whether — for a small, mercury-sensitive segment of the population — the measles vaccine, perhaps in conjunction with mercury or other environmental toxins, may trigger "autism-spectrum disorders" ranging from learning disabilities and attention-deficit disorders on the mild end to autism on the severe end.

The American Medical Association (AMA) recently said that up to 20 percent of children have one of a spectrum of neurodevelopmental conditions that includes autism, learning disorders and attention-deficit/hyperactivity disorder. In California, autism diagnoses soared 273 percent and diagnoses of related disorders skyrocketed 1,966 percent between 1987 and 1998. Maryland reported a 513 percent rise in autism between 1993 and 1998, and several dozen other states have reported increases of 300 percent or more.

Mercury, a potent neurotoxin linked to mental retardation, cerebral palsy and central nervous system disorders, has been used in vaccines since the 1930s, in a preservative called thimerosal. Thimerosal is present in more than 50 vaccines and other medicines, even though it has been banned in many over-the-counter medications since the 1980s.

Because children in the past decade have begun receiving more vaccines at earlier ages — often multiple vaccines in a single day — concerns have arisen about how much mercury infant brains are being exposed to from vaccines.

"My grandson received vaccines for nine different diseases in one day," said House Government Reform Committee Chairman Dan Burton, R-Ind., who said the child is now autistic. "He may have been exposed to 62.5 micrograms of mercury in one day through his vaccines. According to his weight, [that] is 41 times the amount at which harm can be caused." And Burton added, "These vaccines are still in use."

Lyndale Redwood, a nurse from Atlanta, told the hearing that her autistic 2-month-old son had received 125 times his allowable daily exposure of mercury after getting two infant vaccines in one day. "These large exposures

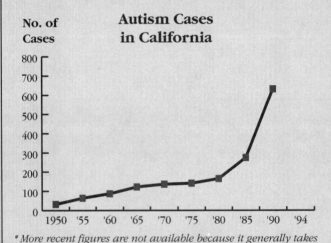

Cases of Autism Rose Sharply

*The number of autistic children seeking state services in California more than doubled in the 1980s and nearly doubled again in the first half of the 1990s.**

No. of Cases

Autism Cases in California

800
700
600
500
400
300
200
100
0

1950 '55 '60 '65 '70 '75 '80 '85 '90 '94

* More recent figures are not available because it generally takes several years after birth to determine if a child is autistic.

Source: California Department of Developmental Services

...Blame Mercury Poisoning

continued at 4, 6, 12 and 18 months," she said. She also discovered that the injections she received during the first and third trimesters of her pregnancy and an hour after delivery to prevent RH blood incompatibility also contained mercury. An analysis of her son's hair revealed that he had five times more mercury than was considered safe.

Mercury is extremely toxic to developing fetal brains. In many parts of the country, pregnant mothers are advised not to eat canned tuna fish, which contains high levels of mercury. Emissions from coal-fired power plants are another major source of mercury contamination.

Parents at the hearing were particularly concerned about the impact of mercury on the brains of hours-old newborns, who, since 1991, have been immunized with a thimerosal-containing hepatitis B vaccine before they leave the hospital. They angrily demanded to know why federal agencies had not banned the use of mercury.

William Egan, acting director of the Food and Drug Administration's (FDA) Office of Vaccine Research and Review, said, "There is no convincing data or evidence of any harm caused by the low levels of thimerosal that some children may have encountered in following the existing immunization schedule." Furthermore, the federal guidelines for mercury exposure include margins of safety, and most vaccine exposure is within that margin of safety, he said.

Benjamin Schwartz, acting director of epidemiology and surveillance for the Centers for Disease Control and Prevention's (CDC) National Immunization Program (NIP), says "There's a difference between chronic, daily exposure and what a child can be exposed to on any given day." The agency interprets the mercury guidelines as how much a person can be exposed to over six months.

Nevertheless, Egan said, even though the threat from mercury is only "theoretical," the government last year asked manufacturers to voluntarily remove or significantly reduce by next spring the thimerosal from all vaccines routinely administered to infants. It was not banned outright in order not to disrupt the nation's vaccine supply, he said.

As a result, said Roger H. Bernier, associate director for science at the NIP, the amount of mercury an infant may be exposed to from routine immunizations has been reduced by 60 percent in the past year. Plus, responding to concerns about newborns, the CDC recommended that physicians temporarily discontinue giving them the hepatitis B vaccine at birth until a mercury-free vaccine was available. Mercury has since been removed from the vaccine, and it is again given routinely to newborns.

Redwood also cited a West Coast study of the mercury exposure of 120,000 children, which showed a "statistically significant (albeit weak) association" between thimerosal exposure and attention deficit disorders, tics, speech and language delay and neurodevelopment delays in general."

But Bernier said the CDC duplicated the study but did not get the same results. "These results require further scrutiny," he said, "but the direction of the findings is reassuring."

However, Neal Halsey, director of the Institute for Vaccine Safety at Johns Hopkins University, said, "Uncertainties rising from the new data do not resolve any of the controversies or differences of opinion regarding the potential risks from thimerosal in vaccines," he said. "Additional studies need to be conducted." [1]

Bernier said the CDC is studying whether autism is related to the measles vaccine. The agency is also collaborating with the National Institutes of Health (NIH) on a study of autistic regression and vaccination. Finally, the CDC, NIH and Institute of Medicine (IOM) have recently established a standing committee on vaccine safety, which will assess new evidence about possible adverse health effects — including autism — from vaccines.

But pediatricians like Stephanie Cave of Baton Rouge, La., are not waiting for any more studies. She says she is seeing major improvements using timed-release chelation therapy to remove mercury and other heavy metals from autistic and learning-disabled children's bodies. "As the treatments progress," she says, "we're seeing eye contact, socialization and speech. The children are literally turning around."

But she and other researchers do not think that mercury is the only culprit. She thinks the mercury may compromise babies' immune systems, so that when babies get their measles, mumps, rubella (MMR) vaccines at age 15 months, the body may not be able to fight off the viruses as well as it should.

A related theory set off a firestorm two years ago, when a report appeared in the influential British medical journal *Lancet* arguing that the MMR vaccine might trigger a bowel disorder that may allow toxins like mercury to cross from the blood into the brain, causing regressive autism. The report was widely criticized as methodologically flawed, and at least two subsequent epidemiological studies did not find a link. Additional studies are being conducted.

But Rick Rollens, a Granite Bay, Calif., parent whose child developed late-onset autism following vaccines, thinks independent studies must be done on this subject, without influence from either the vaccine industry or the public health agencies. Prodded by Rollens and the parents of other autistic children, the California legislature appropriated $34 million for a study of neurodevelopmental disorders at the University of California at Davis.

"Asking the public health community to investigate the role of vaccines in the development of autism is like asking the tobacco industry to investigate the link between lung cancer and smoking," Rollens says.

---

[1] From the Institute for Vaccine Safety Web site, www.vaccinesafety.edu/ACIP-thim-0621.htm.

At Issue:

Do vaccines cause autism?

DR. BERNARD RIMLAND

Director, Autism Research Institute, San Diego, Calif.;
www.autism.com/ari

FROM *LOS ANGELES TIMES*, APRIL 26, 2000

*f*irst, do no harm. If the multibillion-dollar vaccine industry had heeded Hippocrates' ancient dictum and concentrated on making vaccines safe, the 300-500 percent nationwide increase in autism probably would not have occurred.

Concern for vaccine safety might have prevented the simultaneous sharp rise in other chronic and debilitating diseases such as asthma, allergies, attention deficit/hyperactivity disorder [ADHD], learning disabilities and arthritis.

The cause of the skyrocketing rates of these disorders, like the rise in autism, has mystified the experts. Many thoughtful and informed people believe that medical overexuberance has resulted in an unintended trade-off: Vaccination against acute diseases such as measles and rubella has increased susceptibility to chronic disorders such as autism, asthma, arthritis and ADHD. . . .

We learned in the latter half of the 20th century that one must be careful in tinkering with Mother Nature. Those marvelous pesticides, herbicides, gasoline additives and other miracles of modern chemistry have a downside. While we now know that toxic pollution of the environment is bad news, we are just beginning to learn that pumping toxins — viruses, bacteria, mercury, aluminum and formaldehyde, for example — into the body in the form of vaccinations for immediate gain may prove to be costly in the long term.

Those who share my view do not oppose vaccines. What we oppose is overvaccination and unsafe vaccines. . . .

In 1965, parents began telling me that their children became autistic upon getting the DPT (diphtheria, pertussis, tetanus) shot — a triple vaccine. When another triple vaccine, MMR (measles, mumps, rubella), was introduced in the 1980s, the alarming reports from parents and the prevalence figures for autism rose sharply. Corroborating evidence is plentiful.

In his testimony before the House Government Reform Committee, Paul Offit, the chief of infectious diseases at Children's Hospital of Philadelphia — who acknowledged at the hearing that he also is paid by the Merck Co. to educate doctors about vaccines — attacked the "notion" that giving three vaccines at once is unsafe. . . .

Don't just tell us vaccines are safe. Where are the scientific data? There are none. It is no secret that . . . doctors report only 1-10 percent of the adverse reactions they learn about. We cannot afford to deny, dismiss or sidestep the issue of vaccine safety. Research on this critical problem must be undertaken as the highest priority.

REP. HENRY A. WAXMAN, D-CALIF.

FROM *LOS ANGELES TIMES*, APRIL 17, 2000

*r*ep. Dan Burton, R-Ind., chairman of the House Government Reform Committee, held a hearing this month to publicize his conviction that childhood vaccines cause autism. We heard heart-rending testimony from parents of autistic children who sincerely believe that vaccines caused their children's condition. And a few hand-picked researchers lent a scientific veneer by testifying that they believe vaccines may cause autism.

This is the kind of news that can alarm millions of families. That's why it's essential that parents know that the American Medical Association, the American Academy of Pediatrics, the Centers for Disease Control and Prevention and virtually every medical expert around the world have reached a different conclusion: Scientific evidence does not support a causal association between vaccines and autism.

Disregarding this evidence or overstating the dangers of childhood immunization runs the risk of needlessly scaring parents from vaccinating their children. Failing to immunize our children exposes them to risks of serious illness, disability and death. Every year, 2.5 million children die and 750,000 are crippled worldwide from childhood diseases. Once common and now rare in our country, rubella causes deafness, blindness and mental retardation. Measles, mistakenly viewed by some as an innocuous childhood illness, caused 11,000 hospitalizations and 120 deaths in our country during a 1989-91 epidemic. . . .

The dangers of a vaccine-autism scare are real. In 1998, British surgeon Andrew Wakefield published a preliminary report alleging that autism in 12 children was associated with the measles-mumps-rubella vaccine. The resulting hysteria quickly drove measles immunization rates in Britain below the level experts say is necessary to avoid an epidemic. . . .

Large-scale studies in Sweden, Finland and Britain have found no causal connection between vaccines and autism. The British government has reviewed and refuted the allegations, concluding — most recently on April 3 — that "there is no new evidence to suggest a causal link between MMR vaccination and autism."

Everyone agrees that more autism research is essential. . . . Yet as we increase research, we must also make sure that every parent knows that the best available science does not support a link between vaccines and autism. Nothing could be more harmful than to mislead parents about these facts and to encourage an unwarranted mistrust of vaccines, leaving our children defenseless before terrible childhood diseases.

At Issue:

Should vaccinations be mandatory?

SAMUEL L. KATZ, M.D.
American Academy of Pediatrics (AAP), Infectious Disease Society of America (IDSA)

FROM TESTIMONY BEFORE HOUSE COMMITTEE ON GOVERNMENT REFORM, AUG. 3, 1999

*i*t is true that despite all that vaccines have done to improve the health of individuals and communities in the United States and throughout the world, they are not perfect. However, one simple fact cannot reasonably be disputed — the benefits of immunizations far outweigh any possible risks.

I would just like to remind you of a few anecdotal events. Where were the last big measles outbreaks in older youngsters in this country? In a school for Christian Science college students where there were deaths due to measles because they don't follow immunization. . . .

The last epidemics of polio in this country [were] in a boys' school in Greenwich, Conn. for a religious group who do not practice immunization; among an Amish population in Pennsylvania and several other states because they do not practice immunization. Should we allow our community immunity to wane, we will negate all the progress we have made and allow our communities to be at risk from threats that are easily prevented. . . .

Immunization has a clear community benefit in addition to its benefit to the individual patient. An individual's freedom to ignore a stop sign, to pollute the environment . . . or to spread disease do not serve the public good ultimately. We do place certain restraints on individual freedom because of our belief in the greater social well-being. . . .

Ongoing vaccine safety efforts and continuous monitoring of adverse events, be they alleged, potential, or real, are crucial to our nation's childhood immunization program. As science and resources allow, we are obligated to continue to improve the effectiveness of these safety-monitoring measures.

The AAP and the IDSA have seen allegations that a variety of illnesses may be caused by various vaccines. It's easy to understand how a family with a tragedy can believe that a vaccine caused the sudden, unexpected death of a child or the appearance of autism. . . . We give vaccines in the first two years of life, when all of these disorders have their common onset, so that guilt by temporal association is very difficult to separate from guilt by causality.

A robust system of checks and balances exists to monitor the safety and effectiveness of our vaccines, a system that we strive continuously to perfect. These efforts are designed to ensure that our recommendations about immunization and procedures reflect the best available science.

DAWN RICHARDSON
President, Parents Requesting Open Vaccine Education (PROVE), Cedar Park, Texas; prove@vaccineinfo.net; www.vaccineinfo.net

*p*arents love their children and want to protect them. But vaccines, like the diseases they are designed to prevent, carry an unpredictable risk of injury or death. Parents should be free to make their own informed, voluntary vaccination decisions without being subjected to government sanctions.

All diseases and vaccines are not the same, and neither are all children. Yet current mandatory-vaccination laws treat chickenpox like smallpox. Over 200 new vaccines being developed for everything from cocaine addiction to sexually transmitted disease (STD) will be candidates for mandates. Additionally, some children are at greater biological risk than others for reacting to vaccines. "One-size-fits-all" mass vaccination policies don't take these differences into account and fail to minimize the risk of vaccine-induced injury and death for too many children.

Annually, 12,000-14,000 reports of hospitalizations, injuries and deaths following vaccinations are made to the federal Vaccine Adverse Event Reporting System (VAERS), but only 1-10 percent of doctors report. More than $1 billion has been paid out under the federal vaccine-injury compensation program, but three out of four applicants are turned away and left to cope on their own.

Recent congressional hearings have raised eye-opening questions about inadequate vaccine licensing and safety standards; conflicts of interest between drug companies and vaccine policy-makers; and huge gaps in scientific knowledge about how vaccines impact the body.

Health officials measure public health in terms of high vaccination rates and low infectious-disease rates, and yet the rate of chronic disease and disability in children is at an all-time high. With children now getting as many as 39 doses of 12 different vaccines by school entry — while the brain and immune system are developing at the most rapid rate — nobody knows whether over-vaccination has contributed to the dramatic increases in asthma, allergies, learning disabilities, autism, attention-deficit disorder, diabetes and other chronic neuroimmune illnesses. Yet, the Centers for Disease Control and Prevention (CDC) insists all children, regardless of their personal disease risk, must get every government-mandated vaccine for the theoretical "greater good."

Because vaccination is a medical procedure that carries an inherent risk of injury or death, informed consent to vaccination should be the right of every American. Every parent deserves to be given truthful, unbiased information about diseases and vaccines and be allowed to make informed, voluntary, vaccination decisions for their children.

1978-79 study sponsored by the FDA and the University of California at Los Angeles (UCLA), which found that an alarming number of children receiving the DPT shot, one in 1,750, was at risk of suffering from "collapse shock" and an equal number of having convulsions.

Yet by 1990, after having received a $400,000 grant from Lederle, he declared in the *Journal of the American Medical Association* (JAMA) that severe brain damage caused by the vaccine was a "myth." By 1993, Lederle had given Cherry and UCLA an additional $834,000 for pertussis research and expert testimony in lawsuits brought by parents of injured children. [20]

Meanwhile, Congress in 1986 limited the liability of manufacturers of mandated vaccines and health practitioners who administer them. The National Childhood Vaccine Injury Compensation Act also:

• Established a "no-fault" system of compensation for injuries or deaths reasonably associated with the administration of childhood vaccines;

• Ordered CDC to set up a centralized system for reporting adverse reactions to vaccines; and

• Required periodic independent reviews of the scientific evidence on adverse events.

Immunizations Lag

By the late 1980s, immunization rates were slipping again. Then, in the first years of George Bush's presidency, the nation got a wake-up call on the dangers of incomplete immunization: A major measles epidemic in 1989-91 killed at least 132 persons.

Concentrated in Chicago, Houston, Los Angeles, New York and Philadelphia, the outbreak had infected 18,000 people by 1989. More than three-fourths of the cases involved unimmunized preschool children, mostly blacks and Hispanics.

"Everyone knows that when immunization levels drop, it is just a matter of time before you get an epidemic," said Philip A. Brunell, former chairman of the AAP Committee on Infectious Diseases. [21]

In recent years, concern about vaccines has deepened as officials have begun adding new vaccines for non-epidemic diseases to the mandatory schedule, and as enforcement of mandatory vaccinations has begun to tighten. (*See graph, p. 72.*)

Some doctors, rewarded by managed-care companies for achieving high inoculation rates, won't treat patients who refuse vaccination.

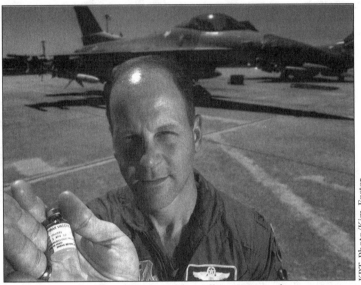

The U.S. military's push to inoculate all service members against anthrax spread by germ warfare has been highly controversial. Many service members quit rather than take the vaccine or were court-martialed for refusing to take it.

KRT Photo/Kim Foster

States, which receive federal grants for achieving high inoculation rates, are pressuring local health departments to improve inoculation rates. And welfare mothers in some states are having their checks reduced if their kids don't get vaccinated.

The Clinton administration has won legislation to extend vaccination programs to the poor and has recommended new legislation to improve vaccination levels. Since 1994, the Vaccines for Children program has allowed the government to provide free pediatric vaccines for low-income children.

In addition, the federal government is overseeing establishment of a network of state electronic vaccine-tracking registries. So far, 22 states have set up or are in the process of establishing such registries, whereby all children are enrolled at birth. One state is using the database to contact parents of children who have not received all their federally mandated vaccines. ∎

CURRENT SITUATION

Compensation Law

Debate over implementation of the 1986 vaccine-injury compensation law heated up during congressional hearings last September, when critics claimed the administration had turned lawmakers' intent on its head. [22]

"We were betrayed," says the NVIC's Fisher, whose group helped draft the original legislation. Fisher had been promised the system would be fair and non-confrontational, she says, but instead it has become "highly adversarial," rejecting three out of four claimants.

However, program Director Thomas E. Balbier Jr. told the subcommittee that 42 percent of petitions have been awarded compensation. "This compares to a compensation rate of only 23 percent for those who file medical malpractice lawsuits through the usual tort system."

The law set up a "no-fault" system to compensate parents of vaccine-injured children "quickly, easily and with certainty and generosity." The program was to replace the expensive product-liability and medical-malpractice suits that were becoming so burdensome in the mid-1980s that pharmaceutical companies threatened to stop manufacturing vaccines.

Unique in U.S. law, the compensation system is supported by a 75-cent surcharge on each mandatory vaccine and is administered by special masters at the U.S. Court of Claims. The law listed conditions covered for each vaccine and the time period following vaccination when the condition must occur.

As of Aug. 3, 1999, more than 1,400 families had received awards totaling over $1 billion, most for injuries suffered following the whole-cell DPT shot.

But in 1995, Health and Human Services (HHS) Secretary Donna Shalala tightened the requirements for several compensable conditions, including encephalopathy, or brain damage, one of the most common conditions claimed by DPT vaccine-injury victims. Under the new terms, a child would have to suffer a "diminished level of consciousness" for more than 24 hours before being compensated. Plus, residual-seizure disorder, another DPT-related side effect, was removed from the compensable-injuries table.

In dramatic testimony, Michelle Clements, a parent from Milwaukee, told the subcommittee how the changes had affected her. Several hours after her 7-month-old son Andrew received his third DPT shot in 1992, he went into convulsions — and continued to have them over the next three years. Then on Sept. 8, 1995, he suffered a convulsion lasting four and a half hours and his temperature climbed to 108.8 degrees. When doctors finally allowed the Clements to see their son, "We saw a child double the size he was when he came into the hospital."

Today he cannot walk, talk, eat or drink. He is fed through a tube in his stomach. "His body is 7 years old but his brain is like a 3-month-old," she told the panel.

Yet the family was turned down for compensation. "The special master told us that if we had applied a year earlier, she would have found in our favor, but because of the changes in the injuries table, she had to find for the government."

"The government forces us to give our children these vaccines," Clements said, "and then when something goes wrong — too bad — you're on your own." She was especially furious when she learned that a safer DPT shot existed in 1992, but the government had waited until 1996 to recommend that doctors use it.

Ironically, parents who helped write the compensation law had understood that Congress granted the HHS secretary broad discretionary authority to alter the injuries table primarily to expand the list of compensable events and make the system more, not less, inclusive. Instead, the secretary has used her discretionary authority to remove or "redefine permanent injuries long recognized by the medical community as being associated with vaccine reactions," Fisher says.

The General Accounting Office pointed out last December that while Shalala did add some injuries to the table, most parents would find it harder to receive compensation with the new changes, because "far more claims have historically been associated with injuries HHS removed from the table than for injuries HHS added to it." [23]

Although a group of injured parents sued HHS in 1995, claiming Shalala had overstepped her authority in changing the table, a judge disagreed with them.

Other witnesses complained that because Justice Department lawyers have made the process so adversarial, cases can take up to nine years, compared with the nine months envisioned by Congress. Moreover, Clifford J. Shoemaker, an attorney who has represented vaccine victims for over 20 years, told the subcommittee that even when the court rules in the parents' favor, it can take years to receive compensation. Shalala's changes "effectively devastated the program," he said.

Compensation program Director Balbier defended Shalala's revisions, saying that the law mandated that the secretary should modify the table to "bring it in line with science." "The program was never intended to serve as a compensation source for a wide range of naturally occurring illnesses and conditions," he said.

Fisher told the committee that the latest IOM studies support the connection between encephalopathy and the DPT vaccine.

But Balbier says the changes were approved by the program's advisory committee after several months of public comment and deliberation, and were based on scientific evidence available at the time. The definition of encephalopathy that was finally adopted was actually broader than some of the scientific advisers thought it should be, Balbier says, but "it was decided that we should give the plaintiffs the benefit of the doubt."

But pediatric neurologist Kinsbourne, who has testified as an expert witness in many vaccine-injury cases, told the subcommittee that the government now puts the burden of proof on the victims. Instead of presuming the injury was caused by the vaccine, as the original law intended, he said, the secretary now requires the plaintiff to prove the injury was definitely caused by the vaccine.

Because DPT vaccine injuries have become so difficult to prove under the compensation program, some lawyers are threatening to go back to civil court to pursue lawsuits against the manufacturers, exactly what the act was intended to prevent.

"We're going back to war," said Boston attorney Michael Hugo. "The vaccine program is an abysmal failure. It is an uncertain, slow, horrible system." [24] ■

OUTLOOK

New Vaccines

A flood of new vaccines, many of them genetically engineered, soon may be in use for diseases from pneumonia and tuberculosis to chlamydia and genital herpes. About 100 new vaccines are already in clinical trials.

All are not aimed at children, but scientists at the Children's Vaccine Initiative (CVI), a global organization of private and government groups, are working on a genetically engineered "supervaccine." To be given orally at birth, it would protect against childhood diseases as well as pneumonia, typhoid,

encephalitis, diarrhea, strep and influenza. The project is spurred by estimates from the WHO that up to 8 million children around the world die each year from preventable diseases.

Researchers are also examining novel ways of delivering vaccines, such as nasal sprays and genetically engineered fruits and plants. "An edible vaccine could be easy to produce, safe, affordable and effective," said Carol O. Tacket, a University of Maryland medical professor. "This novel approach to developing vaccines [could] protect individuals around the world, especially in regions where injected vaccines are less practical." [25]

But some critics fear that the lure of profits may be more powerful than safety considerations. "With every child (and possibly adult) on Earth a potential required recipient of multiple doses and every health-care system and government a potential buyer, it is little wonder that countless millions of dollars are spent nurturing the growing multibillion-dollar vaccine industry," writes Alan Philips, director of Citizens for Healthcare Freedom, in Durham, N.C. [26] "Without public outcry, we will see more and more new vaccines required of us and our children. And while profits are readily calculable, the real human costs are being ignored."

"We must have more scientific information to make sound medical policy on different vaccines — especially if vaccines are to continue to be mandated," says molecular biologist Bonnie S. Dunbar of the Baylor College of Medicine in Houston.

Surgeon General Satcher told Burton's subcommittee on Aug. 3, 1999, "As the number of vaccines available for our use increases, an improved safety-assessment program will be critical, and effective risk communication will be essential."

But critics say pediatricians rarely provide parents with the vaccine risk-benefit information sheets that they are required by law to provide.

"If we had informed-consent protections in place, the public could exert economic pressure on the companies to improve existing vaccines by refusing to use them if they prove to be too dangerous," Fisher says. "But that system is not in place, and the drug companies continue to profit while taking no financial responsibility for vaccine injuries and deaths."

Critics also fear that the government's zeal to immunize every American child may soon begin to seriously infringe on privacy rights and constitutional protections. They are particularly fearful that new computerized vaccine-tracking systems could lead to harassment of parents of unvaccinated children.

Some vaccine "choice" advocates worry that the vaccine registries may be used to force universal vaccination against the AIDS virus, once a vaccine is developed. "Any effort to try to make the HIV vaccine mandatory will run into one heck of a battle," consumer lawyer Turner says. "There are so many better ways to control HIV without a vaccine. It's not necessary to vaccinate the entire population."

Meanwhile, some scientists have begun to question the wisdom of trying to eradicate every childhood disease since some studies indicate that childhood infections may actually increase the body's ability to fend off chronic diseases, such as diabetes and asthma.

Parent advocates say more oversight and accountability is needed over public health policies that could have such long-term impacts on society.

Some health-care professionals fear that if the impending wave of vaccinations is aggressively promoted at the same time that public trust in vaccines is eroding, many of the public health gains made in the last century could be undermined. Noncompliance might be driven underground, creating even greater danger of disease outbreaks.

"When I was a young doctor and was faced with a ward full of polio victims, or 1,000 children damaged by congenital rubella, the benefits of vaccines were very compelling," recalls Louis Cooper, vice president-elect of the American Academy of Pediatrics.

"But in the 21st century, with those kinds of epidemics fading into memory, and with so many new vaccines in the pipeline, many of us are looking at what kinds of vaccines should be mandated, what should be recommended and what should be optional," Cooper says.

"A lot of thoughtful people are saying it's time to develop some principles for dealing with the new era of vaccination." ■

Notes

See CDC report "Six Common Misconceptions about Vaccination," at www.cdc.gov/nip/publications/6mishome.htm.

For background, see Craig Donegan, Gene Therapy's Future," *The CQ Researcher*, Dec. 8, 1995, pp. 1089-1112.

Quoted in Susan Fenelon Kerr, "Poor health among children confounds parents, doctors," *Union News, Sunday Republican*, July 30, 2000. The Web site is: www.gval.com

For details on the DPT vaccine controversy, see Andrea Rock, "The Lethal Dangers of the Billion-Dollar Vaccine Business," *Money*, December 1996.

Kathleen R. Stratton et al, "DPT Vaccine and Chronic Nervous System Dysfunction: A New Analysis" (1994).

Quoted in Brian Wallstin, "Immune to Reason," *Houston Press*, June 3-9, 1999.

Ibid.

Testimony before House Government Reform Committee, July 18, 2000.

Neal A. Halsey, "Limiting Infant Exposure to Thimerosal in Vaccines and Other

Sources of Mercury," *Journal of the American Medical Association*, Nov. 10, 1999.

[11] For background, see Adriel Bettelheim, "Managing Managed Care," *The CQ Researcher*, April 16, 1999, pp. 305-328.

[12] From Susan S. Ellenberg and Robert T. Chen, "The Complicated Task of Monitoring Vaccine Safety," *Journal of the U.S. Public Health Service, Public Health Reports*, January/February, 1997; Vol. 112, No. 1; pp. 10-20.

[13] *Jacobson v. Massachusetts* 197 U.S. 11 (1905).

[14] For background, see Kenneth Jost, "Childhood Immunizations," *The CQ Researcher*, June 18, 1993, pp. 529-552.

[15] For background, see Mary H. Cooper, "Combating Infectious Diseases," *The CQ Researcher*, June 9, 1995, pp. 489-502.

[16] Rock, *op. cit.*, p. 153.

[17] Harris L. Coulter and Barbara Loe Fisher, *A Shot in the Dark* (1991), p. 209.

[18] "Industry Perspective: An Interview with Dr.

Stanley Plotkin," *IAVI Report*, June 1996. p. 7.

[19] Katz's comments were made in testimony Aug. 3, 1999, before the House Government Reform Committee.

[20] Rock, *op. cit.*, p. 153.

[21] Jost, *op. cit.*, p. 540.

[22] The hearings were before the House Subcommittee on Criminal Justice, Drug Policy and Human Resource, Sept. 28, 1999.

[23] "Vaccine Injury Compensation: Program Challenged to Settle Claims Quickly and Easily," *Letter Report*, GAO, Dec. 22, 1999.

[24] John Hanchette and Sunny Kaplan, "National Vaccine Compensation Program For Children Draws Fire," Vaccination Nation, Gannett News Service, Aug. 11, 1998.

[25] Quoted in Ronald Kotulak and Jon Van, "Discoveries," *Chicago Tribune*, July 30, 2000.

[26] Philips' comments appeared on the group's Web site: www.UNC.edu/~aphilip/www/chf/

[27] For details, see "Plagued by Cures," *The Economist*, Nov. 22, 1997.

FOR MORE INFORMATION

Autism Research Institute, 4182 Adams Ave., San Diego, Calif. 92116; (619) 281-7165; www.autism.com/ari/. This nonprofit, established in 1967, conducts research on autism and disseminates its findings to medical personnel and to parents.

Immunization Action Coalition, 1573 Selby Ave., Suite 234, St. Paul, Minn. 55104; (651) 647-9009; www.immunize.org. The coalition works to boost immunization rates. Receives some funding from vaccine manufacturers.

National Network for Immunization Information, www.infoinc.com/imnews2/ Web site operated by the Infectious Diseases Society of America, the Pediatric Infectious Diseases Society, the American Academy of Pediatrics and the American Nurses Association. Funded by the Robert Wood Johnson Foundation, it receives no funds from the vaccine industry.

National Vaccine Information Center, 512 W. Maple Ave., Suite 206, Vienna, Va. 22180; (703) 938-3783; www.909shot.com. The center, the oldest and largest national group advocating reform of the vaccination system, provides assistance to parents of children who have experienced vaccine reactions.

National Immunization Program, Centers for Disease Control and Prevention, 1600 Clifton Rd., Mailstop E-05, Atlanta, Ga. 30333; (800) 232-2522; www.cdc.gov/nip. This government program plans, coordinates and administers immunization activities nationwide.

Bibliography

Selected Sources Used

Books

Coulter, Harris L. and Barbara Loe Fisher, *A Shot in the Dark: Why the P in the DPT Vaccination May Be Hazardous to Your Child's Health*, **Avery Publishing Group Inc., 1991.**
This book documents the dangers of the DPT vaccine by tracing the history of its development and use. Coulter, a medical historian, and Fisher, president of the National Vaccine Information Center whose son suffered vaccination damage, provide parents with important questions to ask their child's physician about vaccines.

Murphy, Jamie, *What Every Parent Should Know about Childhood Immunization*, **Earth Healing Products, 1993.**
Decidedly anti-vaccine, this medical researcher tells parents "more about the risks [of childhood vaccines] than your pediatrician wants you to know." He describes the toxic chemicals in vaccines and cites numerous medical journal articles describing adverse reactions to childhood vaccines. He advises parents how to legally avoid vaccinating their children.

Offit, Paul A., and Louis M. Bell, *Vaccines: What Every Parent Should Know*, **IDG Books, 1999.**
This pro-vaccine parents' guide, written by two doctors from Children's Hospital of Philadelphia, has a chapter on each childhood vaccine in which the authors discuss the risks and benefits of each shot.

Oldstone, Michael B. A., *Viruses, Plagues and History*, **Oxford University Press, 1998.**
The author, director of the viral immunobiology laboratory at the Scripps Research Institute and an editor at the medical journal *Virology*, traces the long-term medical campaigns to eradicate diseases that have long tormented humankind: measles, smallpox and polio. He also discusses efforts to tame modern plagues caused by the Ebola virus, Hantavirus and AIDS virus.

Articles

Ellenberg, Susan S. and Robert T. Chen, "The Complicated Task of Monitoring Vaccine Safety," *Journal of the U.S. Public Health Service, Public Health Reports,* **January/February 1997; Vol. 112, No.1.**
This article describes the history of vaccines, as well as the method by which their safety is monitored today.

Goodwin, Jan, "The Trouble With DPT," *Redbook*, **August/September, 2000, pp. 158-175.**
This article chronicles the case of a New York anesthe-

siologist convicted of manslaughter after his daughter died of what prosecutors said was "shaken baby syndrome" but what several doctors testified was actually a vaccine reaction. It says a growing number of parents are being blamed for the side effects of vaccines given to millions of babies each year.

Halsey, Neal A., "Limiting Infant Exposure to Thimerosal in Vaccines and Other Sources of Mercury," *Journal of the American Medical Association*, **Nov. 10, 1999.**
The director of the Vaccine Safety Institute at Johns Hopkins University argues for limited the exposure of infants to thimerosal until vaccines free of this mercury-laden preservative are available.

Hanchette, John and Sunny Kaplan, "National Vaccine Compensation Program For Children Draws Fire," *Vaccination Nation*, **Gannett News Service series, June, 1998.**
Silver bullet vaccines have nearly wiped out many childhood diseases. But this five-part series uses government documents to disclose how some vaccines trigger dangerous reactions resulting in lifelong disability or even death.

Rock, Andrea, "The Lethal Dangers of the Billion-Dollar Vaccine Business," *Money*, **December 1996, pp. 148-163.**
This article exposes the politics and economics behind the billion-dollar vaccine industry and explains why safer versions of certain vaccines took so long to replace the standard-issue shots.

Reports and Studies

"Vaccine Injury Compensation: Program Challenged to Settle Claims Quickly and Easily," *Letter Report* **GAO, Dec. 22, 1999.**
The General Accounting Office last December pointed out that while Health and Human Services Secretary Donna Shalala added some injuries to the list of those the government compensates vaccine-damaged children for, most parents would find it harder to receive compensation because "far more claims have historically been associated with injuries HHS removed . . . than for injuries HHS added."

Stratton, Kathleen R., et al., "Adverse Events Associated with Childhood Vaccines: Evidence Bearing on Causality," **Institute of Medicine, National Academy Press, 1994.**
In a study mandated by Congress, the IOM examined possible links between pertussis and rubella vaccine and adverse reactions in children.

96   **Illness, Treatment, and Health Policy**

6 Patients' Rights

KENNETH JOST

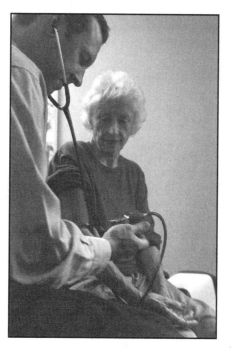

Minnesota computer executive Patrick Shea thought he should see a cardiologist. He had been experiencing shortness of breath and dizzy spells. And heart disease ran in his family.

But Shea's physician assured him a specialist wasn't necessary and refused to give him the written referral required by his health plan. Instead, he told Shea that his problems were stress-related and that he was too young to have heart problems.

Later, while on an overseas business trip, Shea suffered chest pains so severe that he was hospitalized and had to return home. But his doctor still dismissed his concerns.

Shea never saw a specialist. He died in March 1993, less than a year later, leaving his wife Dianne with two young children and troubling questions. He was 40. An autopsy disclosed that Shea had suffered from arteriosclerosis — blocked arteries — which might have been corrected with cardiac bypass surgery.

"We repeatedly asked for referral to a cardiologist," Dianne later told a Minnesota legislative committee. "Not only were our pleas ignored, we were assured time and time again that our fears were unfounded."

In the months that followed, Dianne sought to discover how a man who had always followed his doctor's advice could die of an undiagnosed disease. What she found shook her confidence not only in their own doctors but also in the health care that more than 150 million Americans receive today from so-called managed-care systems: health maintenance organizations (HMOs) and similar network health-care plans. [1]

Supporters say managed care helps provide affordable, high-quality health care at a time when patients,

Updated by Adriel Bettelheim, December 1, 2000. Originally published February 6, 1998.

health-care providers, insurers and employers are all straining to keep down costs. But Dianne became convinced from the inquiry she and her lawyers made that cost controls helped kill her husband.

She claims in a wrongful death lawsuit that Shea's doctor had an undisclosed financial conflict of interest in refusing to refer him to a cardiologist because he received extra compensation from their HMO, Medica, for not sending patients to specialists.

The defendants in the federal court suit — Shea's doctors, their HMO clinic and Medica — deny that the doctors' compensation in any way depended on rejecting Shea's request to see a specialist. "Sheer speculation," Medica's lawyers say. The defendants also deny they were negligent in failing to diagnose Shea's heart disease. A trial in the case is expected later this year. [2]

Dianne Shea, meanwhile, has begun advocating reform of managed care. She urged the Minnesota Legislature to require health insurers to

disclose their "payment methodology" — information she says that might have prompted Shea to ignore his doctor's advice and see a cardiologist. "People have to understand that health care is a business," she says. "Just as we would never buy an investment blindly, we just cannot trust our doctors blindly."

The state Legislature last year passed a weakened version of Shea's proposal, requiring disclosure of the financial arrangements only on the patient's request. Minnesota thus became one of more than 30 states to pass legislation in the past three years aimed at strengthening the rights of patients enrolled in managed care — by far the dominant form of health care in the United States. *(See chart, p. 100.)*

Congress is also considering legislation that would impose far-reaching regulations on managed-care systems and possibly make it easier to sue health insurers for malpractice. Consumer and patient advocacy groups as well as the American Medical Association (AMA) are generally backing the proposals as part of an envisioned "Patients' Bill of Rights." However, the proposals are strongly opposed by health-care insurers and employers, who so far have thwarted any large-scale reform effort.

The efforts reflect a widespread belief that patients are being harmed in the shift away from traditional "fee-for-service" health insurance, which gave consumers greater freedom in choosing their own doctors and doctors greater freedom in prescribing treatment that insurers would pay for.

"Patients feel less personally taken care of, that they have interactions with too many health-care providers, that there's too much red tape in getting access to the specialists," says Myrl Weinberg, president of the National Health Council, a coalition

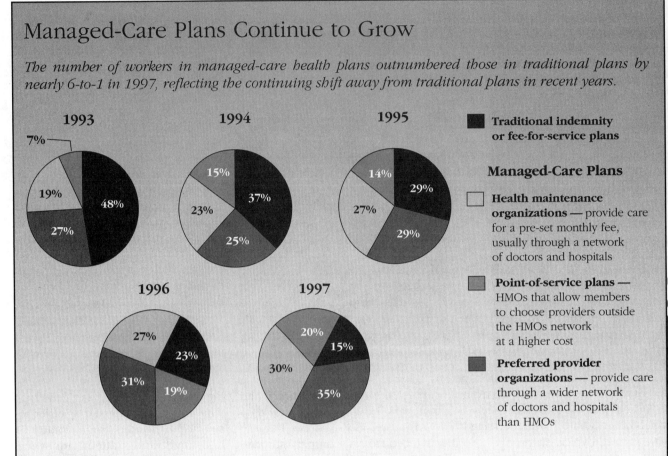

Managed-Care Plans Continue to Grow

The number of workers in managed-care health plans outnumbered those in traditional plans by nearly 6-to-1 in 1997, reflecting the continuing shift away from traditional plans in recent years.

1993
7% · 19% · 48% · 27%

1994
15% · 37% · 23% · 25%

1995
14% · 29% · 27% · 29%

1996
27% · 23% · 31% · 19%

1997
20% · 15% · 30% · 35%

Traditional indemnity or fee-for-service plans

Managed-Care Plans

Health maintenance organizations — provide care for a pre-set monthly fee, usually through a network of doctors and hospitals

Point-of-service plans — HMOs that allow members to choose providers outside the HMOs network at a higher cost

Preferred provider organizations — provide care through a wider network of doctors and hospitals than HMOs

Note: Percentages do not add up to 100 because of rounding. The survey includes all employers with 10 or more employees.

Source: Mercer/Foster Higgins "National Survey of Employer-Sponsored Health Plans," 1997.

of more than 40 patient advocacy groups, such as the American Cancer Society and American Heart Association, as well as major drug manufacturers and health insurers.

But health insurance industry officials insist that patients actually receive better care under managed-care plans.

"There's a tremendous possibility [with HMOs] to receive better, more integrated care," says Karen Ignagni, president of the American Association of Health Plans (AAHP). She says greater coordination among health-care providers also enhances

accountability. "We've put in place the beginnings of quality measurement so that we can ensure significant improvements," she says.

Critics of managed care generally stop short of blaming it for an overall decline in the quality of health care. "For the most part, the studies have shown that the care is relatively the same," says Thomas Reardon, an Oregon physician and chairman of the AMA's Board of Trustees.

But the critics cite cases like Shea's to argue that managed-care plans have an incentive to skimp on care at the patient's expense. "There are

pluses and minuses," says Adrienne Mitchem, legislative counsel for Consumers Union. "Some of the minuses are the overriding cost pressures. With traditional fee-for-service, you had the financial incentives to overtreat. With managed care, you have the financial incentives to undertreat."

Managed-care advocates indeed take credit for helping contain health care cost increases, which rose a double-digit rates in the late 1980 and early 1990s — and now fee unjustly blamed for the difficultie that patients and providers face ir adjusting to the changes.

"The public said to do something about health-care inflation, and we've been largely successful in doing that," says former Rep. Bill Gradison, R-Ohio, president of the Health Insurance Association of America (HIAA), which includes companies offering both managed care and fee-for-service insurance.

"Now, patients are saying, 'Hold on, we don't like the way you're doing it,'" Gradison continues. "The pace of change is bewilderingly fast and off-putting to a lot of people, and I mean not just the patients but the providers as well."

Gradison warns that new regulations "run the risk of increasing the cost of health plans and discouraging innovation." But critics say some changes are needed. "Managed care can do a lot of things well, but it needs to be regulated differently than we're now regulating it," says Lawrence Gostin, a health-law expert at Georgetown University Law Center.

The proposal with the most bipartisan support in Congress is a managed-care bill sponsored in the House by Reps. Charlie Norwood, R-Ga., and John Dingell, D-Mich. Norwood, a dentist, says he wants to "reverse what's going on in this country in health care." But while the measure won the support of 68 Republicans in 1999, Republican leaders have refused to endorse it.

"We've gone from patients having the right to choose their own doctors to patients being denied care and being denied the right to choose their own doctors to save money," Norwood says. "I don't oppose managed care, but I think there needs to be rules and regulations."

President Clinton also strongly endorsed managed-care reform. "Medical decisions ought to be made by medical doctors, not insurance company accountants," Clinton said in his 1998 State of the Union address. The line drew bipartisan applause from lawmakers that continued as Clinton spelled out his proposal:

"I urge this Congress to reach across the aisle and write into law a consumer bill of rights that says this: 'You have the right to know all your medical options, not just the cheapest. You have the right to choose the doctor you want for the care you need. You have the right to emergency room care, wherever and whenever you need it. You have the right to keep your medical records confidential.' Now, traditional care or managed care, every American deserves quality care."

Clinton's plea covered the main parts of a "Patients' Bill of Rights" issued by a 34-member commission he created in 1997. But he made no specific reference to one of its most contentious recommendations: a proposal to give patients greater ability to contest decisions by health plans to deny coverage for medical treatment.

Earlier, the administration also proposed separate legislation aimed at protecting patients' medical information. The privacy issue has become increasingly worrisome as computers have become more capable of accessing the most personal information. But the administration's proposals were widely criticized as too weak — in particular for giving law enforcement agencies broad discretion to obtain medical records without a patient's consent (see p. 102).

When Congress and state legislatures continue to ponder managed-care reform, these are some of the questions likely to be considered:

Should managed-care health plans be required to make it easier for patients to see specialists outside the plan's network of physicians?

The most visible difference between managed-care health plans and traditional fee-for-service insurance involves choosing a doctor and deciding when to seek treatment. Traditional insurance plans leave those choices to the patient; managed-care plans limit the patient's options.

Typically, a patient who enrolls in an HMO, like Patrick Shea, selects a "primary-care provider" from its network of doctors. That doctor then functions as a "gatekeeper" — overseeing the patient's health care and deciding when the patient needs to be referred to a specialist. [3]

The earliest group-health plans, in the 1920s and '30s, centralized medical decisions both to improve health care and lower costs. But since the federal government began promoting HMOs in the '70s, and later as for-profit managed-care plans came to dominate the industry, the emphasis increasingly has been on cost.

Critics, including patients, doctors and some outside observers, say the result has been to deny patients needed care in some cases. "Obviously, you can cut costs by cutting services," says George Annas, a professor of health law at Boston University, "but that wasn't the idea."

Managed-care health plans do take credit for helping hold down costs, but they insist that the quality of care has not suffered. "I don't know of many physicians who are devoted more to controlling costs than to care delivering," says AAHP President Ignagni.

Access to specialists is the most frequent source of friction between patients and health plans. Health plans control costs by limiting the number of specialists in the plan and the number of referrals to specialists outside the plan; they may pay their primary physicians in ways that create incentives to minimize the number of referrals. For patients, those incentives may create minor burdens — for example, a woman's need to get a referral for routine obstetric care — or more serious disputes.

Critics say the industry has been

States Where Patients Get Special Treatment

Specialist care — *At least thirty states make it easier for people in managed-care health plans to see certain specialists; all but Kentucky allow women either to designate an obstetrician-gynecologist as their primary-care provider or see an ob-gyn without a referral:*

Alabama, Arkansas*, California, Colorado, Connecticut, Delaware, Florida**, Georgia***, Idaho, Illinois, Indiana, Kentucky****, Louisiana, Maine*****, Maryland, Minnesota, Missouri, Mississippi, Montana, Nevada, New Jersey, New Mexico, New York, North Carolina, Oregon, Rhode Island, Texas, Utah, Virginia and Washington

External review — *Eleven states allow health-care patients to appeal coverage decisions to outside bodies:*

Arizona, California, Connecticut, Florida, Minnesota, Missouri, New Jersey, Rhode Island, Texas, New Mexico and Vermont

Post-mastectomy care — *Thirteen states require coverage of post-mastectomy inpatient care:*

Arkansas, Connecticut, Florida, Illinois, Maine, Montana, New Jersey, New Mexico, New York, North Carolina, Oklahoma, Rhode Island and Texas

Gag-rule ban — *Thirty-six states bar insurers from limiting doctors' communications with patients about treatment options:*

Arkansas, California, Colorado, Connecticut, Delaware, Florida, Georgia, Idaho, Illinois, Indiana, Kansas, Maine, Maryland, Massachusetts, Minnesota, Missouri, Montana, Nebraska, Nevada, New Hampshire, New Jersey, New Mexico, New York, North Carolina, Ohio, Oklahoma, Oregon, Rhode Island, South Carolina, Tennessee, Texas, Utah, Vermont, Virginia, Washington and Wyoming

* also covers optometrist or ophthalmologist; ** also covers chiropractor, podiatrist, dermatologist; *** also covers dermatologist; **** only covers chiropractor; ***** also covers nurse-practitioner, nurse-midwife

Sources: American Association of Health Plans, National Conference of State Legislatures.

physician and network of specialists — actually simplifies decisions for patients. "Unlike the old days, where you went to the phone book, now you have the ability to seek care through a network of professionals working together," Ignagni says.

Moreover, she points out that many plans in recent years have given consumers more options — for example, "point-of-service" (POS) plans that allow enrollees to see physicians outside the plan's network if they pay part of the cost through a higher deductible or a percentage of the fee. "We recognize that [a closed-plan HMO] doesn't meet the needs of all consumers," she says, "and that's why these other products have been developed."

Still, state and federal legislators are seeking ways to assure patients easier access to specialists. Some 30 states require health plans to give women the option of selecting an obstetrician as their primary-care provider. (*See table, at left.*) A number of states are considering bills to establish a procedure for a "standing referral" to a specialist for patients with chronic or life-threatening diseases or conditions. In Congress, Norwood and a number of other lawmakers have endorsed similar provisions.

Annas says health plans should be required to pay specialists whenever a subscriber must go outside the network. "I don't think that would happen very often," he says. "But it's not really a health plan if it doesn't offer the full range of medical services."

Norwood's bill, as well as some bills in the states, also includes a provision requiring health plans to offer a "point-of-service" option. Some critics say that would harm patients by undercutting the ability of HMOs to control costs and reduce premiums.

"The way HMOs keep costs down is by hiring physicians who practice conservatively" and don't order a lot of tests, says John Goodman, president of the National Center for Policy

making it more difficult for health-plan subscribers to see specialists. "Managed-care plans are increasingly using payment systems that discourage providers from referring patients to specialized care," John Seffrin, president of the American Cancer Society and chairman of the National

Health Council, told the president's patients' rights commission last year.

"For the patient, it is difficult to know what they need to do" to see a specialist, agrees Weinberg, the council's president.

Industry officials, however, say that managed care — with its "gatekeeper"

Analysis, a free-market think tank in Dallas. "You can lower your premiums by joining an HMO that employs doctors who practice conservative medicine. If you take away the HMO's ability to do that, you take away one of the options that people have."

For their part, industry officials argue against any regulatory requirements, saying that market forces will drive health plans to give patients more choices for getting to a doctor of their choice. "Many plans are moving in that direction," Gradison says. "The question is whether the law should require that in every case, and my answer would be no."

But Paul Starr, a professor of sociology at Princeton University and author of a well-regarded history of the medical profession, says the industry cannot be counted on to give patients adequate choices for health care.

"We need legislation because whatever they're doing today doesn't guarantee what they'll do tomorrow," says Starr, who was an adviser for President Clinton's unsuccessful national health-care initiative in 1993 and '94. "They can just as easily withdraw access as provide it."

Should health plans be subject to medical malpractice liability?

When Ron Henderson died in a Kaiser Permanente hospital in Dallas in 1995, his family sued the HMO and several of its doctors for not diagnosing his heart disease.

Kaiser denied any wrongdoing and depicted Henderson as an overweight smoker who had ignored doctors' instructions. But the family's lawyers turned up embarrassing evidence of Kaiser's efforts to control costs by limiting hospital admissions in cardiac cases. In December 1997, Kaiser settled the case for $5.3 million. [4]

Kaiser was subject to a malpractice suit because, unlike most HMOs, it directly employs the physicians and nurses in its clinics. Courts have held

that HMOs that contract with individual doctors or medical groups are shielded from malpractice suits on the theory that the doctor rather than the health plan is actually providing the care. But a new Texas law seeks to erase that distinction. [5]

"I can see no reason why a private, very profitable enterprise ought not be held accountable for mistakes that are made when everybody else is," says Texas state Sen. David Sibley, a conservative Republican and oral surgeon.

The new Texas law, which took effect on Sept. 1, was strongly pushed by the state medical association but vigorously opposed by health insurers. Geoff Wurtzel, executive director of the Texas HMO Association, called the law "bad policy" and blamed its enactment on what he termed "medical politics."

"In 1995, the Legislature overwhelmingly agreed that the threat of being sued didn't produce a better standard of care," Wurtzel said, referring to a restrictive malpractice law passed that year. "But all of a sudden, if it was HMOs, liability was OK."

Texas was the only state to directly subject health plans to malpractice liability. But Missouri opened the door to malpractice suits against HMOs by repealing a law that gave health plans a defense against malpractice. And Rhode Island and Washington, among others, have created commissions to study the issue.

The Texas law was challenged in federal court by the Aetna insurance company on the grounds that it is pre-empted by the federal law that governs employee benefits, including health insurance.

That law — known as ERISA, short for the Employee Retirement Income Security Act — is also now at the center of the legislative debate in Congress. Reform bills such as the one proposed by Norwood and Dingell would provide that ERISA does not pre-empt state laws dealing with malpractice liability,

as some federal courts have held. Those courts have held that health-plan subscribers who feel they were wrongly denied medical care can sue the plans only for reimbursement of the value of the care they did not receive. [6]

Norwood says there is no justification for shielding health plans from malpractice suits. "If you're a health-plan accountant or administrator and you want to make decisions about medical necessity," Norwood explains, "then you have to be responsible about those decisions in a court of law."

The AMA, a strong supporter of limiting medical malpractice suits in the past, supports the change. "When I make a decision, I as a physician accept accountability and liability," says Reardon. "When the plan makes a decision to provide or not to provide treatment, they should have the same responsibility and liability, especially when they're overriding a recommendation from the treating physician."

But the health insurance industry is adamantly opposed. "That's a perfect example of raising the costs of insurance with little, if any, discernible effect on the quality of the care," says the HIAA's Gradison. "It's a boon for the trial lawyers; I don't think it's a boon for the patients at all."

"All of the data suggest that consumers are not the beneficiaries of the current system," says AAHP President Ignagni. "We don't do families very much good if we provide them in the end with a situation that is designed to maybe provide compensation, maybe not, vs. trying to set up a situation that is built on quality improvement in which injuries don't occur in the first place."

One patients' group voices a similar interest in improving medical care without resorting to litigation. "We feel [litigation] is not necessarily the most productive way to resolve problems," says Weinberg of the National Health Council. Instead, Weinberg

The Downside to Managed Care

A majority of Americans believe health maintenance organizations (HMOs) and other managed-care plans have had some adverse effects on health care, according to a 1997 survey. Overall, though, two-thirds of the respondents in managed care gave their plans an A or B, compared with three-fourths of the people with traditional health insurance coverage.

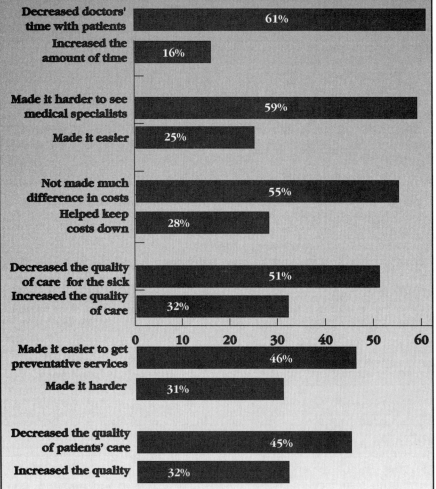

Percent of Americans who say HMOs and other managed-care plans have . . .

- Decreased doctors' time with patients — 61%
- Increased the amount of time — 16%
- Made it harder to see medical specialists — 59%
- Made it easier — 25%
- Not made much difference in costs — 55%
- Helped keep costs down — 28%
- Decreased the quality of care for the sick — 51%
- Increased the quality of care — 32%
- Made it easier to get preventative services — 46%
- Made it harder — 31%
- Decreased the quality of patients' care — 45%
- Increased the quality — 32%

Note: Percentages do not add up to 100 because "No effect" and "Don't know" responses are not shown.

Source: "Kaiser/Harvard National Survey of Americans' Views on Managed Care," November 1997.

says her group favors strong complaint-resolution procedures, such as the use of ombudsmen.

Other consumer groups go further and call for some independent external review of treatment decisions. "When a patient is denied coverage, it's ludicrous to think that they can appeal to the same system that denied them," says Mitchem of Consumers Union. But her group also favors malpractice liability for health insurers. "We want to ensure that there's some type of remedy that consumers can have access to," she says.

Health insurers are balking at any requirement for outside review procedures. "Some plans are doing this," Gradison says. "The question is whether it should be required by law."

Experts differ sharply on the potential effects of subjecting HMOs to malpractice liability. "If you apply tort liability to HMOs, you'll force them to do things that are not cost-effective," Goodman says. "You'll force them to waste money."

But Barry Furrow, a professor of health law at Widener University School of Law in Wilmington, Del., says that the threat of liability would result in better medical care by forcing managed-care administrators to focus more on quality than on costs. "You want to shift the competition more away from price and toward quality," Furrow says.

Are stronger safeguards needed to protect the privacy of patients' medical records and information?

The ongoing transformation from a paper-based health-care system to one that relies on electronic records has spawned an intense debate over who has access to individuals' medical histories and whether the information could be used to deny employment or health insurance. Recent cases of identity theft, hacker attacks on commercial Internet sites and more innocent technological snafus have reinforced a perception that personal information is not secure.

The Department of Health and Human Services (HHS) was expected at the end of 2000 to release guidelines that will allow government agencies, law enforcement and government researchers expanded access to medical databases. The guidelines stem from the Health Insurance Portability and Accountability Act of 1996, which, among other things, mandated Congress to develop national medical privacy standards by August 1999. When lawmakers missed the deadline, the task fell to HHS, which says its standards also will address consumer rights to see medical records and outline penalties for violating patient privacy. Privacy groups, such as the Andover, Mass.-based Coalition for Patients' Rights say the draft rules will not give patients any meaningful control over their medical histories and may allow doctors, insurers and other parties to share information without prior consent.

An early Clinton administration patient-privacy proposal, developed in 1997, spends nearly 40 pages detailing and justifying exceptions to the general rule prohibiting disclosure of patient records without the patient's consent. The list includes exceptions to disclose information necessary for the patient's health care, for payment and for internal oversight of the patient's treatment. The recommendation also calls for permitting disclosure of individually identifiable information to public health authorities for "disease or injury reporting, public health surveillance or public health investigation or intervention."

Most controversially, the administration also said that law enforcement or intelligence agencies should be able to obtain such information, without a court order, if needed for "a legitimate law enforcement inquiry" or — in the case of intelligence agencies — if needed for "a lawful purpose."

HHS Secretary Donna E. Shalala disputed advance reports that the proposal broadened law enforcement access to patient information. [7] She said the provision simply restated existing law. But Sen. Tim Hutchinson, an Arkansas Republican, said the proposal gave patients less privacy than existing federal law for bank records, cable television and video store rentals. Sen. Patrick J. Leahy of Vermont, the committee's ranking Democrat, was also critical. "There is divided opinion in the administration," Leahy said, "and right now the anti-privacy forces are winning on the key issue of law enforcement access to medical records." [8]

"HHS completely dropped the ball" on the issue, says Georgetown's Gostin. "They made an unforgivable mistake."

Gostin also faulted the privacy recommendations from the president's commission, issued two months after Shalala's testimony on Capitol Hill. The report called for permitting disclosure of patient information for purposes of "provision of health care, payment of services, peer review, health promotion, disease management and quality assurance." It addressed law enforcement only obliquely, saying law enforcement agencies "should examine their existing policies to ensure that they access individually identifiable information only when absolutely necessary."

"Everybody's in favor of privacy," Gostin says. "But the devil's in the details, and these don't provide any details. It basically does nothing."

For their part, however, health industry and business groups saw the administration's proposals as unduly restrictive. "The industry is very concerned about interrupting the flow of health information," said Heidi Wagner Hayduk, a consultant on privacy issues for the Healthcare Leadership Council, a coalition of major insurers, hospitals and drug companies. Medical innovation would be "stifled," she warned, if health-care providers and researchers were required to obtain patient authorization "every time information changes hands." [9]

Health-care industry groups also said federal legislation should pre-empt any state laws setting stricter protections for patient privacy. The administration's proposal would leave state laws unaffected, as would a stricter bill introduced by Leahy. But Sen. Robert F. Bennett, a Utah Republican, has introduced a bill that would set a single federal standard on the issue.

The administration also has endorsed a separate privacy proposal affecting the health insurance industry: a bill to bar health insurance companies and managed-care plans from discriminating against people on the basis of their genetic make-up. [10] The proposal has been pushed by a number of bioethics and privacy-advocacy groups, which point to studies documenting instances of genetic discrimination by, among others, employers and insurers.

The genetic privacy bill has languished in Congress for several years. Vice President Al Gore announced the administration's support for also banning genetic discrimination in the workplace. [11]

The administration's medical-records privacy proposal drew additional criticism at a second Senate Labor Committee hearing on the issue. Two medical groups, the AMA and the American Psychiatric Association, both called for stronger protection than the administration supported, while witnesses representing drug manufacturers and the American Hospital Association said the proposal went too far.

Such praise as the administration received for its proposal has been typically begrudging, at best. Boston University's Annas says the administration deserved credit for proposing a federal law guaranteeing patients the right to see their own records. And Robert Gellman, a privacy consultant who led Shalala's outside advisers on the recommendations, stressed that the package would be "stronger than any comparable state law." [12] But both men also faulted the law enforcement provisions, among other exceptions. "The administration," Annas concludes, "has a long way to go." ∎

BACKGROUND

Health Insurance

H ealth care became widely available to most Americans, and a financially secure profession for most doctors, only in the recent past. [13] Well into the 20th century, routine health care was a luxury available only to well-to-do Americans. And many doctors had only modest incomes, since they did not see enough patients often enough to have a lucrative practice.

Two 20th-century developments changed the face of health care in the United States: widespread private health insurance and government-funded medical programs. Together, the two developments produced the mythic image that forms the backdrop of today's debate over medical care. In that idealized vision, most Americans enjoyed the services of a family doctor, a Marcus Welby figure who gave skilled and compassionate care from birth to death with little concern about fees. And the government stepped in to provide care for those few who could not afford medical services. But the two developments also contained the germs of the cost problems that beset the health-care system today.

Private insurance entered the health field tentatively, limited at first to covering accidental injury and death. By the late 19th and early 20th centuries, however, many employers were providing limited medical care for their workers — motivated as much to reduce absenteeism caused by illnesses as to promote their employees' welfare.

The labor scarcities of World War II prompted some employers to begin offering health insurance as a benefit for workers. Labor unions, strengthened by New Deal legislation in the 1930s, included demands for health benefits in contract negotiations. And the postwar economic boom allowed major U.S. corporations to grant the demands.

Through the 1950s, more and more big corporations were including health benefits in union contracts; other employers followed suit. By the end of the decade, around two-thirds of the population at least had hospitalization insurance. [14]

The bill for these benefits was largely invisible. The expense was not a big cost item for employers, at least initially. For employees, the benefits were not taxed: In fact, the amounts did not even appear on pay stubs. As a result, many critics and observers contend, no one — neither business, labor, insurers nor health-care providers — had much incentive to watch the bottom line.

A second problem — access to care — was also somewhat obscured. With so many Americans sharing in the widened availability of health care, it was easy to overlook those who were not: the elderly, the poor and the uninsured.

Government's Role

T he government's initial moves to help provide health care were also tentative and limited. Some local governments began including medical benefits for the poor in general welfare programs in the early 20th century, and a New Deal program helped bring health care to some rural areas during the Depression. Throughout the century, progressives and labor interests called for compulsory national health insurance, but the efforts were blocked by business interests and, most important, the medical profession.

The two big federal health programs, Medicare and Medicaid, were enacted over the continuing opposition of the medical profession in the brief moment of liberal triumph in the 1960s. Congress had passed a limited bill to provide health insurance for the elderly poor in 1960, but the program proved to be unpopular. President Lyndon B. Johnson put the issue of health care for the elderly at the top of his Great Society agenda and pushed legislation through the overwhelmingly Democratic Congress in 1965.

As enacted, Medicare included the original idea of a contributory insurance program to cover hospitalization for the elderly (Part A) plus a similar plan for doctors' services (Part B). In addition, the law established the framework for Medicaid, the federal-state health-care program for the poor and the disabled.

Some doctors talked of boycotting Medicare, but they quickly realized that the program was — as Starr writes — "a bonanza," guaranteeing payment for medical services that

Chronology

Before 1950

Earliest forms of managed care are organized; employers begin to offer hospitalization insurance to workers.

———— • ————

1960s Federal government establishes free health insurance for the elderly (Medicare) and a joint state-federal program to provide health care for low-income persons (Medicaid).

———— • ————

1970s The Nixon administration backs the creation of health maintenance organizations (HMOs) to control health-care costs.

1973
The Health Maintenance Organization Act provides funds and regulatory support for HMOs, but also includes some coverage mandates that slow their growth.

1976
Congress eases some regulations on HMOs; two years later, Congress votes increased funding.

———— • ————

1980s HMOs grow rapidly, gaining support from employers and consumers worried about spiraling increases in health-care costs.

1985
Supreme Court rules that Employee Retirement Income Security Act (ERISA) supersedes state laws regulating private employers' health plans (*Massachusetts Mutual Life Insurance Co. v. Russell*); some lower federal courts interpret decision as barring malpractice suits against managed-care plans.

———— • ————

1990s Backlash against managed care grows.

1993
President Clinton proposes National Health Security Act, aimed at providing health insurance for all Americans; plan is assailed by business interests, medical lobby and Republicans.

1994
Clinton health-care plan dies in Congress.

1995
Many states pass laws requiring managed-care plans to allow women to designate ob-gyns as their primary-care provider.

Aug. 21, 1996
Clinton signs law making it easier for people to keep their health insurance when they lose or change jobs, start their own business or get sick; bill includes provision to facilitate sharing of patient information among health-care providers, but also requires government to develop privacy-protection guidelines by 1999.

September 1996
Congress responds to criticism of "drive-through deliveries" by requiring health insurance plans to cover at least 48 hours of hospital care for new mothers.

May 1997
Texas enacts legislation subjecting health maintenance organizations to medical malpractice liability; Aetna insurance company challenges law in federal court as pre-empted by ERISA.

July 1997
House and Senate conferees agree on provision in budget bill to bar Medicare-eligible HMOs from imposing "gag rules" on doctors by preventing them from discussing treatments or specialists that the plan would not pay for.

Sept. 11, 1997
Health and Human Services Secretary Donna E. Shalala presents medical-information privacy legislation to Congress; proposal is faulted by lawmakers, advocates and experts.

October 1997
Two House subcommittees hold hearings on Patient Access to Responsible Care Act sponsored by Rep. Charlie Norwood, R-Ga.

Nov. 19, 1997
Proposed "Patients' Bill of Rights" is issued by President Clinton's Advisory Commission on Consumer Protection and Quality in the Health Care Industry.

January 1998
Managed-care plans continued to grow in 1997 despite complaints about their services; coalition of health insurance and business lobbies announces plans for advertising campaign against managed-care reform legislation; Clinton urges Congress to pass consumer bill of rights.

June 2000
Supreme Court rules patients cannot sue managed-care plans for malpractice under ERISA.

Are Elderly Americans "Trapped" by Medicare?

Lawmakers and rival interest groups are clashing over the ability of senior citizens to see the physician of their choice outside the federal Medicare system. [1]

Conservatives want to get rid of a policy that largely prevents doctors and patients from arranging for Medicare-covered services outside the system's reimbursement scheme. They view the issue as a simple question of patients' rights.

"When you're sick, the federal government should not stand in the way of your getting the medical treatment you want," says Sen. Jon Kyl, an Arizona Republican who took up the issue after a constituent's complaint last year and forced a limited amendment to the law through Congress.

But the Clinton administration, Democratic lawmakers and the nation's largest senior citizens' group all argue that totally lifting the restriction would create the risk of gouging senior citizens and threaten the viability of the federal government's 33-year-old health insurance program for the elderly.

Seniors "would lose much of the financial protection that they are currently provided under Medicare" if the policy were eliminated, according to Rep. Pete Stark, a California Democrat and veteran legislator on health-care issues.

The dispute stems from a policy adopted by the Health Care Financing Administration (HCFA), the Health and Human Services agency that administers the Medicare program. For many years, the HCFA has prohibited doctors participating in the Medicare program from letting patients pay them out of their own pockets for services covered by Medicare.

Defenders of the policy say Medicare is acting just like any other insurer by requiring participating doctors to limit their fees to its schedule for reimbursements. Medicare reimbursements are sometimes markedly lower than prevailing fees for some services.

"Private payment would undermine the whole rationale for the Medicare fee schedule," says John Rother, legislative director of the American Association of Retired Persons (AARP). The 30-million-member organization strongly opposes lifting the ban.

Critics say the ban is bad for senior citizens and also bad for the Medicare program. They say it prevents senior citizens who can afford it from picking a particular doctor, for example, or from getting treatment without going through government red tape.

As for Medicare itself, these critics say that letting well-off seniors pay for some services themselves would strengthen the financially beleaguered insurance program. Supporters counter that lifting the ban would result in a two-tiered system — with one group of doctors for well-to-do seniors and another for Medicare patients.

Kyl won Senate passage on a party-line vote of an amendment to narrow the policy last summer as part of the Medicare reform provisions of the balanced-budget bill. [2] But the Clinton administration reportedly threatened to veto the entire bill over the issue. The result was a limited compromise that allows physicians to accept private payments for Medicare-covered services if they "opt out" of the Medicare program for two years. Critics say that few doctors could afford to drop out of the Medicare program.

A conservative senior citizens' organization is challenging that law in federal court in Washington. [3] United Seniors Association, a 60,000-member group founded in 1992, claims the law violates senior citizens' constitutional rights.

United Seniors President Sandra Butler says the new law makes health care less accessible for senior citizens. "Because seniors will be barred from contracting privately, many health- and life-saving services will be difficult for them to obtain, if they could obtain them at all," Butler says.

But Rother says few seniors agree. "I don't think I have a single letter in my file asking for the privilege of paying more for the services that Medicare already covers," he says. "This is not a patient-driven concern."

Medical groups are also divided on the issue. The American Medical Association (AMA) strongly supports Kyl's effort this year to repeal the restriction on private payments. "Medicare patients deserve the same rights as other patients to purchase health care directly from their physicians — without interference from the federal government," the AMA says.

But the American College of Physicians, which represents about 100,000 internists, opposes Kyl's bill. It says the measure "could threaten the viability of Medicare as an insurance program that offers accessible, affordable high-quality care."

[1] For background, see *USA Today*, Nov. 26, 1997, p. A6 and "Retiree Health Benefits," *The CQ Researcher*, Dec. 6, 1991, pp. 930-953.

[2] See *Congressional Quarterly Weekly Report*, June 28, 1997, p. 1529.

[3] The case is *United Seniors Association v. Shalala*, pending before U.S. District Judge Thomas F. Hogan.

many doctors had previously provided for free or for reduced fees. [15] Medicare and Medicaid closed the biggest gaps in health-care access, but liberals still said health care was too costly and favored broader national health insurance to ensure access for all.

Under President Richard M. Nixon, however, the federal government took a different tack to deal with the intertwined issue of access and costs. It backed a free-enterprise solution to the problems: a scheme being pushed by a physician-turned-health-care reformer in Minnesota that came to be called a "health maintenance organization" or HMO.

Rise of Managed Care

Managed care had its origins in ideas pushed by socially conscious health-care reformers in the early 20th century. [16] In one form — known as cooperative or prepaid group health plans — consumers paid a modest annual fee to one or more doctors to cover their families' preventive and sick care. The medical profession opposed the idea, however, and succeeded in getting laws passed in many states to bar consumer-controlled cooperatives.

Then during World War II, California industrialist Henry J. Kaiser set up two prepaid group health plans for his company's employees, known as Permanente Foundations. Unlike the health-care cooperatives, Kaiser's plans flourished — and served as the forerunner for what is today the country's largest HMO, Kaiser Permanente.

The Nixon administration saw in HMOs an appealing alternative to the liberal-backed national health insurance plans. Administration officials were sold on the idea by Paul M. Ellwood, today regarded as the father of managed care. Ellwood, a Minneapolis physician, argued that the traditional fee-for-services system penalized health-care providers who returned patients to health. He met with the administration's key health policy-makers on Feb. 5, 1970, to make his case for organizations to provide members comprehensive care for prepaid amounts. At that meeting Ellwood coined the phrase "health maintenance organizations." [17]

Financial and regulatory help were needed to put the idea into effect. The administration initially found money to help launch HMOs beginning in 1970, without specific congressional authorization, even as it was asking Congress to pass a law to promote the plans. The law enacted three years later — the Health Maintenance Organization Act of 1973 — provided more money, $375 million over five years, for grants and loans to help start up HMOs. [18] More important, the law required all businesses with more than 25 employees to offer at least one HMO as an alternative to conventional insurance if one was available.

At the same time, though, the act established requirements that proved to be regulatory obstacles to the growth of HMOs. It required HMOs to offer not only basic hospitalization, physicians' services, emergency care and laboratory and diagnostic services but also mental health care, home health services and referral services for alcohol and drug abuse.

These requirements, combined with the government's delay in promulgating regulations to implement the law, stunted the growth of HMOs, according to Starr's account. At the same time, the medical profession viewed the idea with skepticism or hostility. But Congress eased some of the burdens in 1976, and then provided another shot of money in 1978: $164 million over three years. [19] By then, HMOs were starting to take off in the market. At the end of the decade, HMOs had enrolled 7.9 million members — double the figure in 1970. Still, the number represented only 4 percent of the population and — as of the early 1980s — was expected to grow only to 10 percent of the population by 1990. [20]

In fact, enrollment in HMOs more than tripled over the next decade, reaching about 25 million in 1990. Despite a decade of rapidly rising health-care costs, HMOs had to keep fees down and provide good service in order to attract customers. Most faced business losses, and some went bankrupt. But they were generally regarded as successful in containing cost increases, enough so that traditional fee-for-service health plans began copying some of their practices, such as utilization review, where insurers scrutinized doctors' fees and practices.

Meanwhile, the once comfortable relationship between patients and doctors had become badly frayed. The growth of specialized medicine had weakened the bond with the old-style family doctors — who now likely as not called themselves "internists." The rise in doctors' income created a distance between an increasingly well-to-do profession and its patient-customers. And the increase in malpractice litigation led many physicians to adopt "defensive-medicine" practices to guard against the threat.

Managed-Care Backlash

The 1990s saw managed care reach a dominant position in the health insurance market. By 1993, most workers covered by employer-provided health insurance were enrolled in some form of managed care — either an HMO, a preferred provider organization (PPO) or a "point-of-service" (POS) plan. As of 1995, industry figures estimated a total of 150 million people nationwide were in a managed-care plan. Managed care was also credited with helping to bring down the rate of increase in health-care costs. But the decade also witnessed a growing backlash against managed care as many doctors chafed under cost-cutting pressures from HMO administrators, and many patients complained of delays in receiving — or outright denials of — needed medical care.

The consumer backlash against HMOs manifested itself most dramatically in court. A small number of HMO enrollees won whopping verdicts or settlements in suits claiming that their health plans had wrong-fully denied or delayed necessary medical care. In California, the family of Helene Fox, who died of breast cancer after her HMO, Health Net, refused to pay for a bone marrow transplant, collected a $5 million settlement after a jury awarded her $89 million. In Georgia, Lamona and James Adams won a $45 million jury award in a suit that blamed Kaiser Permanente for the botched handling of a bacterial infection that forced doctors to amputate their infant son's arms and legs; the company later settled for an undisclosed sum. [21]

A mid-decade survey produced statistical evidence of the consumer dissatisfaction with HMOs, at least in comparison with traditional fee-for-service health plans. The survey, conducted for the Robert Wood Johnson Foundation by researchers at Harvard University and Louis Harris and Associates, found that significantly more HMO subscribers than fee-for-service plan subscribers complained about their medical care.

The complaints came only from small minorities: For example, 12 percent of HMO subscribers said their doctors provided incorrect or inappropriate medical care, compared with 5 percent of fee-for-service plan subscribers. Still, the higher levels of dissatisfaction with HMOs prompted a cautionary note from the survey's director. "Consumers need to be aware that all health plans don't treat you the same way when you are sick," said Robert Blendon, chairman of the department of health policy management at Harvard's School of Public Health. [22]

Health-care providers were also voicing dissatisfaction with managed care. In one incident, Massachusetts internist David Himmelstein attacked the HMO that he worked for, U.S. Healthcare, in an appearance on Phil Donahue's nationally syndicated television program in November 1995.

Himmelstein charged that the company rewarded doctors for denying care and forbade them from discussing treatment options with patients. The company — later acquired by Aetna — responded by terminating its contract with Himmelstein just three days after the TV show. But it reinstated him in February 1996 after a storm of criticism and also modified its contracts to permit doctors to discuss payment methods with patients.

Himmelstein's comments reflected the concerns that many doctors and hospital administrators had about managed care. "This is all about cost, not improving patient care," a doctor told *Wall Street Journal* reporter George Anders in a 1994 interview. "You survive in managed care by denying or limiting care," William Speck, chief executive of Presbyterian Hospital in New York, told Anders in June 1995. "That's how you make money." [23]

As the complaints escalated, state and federal lawmakers took up the issues. By mid-decade, hundreds of bills were being introduced in state legislatures around the country. The earliest legislation dealt with specific problems — like allowing women to select an ob-gyn physician as their primary-care provider, or prohibiting health-care plans from imposing "gag clauses" on physicians. Congress in 1996 passed a provision requiring health insurance plans to cover at least 48 hours of hospital care for new mothers — prohibiting so-called "drive-through maternity stays." [24]

Lawmakers also have responded to the growth of Medicare managed care. By the end of 1999, an estimated 6.3 million Medicare beneficiaries, or about 16 percent, were enrolled in some variety of managed-care plan, instead of in a traditional fee-for-service program. The Medicare managed-care option was viewed as attractive by some, because the plans could cover services that the traditional Medicare program

would not, most notably prescription drugs. A program called Medicare+Choice, approved by Congress in 1997 as part of the Balanced Budget Act, allows beneficiaries to choose a managed-care plan that provides all health services for a monthly fee that is set by the Medicare program and sometimes supplemented by a small premium from the beneficiary.

While Medicare+Choice was promoted as a potential boom in health care, the program went into turmoil in the fall of 1998, when health plans — faced with lower-than-expected reimbursements from Medicare — withdrew from the program. Forty-three major health plans quit the program in 1999, in a move that affected some 415,000 seniors, and left 45,000 of them with no managed-care option at all. Another 41 plans left in 2000, affecting about 327,000 beneficiaries. Analysts believe such pullouts will continue in regions where the plans determine they cannot make a sufficient profit. But lawmakers are divided on whether reimbursement rates should be adjusted to reflect higher medical costs, and if so, by how much.

CURRENT SITUATION

Reform Efforts

A June 2000 U.S. Supreme Court decision on patients' rights to sue their health plans clarified one important aspect of the debate over managed-care overhaul, but did little to resolve political differences.

Justices in *Pegram v. Herdrich* ruled that a patient cannot sue a health plan under the Employee Retirement Income Security Act of 1974 (ERISA) because the plan offered bonuses to physicians to hold down costs. Justices said a decision in a patient's favor would have undermined the fundamental structure of the managed-care system, adding that it is up to Congress, not the courts, to set guidelines for insurers and patients. "The federal judiciary would be acting contrary to the congressional policy of allowing (health maintenance) organizations if it were to entertain (a) claim portending wholesale attacks on existing HMOs solely because of their structure," wrote Justice David H. Souter.

The suit stemmed from a claim by a Bloomington, Ill. woman, Cynthia Herdrich, that her physician, Lori Pegram, compromised her treatment in 1991 after she complained of abdominal pain. Instead of immediately sending Herdrich for a diagnostic ultrasound at a nearby clinic, Pegram scheduled the test for eight days later at a less expensive clinic 50 miles away. During the delay, Herdrich's appendix burst. During oral arguments in February 2000, Herdrich's attorney tried to convince justices that they should expand the right of patients to sue under ERISA by allowing Herdrich to claim Pegram failed to meet her duties as a trustee who controlled her health plan's administration of benefits.

The case was closely watched because ERISA — a law primarily designed to protect workers' pension rights — has long been criticized as a liability shield for health insurers. Most courts have held that an individual injured by an ERISA denial of care can only sue in federal court, and then only to recover the cost of the denied benefit and assorted court costs. The high court, in denying the right to sue, explored several other legal possibilities. In a lengthy footnote to the ruling, justices indicated

Managed-Care Reforms Get Qualified Support

Most Americans support several of the frequently mentioned proposals to make managed care more user-friendly. But their support drops when they are asked to consider potential consequences of the changes such as higher premiums.

Percentage of Americans who want health plans to . . .

	Favor	Oppose
Provide more information about how health plans operate	**92%**	**6%**
If higher premiums result	58%	34%
If the government gets too involved	55%	38%
If employers drop coverage	54%	43%
Allow appeal to an independent reviewer	**88%**	**9%**
If higher premiums result	63%	32%
If the government gets too involved	51%	41%
If employers drop coverage	49%	45%
Allow a woman to see a gynecologist without a referral	**82%**	**16%**
If higher premiums result	63%	34%
If the government gets too involved	51%	43%
If employers drop coverage	48%	47%
Allow people to see a specialist without a referral	**81%**	**18%**
If higher premiums result	58%	39%
If the government gets too involved	47%	48%
If employers drop coverage	46%	51%
Pay for an emergency room visit without prior approval	**79%**	**18%**
If higher premiums result	62%	33%
If the government gets too involved	52%	41%
If employers drop coverage	48%	47%
Allow people to sue health plan directly	**64%**	**31%**
If higher premiums result	58%	34%
If the government gets too involved	55%	38%
If employers drop coverage	54%	43%

Note: Percentages do not add up to 100 because all respondents did not answer.

Source: Kaiser/Harvard "National Survey of Americans' Views on Managed Care," January 1998.

that health plans may have a responsibility to disclose details about coverage decisions to their patients — a move that could lead to class-action lawsuits claiming the plans breached their ERISA responsibilities by failing to tell patients about their financial structure.

The decision did little to settle a long-running impasse between congressional Democrats and Republicans over managed-care overhaul. Discussions to merge House and Senate bills fell apart in mid-2000 precisely over the issue of a patient's right to sue and how employers might be liable for an insurer's decision about medical care. However, in an indication of the increased political potency of the issue, Senate Republicans in June 2000 went on record in favor of expanding patients' rights to sue, in limited circumstances, during a vote on an amendment to the fiscal 2001 Labor, Health and Human Services and Education appropriations bill. The move, which came in response to a rival Democratic amendment designed to embarrass the GOP on the issue by making them appear to be protecting insurers, endorsed a limited right to sue managed-care plans for damages — an issue Senate Republicans staunchly opposed when the Senate considered and passed a managed-care bill in 1999.

The concession would allow lawsuits against managed-care companies in two instances: unreasonable delays in essential medical care and the failure to cover treatment that an independent physician deemed necessary and said the plan should cover. Patients could not win punitive damages, but could recover unlimited economic damages and as much as $350,000 for pain and suffering. But GOP and Democratic lawmakers continued to disagree over who should be covered by the new rules. The new proposal would limit most

protections to the approximately 56 million Americans in self-insured health plans that are not covered by state patient protection laws. Democrats and some House Republicans who support the Norwood-Dingell managed-care overhaul bill want broader protections and want the lawsuits to be handled in state courts, not federal courts. They also oppose the $350,000 cap on non-economic damages.

The Senate vote was not enough to revive stalled House-Senate talks on a managed-care overhaul bill. The House-passed provision combined the Norwood-Dingell measure with separate legislation featuring so-called "access" provisions that many Republicans believe will give more people affordable coverage. The provisions include an expansion of a pilot program for medical savings accounts (tax-exempt accounts used for medical expenses) and the creation of insurance-purchasing groups, which supporters believe will allow people to get health coverage for more affordable rates. Many Democrats were skeptical of the provisions, saying they doubted the proposals would reduce the ranks of the uninsured. The House provision also would allow patients to sue in state courts for damages. Health plans would be protected from punitive damages if they passed an external review. The House measure notably would cover all 191 million privately insured Americans.

Disagreements between Democrats and Republicans — and between House and Senate Republicans — doomed prospects for a compromise. Lawmakers said there was the possibility of reviving the measures in the 107th Congress, particularly with Democrats picking up seats and pressing for more health-related legislation.

Norwood says he introduced the original managed-care bill despite his

aversion to federal regulation. "It turns my stomach to turn this over to the Labor Department," he said, referring to the agency that would have principal responsibility for implementing the bill's provisions. "But it makes me even more nervous not to do anything."

Among its major provisions, Norwood's bill would require health plans to give consumers an option to buy "point-of-service" coverage — allowing them to select their own doctor for an additional cost. It would also require adequate access to specialists and emergency care, require internal grievance procedures and subject managed-care companies to medical malpractice liability for negligent treatment decisions.

Despite professed support from a majority of the House, Republican leadership remains unenthusiastic. House Majority Leader Dick Armey of Texas as far back as 1998 wrote a strongly worded letter to GOP members urging opposition to the forthcoming recommendations from President Clinton's health-care commission. Even though Armey did not refer to Norwood's bill, he called for restricting rather than expanding medical malpractice liability and recommended medical savings accounts rather than regulatory changes to give consumers more health-care choices. [25]

For its part, the health insurance industry is gearing up for an all-out lobbying campaign to defeat Norwood's bill or anything much like it. "It's our No. 1 issue," says HIAA's Gradison. "It's very bad public policy."

In a two-page lobbying flier, the AAHP warns that Norwood's bill would represent "the single, largest expansion of tort liability in memory," establish "federal price controls" and make it harder for families to get "affordable" health coverage. But Ignagni also hints at the possibility of supporting some legislative changes. "We intend to be very involved and will provide whatever information that we can," she says.

At Issue:

Has the rise of managed care hurt patients' rights?

ADRIENNE MITCHEM
Legislative counsel, Consumers Union

*a*mericans are experiencing a true crisis in confidence in today's managed-care industry. Consumers' faith is shaken because of signs that managed care may be sacrificing quality health care to boost profits.

As managed care replaced the old fee-for-service system, the financial incentives driving the health-care industry have turned upside down. This revolution, replacing incentives to overtreat patients with incentives to undertreat, has provoked a strong backlash. Nearly three in five Americans in a recent poll believe managed-care plans make it harder for people who are sick to see a specialist.

But this revolution also creates an opportunity to reintroduce a simple and old-fashioned idea: consumer protection laws. Responding to grass-roots uprisings, states have passed laws giving consumers tools to help them be smart shoppers, ensure accountability when costly mistakes are made, provide more access to specialist and emergency care and guarantee a fair system to review patient disputes.

A presidential advisory commission has developed a "Consumer Bill of Rights," spurring a flurry of bill introductions on Capitol Hill and the promise of a healthy debate about nationwide reform. On one side is a multimillion-dollar scare campaign, funded by industry, designed to preserve the status quo. On the other, a coalition of consumer groups and individual Americans who have been burned by the current system and want change.

A scorecard of principles for reform from Consumers Union will help measure who wins:

• The linchpin for consumers is an appeals system that gives patients access to an independent entity to settle disputes over medically necessary care when benefits are denied, terminated or delayed. The current system, where the managed-care company serves as both judge and jury for every appeal, is stacked against patients.

• Another vital component is full disclosure. Plans should be required to provide consumers with information to help them understand all of their alternatives for treatment, not just the cheapest.

• Consumers also want assurance that they will not be holding the bag for medical mistakes. Families shouldn't shoulder the financial burdens of medical negligence because industry is unaccountable for its actions.

* Finally, a consumer bill of rights should set minimum standards for all managed-care plans. Voluntary provisions won't suffice. When you get sick, doctors, not accountants, should call the shots.

Congress can restore consumer confidence in the managed-care system by passing enforceable and loophole-free legislation that includes a fair review process, full disclosure and accountability. Anything less falls short of true reform.

KAREN IGNAGNI
President, American Association of Health Plans

*b*ealth plans have advanced the cause of patients' rights with important patient protections that weren't available under the old system. Health-care practices and procedures have been made far more accountable — ensuring that the great majority of patients get the right care, at the right time and in the right setting — and appeals systems are in place to make sure that any patient who disagrees with a coverage or treatment decision has effective recourse.

Discussions of patients' rights should start with the fact that, from a patient's perspective, all other rights are meaningless without access to care. Under the old system, health care was being priced beyond reach. So one of the most important victories that health plans have won for patients' rights is to make health coverage more affordable for millions of working Americans.

Once assured of coverage, you should have the right to be protected against inappropriate care. Health plans promote quality care by emphasizing prevention and early diagnosis and monitoring practice patterns in order to do away with the wide variations in quality that did so much to make the old system not just costly but often downright dangerous. This commitment to accountability represents a major advance in patient protection.

But what if a conflict arises about what's covered or whether a particular treatment is in order? Despite critics' claims, disputes are rare and are usually resolved satisfactorily. Still, there's room for improvement — and health plans are participating in a nationwide initiative to continually improve care by identifying consumer concerns and developing patient-centered solutions. This, too, represents an unprecedented commitment to patients' rights.

Consumers should be wary of much that is being touted today as "consumer protection." For example, efforts to make health plans liable for individual practitioners' actions would simply clog the courts (at taxpayer expense) and enrich trial lawyers (not patients). At the same time, such efforts would adversely affect care by forcing health plans to act defensively, causing higher costs without producing better outcomes. Does that protect patients' rights? No — it just turns back the clock.

And we can't afford that. The health-care revolution that's in progress today was a necessary answer to the costly flaws of the old system. If the revolution has imperfections, the answer is to correct them — not to roll back progress or micromanage plans. Health plans are fully committed to making sure consumers are informed and their concerns met. That way, we can protect patients' rights without smothering innovative health care under layers of inflexible regulations and unproductive litigation.

Estimated Costs of Reform Vary Widely

Two studies — one funded by an industry group, the other by a patient-consumer coalition — reached dramatically different conclusions about the likely cost impact of the original and most widely supported managed-care reform proposal in Congress. But the industry's substantially higher estimate depends on interpretations of the bill, the Patient Access to Responsible Care Act (PARCA), that its sponsor says are wrong.

A report prepared for the insurance-business Health Benefits Coalition by the Washington consulting firm of Milliman & Robertson projected the bill would raise health insurance premiums by 23 percent.[1]

A study prepared for the Patient Access to Responsible Care Alliance — also known as PARCA — by Muse & Associates predicted a rate increase of between 0.7 to 2.6 percent.[2]

The reports made strikingly similar predictions about the effects of some provisions. Both reports, for example, predict little if any effect from provisions requiring emergency care coverage, easing referrals to specialists or giving consumers a choice between types of managed-care plans.

The industry-funded study, however, predicted substantially higher costs for three provisions in the bill:

• No payments to providers as an inducement to reduce or limit medically necessary services. Milliman & Robertson assumed the provision would prevent health plans from negotiating discount rates with providers and projected a 9.5 percent cost increase as a result. Muse & Associates noted that newly drafted report language specifically denied any intention to bar discounts; on that basis, it predicted no cost impact. Difference: 9.5 percent.

• Equal reimbursement for out-of-network providers. Milliman & Robertson say the provision could have no impact if interpreted to apply only to doctors' fees, but could raise premiums by 11 percent if it prevented point-of-service (POS) plans from requiring enrollees to pay a higher deductible for using an out-of-network provider. The firm then averaged the two figures to produce a "best estimate midpoint" of 5.5 percent. Muse & Associates says

the bill would not bar higher deductibles for using a doctor outside the network. Difference: 5.5 percent.

• No discrimination against health professionals. Milliman & Robertson says the provision could require health plans to cover services of professionals not now covered, such as chiropractors or acupuncturists. Muse & Associates said new report language stipulates the bill will not have that effect. Difference: 5.5 percent.

In addition, the industry-funded study predicted that because of its projected increases, some customers would drop their coverage — raising rates still further for consumers still in plans. The consumer-funded study predicts a much smaller effect. Difference: 4.5 percent.[3]

The Muse study predicted only a slight increase from a provision subjecting group health plans to medical malpractice liability; the Milliman-Robertson study did not analyze the provision.

Milliman & Robertson qualified its study by stating that several of its projections "depend heavily on interpretation of PARCA." For its part, Muse & Associates noted that its study took account of legislative changes made after the Milliman & Robertson study was completed.

Rep. Charlie Norwood, R-Ga., the main sponsor of PARCA, says the industry-funded study is based on a misreading of his bill. "The assumptions made are neither reasonable nor honest," he says.

But the Health Benefits Coalition, the business group that released the study, is standing by its predictions. "We have other studies that show that mandates at the state level have raised rates," a spokeswoman says, "and we expect federal regulation to be even more costly."

[1] Milliman & Robertson Inc., "Actuarial Analysis of the Patient Access to Responsible Care Act (PARCA)," released Jan. 21, 1998.

[2] Muse & Associates, "The Health Premium Impact of H.R. 1415/S.644, the Patient Access to Responsible Care Act (PARCA)," Jan. 29, 1998.

[3] Milliman & Robertson says its individual cost estimates total more than its "composite" prediction of 23 percent because some PARCA provisions overlap.

OUTLOOK

Weighing the Costs

The intense partisanship and narrow margins facing the 107th Congress make it difficult to predict whether any managed-care reform proposals will be enacted into law. Health-insurance groups such as AAHP and HIAA along with big-business lobbies such as the U.S. Chamber of Commerce and National Federation of Independent Businesses continue to argue that sweeping reforms would be bad medicine for patients. Specifically, they say legislation giving patients the expanded right to sue managed-care plans for health decisions will drive up premiums and force some small businesses to drop health insurance coverage for their employees.

Norwood and other reform advocates say such arguments are to be expected. "This is pretty normal,"

Norwood says. "The insurance companies stay in the background and try to push the Chamber of Commerce into the front. Yes, that will be formidable opposition. The problem is that they don't have the people on their side, and we do."

Indeed, studies show the public increasingly supports many provisions included in managed-care bills in Congress and in state legislatures. One 1998 survey by the Kaiser Family Foundation and Harvard University found substantial majorities in favor of such proposals as allowing people to appeal to an independent reviewer, to see a specialist or to sue health plans directly. (See poll, p. 109.)

The survey also indicated, however, that public support for those ideas drops significantly if people are asked about the consequences forecast by opponents, such as higher premiums, and reduced health-insurance coverage. "Support may fall if the public comes to see (the proposals) as part of a larger government health-reform plan that could result in employers dropping coverage of higher health insurance premiums," says Drew Altman, president of the Kaiser Family Foundation. Many of the major companies in the industry have been very profitable during the past decade, but in 1997 some of the biggest — including Kaiser, Aetna and Oxford Health Plans Inc. — reported losses. [26] The pressure on the industry has eased somewhat because of the slowing pace of health-care inflation. Managed-care companies also are finding other places to cut costs — for instance, dropping out of the Medicare program in areas where reimbursements lag far behind actual costs of treatment.

Even so, some insurers are beginning to raise premiums in anticipation of accelerating increases in health-care costs over the new few years. [27] Many of the price hikes are linked to the flood of expensive new drugs hitting the market. The cost debate will turn in part on which side managed to convince the public and lawmakers that it has "credible experts" on its side, experts say. The debate already has produced dueling studies on the issue. (See story, p. 112.) One study prepared for the insurance industry and a coalition of business groups projected a 23 percent increase in health insurance premiums if Norwood's proposal were enacted. A rival study for the Patient Access to Responsible Care Alliance forecast a "slight increase" in managed-care premiums of from 0.7 to 2.6 percent. [28]

In Minnesota, however, Dianne Shea believes that the debate over patients' rights should not turn on costs. "This is the richest country in the world, and we're arguing about how to provide health care for everyone," she says. "Isn't it the right of every American to have health care?"

"We've come up with a solution to every problem in this country," Shea concludes. "I know we can come up with a way to provide good health care to people." ∎

FOR MORE INFORMATION

American Association of Health Plans, 1129 20th St., N.W., Suite 600, Washington, D.C. 20036; (202) 778-3200; www.aahp.org. The trade association represents health maintenance organizations (HMOs) and similar network health-care plans.

American Medical Association, 1101 Vermont Ave., N.W., 12th Floor, Washington, D.C. 20005; (202) 789-7400; www.ama-assn.org. The AMA, with 300,000 members, is the nation's largest physicians' group; it supports some managed-care reform proposals.

Consumers Union of the United States, 1666 Connecticut Ave., N.W., Suite 310, Washington, D.C. 20009; (202) 462-6262; www.consumersunion.org. Consumers Union, publisher of Consumer's Report, lobbies on health issues in Washington and in state capitals.

Health Benefits Coalition, 600 Maryland Ave., S.W., Washington, D.C. 20004; (202) 554-9000. The ad hoc coalition, comprising 31 business trade associations, opposes managed-care reform bills in Congress.

Health Insurance Association of America, 555 13th St., N.W., Suite 600E, Washington, D.C. 20004; (202) 824-1600; www.hiaa.org. This trade association represents 250 of the country's major for-profit health insurance carriers.

Patient Access to Responsible Care Alliance, 1111 14th St., N.W., Suite 1100, Washington, D.C. 20005; (202) 898-2400. The ad hoc coalition of 70 patient, provider and consumer-advocacy groups supports the major managed-care reform bill in Congress — the Patient Access to Responsible Care Act (PARCA).

Notes

[1] The American Association of Health Plans reported that nearly 150 million Americans belonged to managed-care plans at the end of 1995, the most recent year surveyed: 58.2 million in HMOs and 91 million in preferred provider organizations (PPOs). See "1995 AAHP HMO and PPO Trends Report." An annual survey of employer-provided health-benefit plans released last month shows that the percentage of employees enrolled in managed-care plans rose in 1996 and 1997. See Mercer/Foster Higgins "National Survey of Employer-Sponsored Health Plans." In his State of the Union address on Jan. 27, President Clinton said that 160 million Americans are in managed-care plans today.

[2] The 8th U.S. Circuit Court of Appeals ruled on Feb. 26, 1997, in *Shea v. Esensten* that the suit could proceed. The court ruled that Shea could sue her HMO under the federal benefits protection law known as ERISA for failing to disclose its system for reimbursing doctors.

[3] For background, see "Managed Care," *The CQ Researcher*, April 12, 1996, pp. 313-336.

[4] See *The Dallas Morning News*, Dec. 23, 1997, p. 1C and *The Washington Post*, Dec. 20, 1997, p. D1.

[5] For background on the debate over medical malpractice litigation, see "Too Many Lawsuits," *The CQ Researcher*, May 22, 1992, pp. 433-456.

[6] For background, see Barry R. Furrow, "Managed Care Organizations and Patient Injury: Rethinking Liability," *Georgia Law Review*, Vol. 31, winter 1997, pp. 419-509, and Clark C. Havighurst, "Making Health Plans Accountable for the Quality of Care," *ibid.*, pp. 587-647.

[7] See *The New York Times*, Sept. 10, 1997, p. A1.

[8] See *The New York Times*, Sept. 12, 1997, p. A24.

[9] PBS, "The NewsHour With Jim Lehrer," Sept. 16, 1997.

[10] For background, see "Medical Screening Raises Privacy Concerns," *The CQ Researcher*, Nov. 19, 1993, p. 1023. For opposing views on the issue, see *USA Today*, April 19, 1996, p. 13A.

[11] See *USA Today*, Jan. 20, 1998, p. 1A.

[12] Quoted in *The Washington Post*, Sept. 12, 1997, p. A1.

[13] Some background is drawn from Paul Starr, *The Social Transformation of American Medicine: The Rise of a Sovereign Profession and the Making of a Vast Industry* (1982).

[14] See *ibid.*, p. 334.

[15] *Ibid.*, pp. 369-370.

[16] Some of this material can also be found in "Managed Care," *The CQ Researcher*, April 12, 1996, pp. 324-327.

[17] Starr, *op. cit.*, p. 395.

[18] See 1973 *Congressional Quarterly Almanac*, pp. 499-507.

[19] See 1976 *Congressional Quarterly Almanac*, pp. 544-548, and 1978 *Congressional Quarterly Almanac*, pp. 576-580.

[20] Starr, *op. cit.*, p. 415.

[21] Details of the Fox and Adams case, along with citations to contemporaneous news accounts, can be found in George Anders, *Health Against Wealth: HMOs and the Breakdown of Medical Trust* (1996). Health Net had argued in the Fox case that the bone marrow transplant was not covered because it was an experimental procedure; Kaiser contended that it provided proper care in the Adams case.

[22] See "Sick People in Managed Care Have Difficulty Getting Services and Treatment," Robert Wood Johnson Foundation, June 28, 1995.

[23] Anders, *op. cit.*, pp. 42, 47.

[24] See 1996 *Congressional Quarterly Almanac*, pp. 10-85. The provision was included in the fiscal 1997 appropriations bill for the Veterans Administration, Department of Housing and Urban Development and other agencies. For a critical view of the impact of the law, see *Newsweek*, Aug. 4, 1997, p. 65.

[25] For background, see *Congressional Quarterly Weekly Report*, Nov. 22, 1997, pp. 2909-2911.

[26] See *The Wall Street Journal*, Dec. 22, 1997, p. A1 (Kaiser) and *The Washington Post*, Jan. 4, 1998 (Aetna, Oxford).

[27] See *The New York Times*, Jan. 11, 1998, p. A1.

[28] Milliman & Robertson, Inc., "Actuarial Analysis of the Patient Access to Responsible Care Act (PARCA)," released Jan. 21, 1998; Muse & Associates, "The Health Premium Impact of H.R. 1415/S.644, the Patient Access to Responsible Care Act (PARCA)," Jan. 29, 1998.

Bibliography

Selected Sources Used

Books

Anders, George, *Health Against Wealth: HMOs and the Breakdown of Medical Trust*, Houghton Mifflin, 1996.

Anders, a reporter for *The Wall Street Journal*, provides a strongly written, critical account of the impact of health maintenance organizations on patients' rights. The book includes detailed source notes.

Annas, George J., *The Rights of Patients: The Basic ACLU Guide to Patient Rights* [2d ed.], Humana Press, 1989.

This American Civil Liberties Union handbook, updated in 1989, gives an overview of patients' rights in such areas as informed consent, medical records, privacy and confidentiality and medical malpractice. The book includes source notes and an eight-page list of organizations and other references. Annas is a professor of health law at Boston University's schools of medicine and public health.

Goodman, John C., and Gerald L. Musgrave, *Patient Power: Solving America's Health Care Crisis*, Cato Institute, 1992.

Goodman and Musgrave argue strongly that the country's health-care "crisis" calls for free-market solutions — reducing government regulation, diminishing the role of insurance and giving individual consumers and patients greater responsibility for paying for their health care. Goodman is president of the National Center for Policy Analysis, a free-market think tank in Dallas; Musgrave is president of Economics America Inc., a consulting firm in Ann Arbor, Mich.

Patel, Kent, and Mark E. Rushefsky, *Health Care Policies and Policy in America*, M.E. Sharpe, 1995.

The book gives an overview of contemporary health-care issues. It also includes a brief chronology (1798-1995) and a 23-page bibliography. Patel and Rushefsky are professors of political science at Southwest Missouri State University.

Starr, Paul, *The Social Transformation of American Medicine: The Rise of a Sovereign Profession and the Making of a Vast Industry*, Basic Books, 1982.

This widely praised study traces the history of the U.S. medical profession and health-care system from the 1700s through the birth and emerging growth of managed care in the 1970s and early '80s. Starr, a professor of sociology at Princeton University, has been an adviser to President Clinton on health-care policy. The book includes detailed source notes.

White, Joseph, *Competing Solutions: American Health Care Proposals and International Experience*, Brookings Institution, 1995.

White compares the U.S. health-care system with those in other countries, including Australia, Canada, France, Germany, Great Britain and Japan. He is a research associate in governmental studies at the Brookings Institution.

Articles:

Langdon, Steve, "Critics Want More 'Management' of Managed Care Industry," *Congressional Quarterly Weekly Report*, March 15, 1997, pp. 633-640.

The article provides an overview of legislative developments on managed care at the start of the 105th Congress, along with summaries of major bills, legislative activity in selected states and a glossary.

Reports and Studies

Advisory Commission on Consumer Protection and Quality in the Health Care Industry, *Consumer Bill of Rights and Responsibilities: Report to the President of the United States*, November 1997.

The 72-page report by the 34-member commission appointed by President Clinton contains recommendations dealing with such issues as choice of providers and health plans, complaints and appeals and confidentiality of health information. A list of references and selected reading are included.

Computer Science and Telecommunications Board, National Research Council, *For the Record: Protecting Electronic Health Information*, National Academy Press, 1997.

This book-length report details a scientific panel's findings and recommendations on protections for electronic health information. The book includes an 11-page bibliography as well as detailed source notes.

Kaiser Family Foundation/Harvard University, *National Survey of Americans' Views on Managed Care*, Nov. 5, 1997; *National Survey of Americans' Views on Consumer Protections in Managed Care*, Jan. 21, 1998.

The first survey found that majorities of the public are concerned about key aspects of managed health care. The second found majority support for many of the major reform proposals currently being debated, but support dropped when people were asked about potential consequences of changes, such as higher insurance premiums.

7 Managing Managed Care

ADRIEL BETTELHEIM

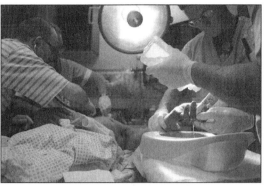

Backlash against managed care usually takes the form of fiery speeches from reform-minded politicians or the telling of horror stories by patients denied access to critical care.

But things took a turn toward the unusual in March, when 15,000 frustrated doctors — average income $166,000 a year — joined a labor union. They pledged to fight managed care companies that they say delay reimbursements, make them work longer hours and excessively meddle in patient care.

"Our major agenda is to organize every employed doctor in this country," said Barry Liebowitz, leader of the dissident physicians.

The odd alliance of affluent professionals and a traditionally blue-collar union reflects the depth of the debate over America's medical system. Managed care companies, which now serve approximately 160 million Americans, are under unprecedented attack by a variety of critics, who say they have sacrificed the quality of medical services by excessively focusing on financial results.

A survey last September by the Kaiser Family Foundation and Harvard University found Americans are increasingly worried about managed care. Sixty-five percent of the respondents favored some government involvement to protect consumers in managed care plans compared with 52 percent the year before. And 73 percent favored giving consumers the right to sue their health plans, compared with 64 percent in 1997.

The debate in the last Congress over managed care regulation and President Clinton's proposed "Patients' Bill of Rights" got sidetracked

From *The CQ Researcher,*
April 16, 1999.

by partisan bickering and the Monica Lewinsky scandal. But with the 2000 elections less than 19 months away and consumer frustration building, lawmakers are again trying to address public concerns. At least a half-dozen members of Congress have proposed competing versions of patients'-rights legislation that would impose new regulations on health insurers and strip away their decision-making power. Several of the measures would amend the Employee Retirement Income Security Act of 1974 (ERISA), which exempts many health plans from state laws and prevents millions of patients from suing managed care firms. [1]

The proposed regulations also deal with more fundamental issues, such as whether managed care "gatekeepers" should continue to decide what procedures are "medically necessary." But Republicans and Democrats remain sharply divided over how far regulations should go, making it unclear whether the two sides will compromise and pass legislation or turn health-care reform into a campaign issue in next year's elections.

"The $64,000 question is what kind of debate does Congress want, and are the problems real, perceived or just designed to protect health-care providers?" says Karen Ignagni, president of the American Association of Health Plans (AAHP). Ignagni argues that new regulations will only drive up health costs by imposing new

layers of red tape, making it more difficult for working people to afford coverage.

Health-provider groups like the American Medical Association (AMA) counter that the time is ripe for reform, citing numerous examples in which, they say, health plans trampled on patients' rights. Many physicians, long bitter over plan administrators' ability to overrule their decisions, want to revert back to something resembling a traditional fee-for-service system, in which insurers agreed to pay for whatever care the doctor ordered.

"There are some good managed care plans out there, but as the opportunity to make a buck increases, a number are cutting here and there and coming up woefully short of what acceptable standards for care should be," says Texas family physician Nancy Dickey, president of the AMA.

The health-care debate comes as more and more Americans are being funneled into managed care plans through their employers. Approximately 60 percent of the population — and 85 percent of Americans with employer-based health insurance — receive their care through managed care. Some 71 million are enrolled in the most prevalent type of managed care program, a health maintenance organization (HMO). Many managed care companies also are angling for retirees covered by Medicare, who have the option of switching from the traditional coverage the government program offers to an HMO.

Polls suggest a majority of plan enrollees are satisfied with the quality of care they receive. But many people complain that they have had problems getting permission from managed care plans to see medical specialists or pay emergency room

Concern About Managed Care Rose

Americans have become increasingly concerned about the quality of managed care and more supportive of consumer-protection proposals, according to a recent survey by the Kaiser Family Foundation.

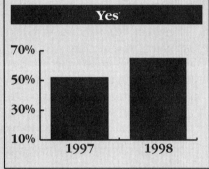

Does government need to protect consumers from not getting the care they need from managed care firms?

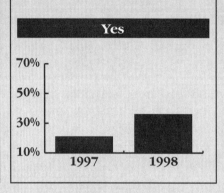

Are managed care plans doing a bad job serving consumers?

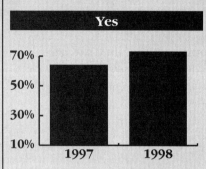

Should consumers have the right to sue their health plans?

Source: Kaiser Family Foundation, "Kaiser-Harvard Survey on Americans' Views on the Consumer Protection Debate," Sept. 17, 1998

bills — and they say they have no place to turn when a claim is denied. They also aren't sure whether they want to pay more for added protections. A recent Employee Benefit Research Institute (EBRI) survey found that 46 percent of respondents favor increasing government regulation of health insurance in theory, but only 20 percent favor drafting more rules if they would increase health insurance costs by $50 per month or more.

Health-care economist Paul Fronstin, who conducted the survey, says Americans are reluctant to pay more for added protection because they treat health insurance differently from other essentials. While they may be willing to spend more to go to a better college or buy a fancier car, they are not willing to pay out-of-pocket for extra services or protection, and thus will accept whatever coverage their employer provides.

The anti-managed care sentiment is ironic to some because most experts give the industry credit for holding down health costs for most of the 1990s. By using their purchasing power to extract price concessions from doctors, hospitals and other health-care providers, plans were able to reverse a trend of double-digit premium increases. The federal Health Care Financing Administration (HCFA) reports that health-care spending growth was 4.8 percent in 1997, the last year for which complete figures are available, compared with a high of 12.2 percent in 1990. [2]

Some economists estimate that, by next year, managed care companies will be saving Americans as much as $300 billion a year on health care. Much of the cost controls came at a time when new diagnostic tests and technologies and a host of novel drugs were exerting upward price

pressure. Indeed, many HMOs kept premiums deliberately low to attract new employer groups, suffering crushing financial losses. Many are expected to raise premiums 6-9 percent this year to firm up their balance sheets.

Despite the cost controls, managed care companies managed to anger many different groups. Uwe Reinhardt, a professor of health-care economics at Princeton University, says health plans unwisely focused on shortening patients' hospital stays, leading to highly publicized incidents, such as mothers being kicked out just one day after delivering their babies.

Plan administrators also were reluctant to provide basic customer information, such as the background of plan physicians and how satisfied current enrollees were with services. Moreover, Reinhardt says industry leaders were slow to spend on information systems that could track key variables — such as the outcomes of treatments — and gauge the quality of care. Some state and federal lawmakers now are demanding the information as part of patient-protection legislation.

The result has been growing consumer dissatisfaction and the perception that health plans are compromising quality for cost. The Foundation for Taxpayer and Consumer Rights recently sued one of the nation's largest HMOs — Kaiser Permanente — alleging its advertising fraudulently portrayed plan doctors as not subject to financial constraints on patient care. [3]

Medical caregivers have also jumped into the managed care fray, accusing HMO gatekeepers of restricting patient access to their services. The 15,000 doctors who recently became members of the AFL-CIO-affiliated Service Employees International Union joined some 600,000 registered nurses, medical technicians and home health aides who had already joined the union in the hope of gaining leverage in negotiating contracts with HMOs and other managed care providers. Some large employers, responding to their workers' complaints, have even begun bypassing managed care companies altogether and contracting directly with doctors and hospitals.

Faced with the public outcry, managed care providers are trying to mollify critics by advocating more external reviews of their decisions. By allowing enrollees to appeal coverage decisions to outside professionals, the plans hope to clean up their image and obtain some legal protection from liability suits. The pace quickened in January after a Superior Court jury in San Bernardino, Calif., ordered Aetna US Healthcare of California to pay the widow of a cancer patient $120.5 million for rejecting a doctor's request to try experimental

Higher Health-Care Costs Predicted

Major U.S. employers predict that their health-care costs will increase by up to 11 percent in 1999, compared with last year's 3.7 percent increase.

Type of Plan	Anticipated Increase	Average Cost Per Employee
Health-maintenance organizations	6–9%	$3,532
Point-of-service plans	6–9%	$4,012
Preferred provider organizations	5–8%	$4,312
Traditional indemnity plans	9–11%	$4,910

Source: Survey by Hewitt Associates of 2,000 health plans and 200 employers.

bone marrow treatment for a rare form of stomach cancer. [4] Plans also are agreeing to help pay the costs of members participating in clinical trials of experimental drugs.

It's unclear whether the changes will affect the calls for federal reforms. Democrats, who have been closely linked to health-care reform since the Clinton administration's failed 1993 health plan and generally score well with the issue in elections, are under pressure to produce some legislation during the current Congress. This time around they may have an easier time exerting influence on Republicans, who hold slim majorities in both the House and Senate and need Democratic support to pass practically any measures.

Many GOP lawmakers believe some reforms are necessary but find excessive regulations don't square with their anti-regulatory leanings. They also are feeling pressure from big business, which believes new regulations will lead to steep premium increases that they will have to pay. To avoid being labeled do-nothings, lawmakers may pass a series of

limited measures dealing with specific proposals — say, expanded emergency-room care or better access to specialists. Another proposal under consideration, sponsored by Rep. Tom Campbell, R-Calif., would give physicians and other health-care providers immunity from antitrust laws so they can negotiate as groups with health plans over fees and services. Campbell says it would give health professionals the same leeway labor organizations now enjoy; critics contend it could immunize anti-competitive activities by the doctors.

"They say it takes seven years to produce legislation that is complex," Rep. Charlie Norwood, R-Ga., a dentist who has proposed bills similar to Democratic plans, mused recently. "This is complex, and we're only in our fifth year."

Interest groups on both sides of the debate are trying to influence the outcome. Managed care reform advocates sponsored a "Patients' Bill of Rights Day" on April 9, featuring rallies around the country pressing for more federal protection for patients. The managed care industry is trying to persuade presidential and congressional candidates in the 2000 elections that managed care reform isn't high on voters' agendas. The AAHP in January polled 300 likely Republican primary voters in New Hampshire, finding 85 percent in managed care plans were satisfied with their coverage. The poll also showed that a candidate's stance on reform ranked low among factors likely to influence voters. [5]

As lawmakers and policy experts debate how to manage managed care, here are some of the questions they are asking:

Should managed care legislation strip away decision-making power from insurers?

For many Americans, the question of who decides what is medically necessary was brought home last June by a declaration from Kaiser Permanente. The powerful HMO told its 9 million members it wouldn't cover the $10 cost of the popular anti-impotence pill Viagra. Barely a month later, HCFA, which administers the Medicare and Medicaid programs, announced that Medicaid, a federal-state program for the poor, must cover Viagra in cases where a doctor believes it's medically necessary to treat erectile dysfunction. [6] The conflicting decisions unleashed a heated debate over which stance was correct and whether Kaiser and other HMOs were letting cost considerations interfere with the quality of care.

Doctors and insurers have long been in conflict over who should decide when health care is medically necessary. Physician groups led by the AMA contend that performance reviews, practice guidelines and other managed care cost controls undermine physicians' autonomy, preventing them from choosing what is right for the patient. The added paperwork justifying decisions to insurers also eats into doctors' incomes.

Seizing on the current anti-HMO sentiment, the doctors are mounting an intense lobbying effort to include medical-necessity provisions in any patient-protection laws that are considered by the current Congress. Such provisions would effectively take away insurers' ability to determine what patient care is necessary.

"Patients are extraordinarily frustrated by the current system of care," says AMA President Dickey. "We should have some guidelines that let health plans demonstrate a [decision by a] physician is out-of-date, or not cost-effective. But to just have a box [on a form indicating coverage is denied without providing a rationale for the decision] really leaves patients hung out to dry."

Doctors complain that a growing number of managed care firms are arbitrarily denying coverage for a wide range of accepted treatments that don't fall within the insurers' guidelines, such as physical therapy for a child with cerebral palsy. Doctors also complain that managed care firms use contracts with carefully worded language that says, in essence, certain good practices are nonetheless not necessary practices. This makes it harder for patients to appeal decisions, the physicians contend.

Sara Rosenbaum, a professor of public health and health services at George Washington University, co-authored a study documenting HMO decision-making practices in the Jan. 21 issue of *The New England Journal of Medicine*. The study describes how medical directors at large HMOs often ignore published medical studies, national experts and guidelines of the Food and Drug Administration and National Institutes of Health when they make coverage decisions. For example, Rosenbaum cites insurers' unwillingness to cover growth-hormone therapy for children with an endocrine disorder even though 96 percent of pediatric specialists approved the treatment. [7]

With public sentiment increasingly tilted against managed care, lawmakers are embracing the doctors' pitch. "Too often, HMOs and other insurance companies deny services that ought to be covered by saying that the services are not medically necessary," Sen. Edward M. Kennedy of Massachusetts, ranking Democrat on the Senate Health, Education, Labor and Pensions Committee, said during a March hearing.

Pending proposals in the Senate and House would prohibit group health plans from "arbitrarily interfering with" covered health services when a physician determines they are medically necessary. The physician may be the patient's primary-care doctor or a specialist to whom the patient was referred. The language was included in legislation proposed by Kennedy and Senate Minority Leader Tom Daschle, D-S.D. It also is part of measures sponsored by Rep. John D. Dingell, D-Mich. Rep. Greg Ganske, R-Iowa, and Sen. John H. Chafee, R-R.I.

Insurers counter that doctors are trying to go back to the unconstrained fee-for-service system that threw health-care costs out of kilter in the 1970s and '80s. With providers interpreting the scope of coverage under a contract, the insurers say they can't assure that health dollars will be spent fairly or equitably on safe and proven medical treatments. Health-plan administrators add that physicians' complaints about autonomy are a red herring, pointing to insurance industry studies that show as many as 97 percent of doctors' recommended courses of treatment are approved by managed care firms. [8]

"These proposals would give virtual carte blanche to treatments that are unnecessary, and sometimes even dangerous," says Chip Kahn, president of the Health Insurance Association of America (HIAA). "The result would be consumers pay higher premiums and receive lower-quality health care."

Kahn says the pending proposals would saddle health plans with legal barriers to challenging coverage, making it easier to file fraudulent claims or undertake risky medical procedures. HCFA estimates that fraud accounts for more than $100 billion of the nation's health-care spending.

And just as managed care foes roll out horror stories about denied coverage, insurers offer examples of doctors who abuse the system — a Pennsylvania physician who was convicted on 59 counts of illegally distributing narcotics to drug abusers and dealers, saying the drugs were "medically necessary," or the New York community center director who stole nearly $1 million by fraudulently billing the state for more than 25,000 psychiatric sessions that never took place. [9]

Ultimately, the dispute over medical necessity could be decided by outside reviews by independent experts. Groups such as the Healthcare Leadership Council — a Washington-based coalition of hospital, pharmaceutical and other health-care industry executives — say they would support legislation that allowed patients to make binding, independent appeals if doctors and insurers have a dispute.

Many health plans already are implementing such appeals procedures, but the industry is opposed to government regulations mandating them. Kahn says consumers can patronize those plans that offer appeal rights. But he adds that health insurers still have a fiduciary responsibility to all customers not to pay for unnecessary care.

Will tougher regulations lead to a rationing of health care?

The fundamental question underlying the managed care flap is the same question that fueled past battles over regulating airlines, telecommu-

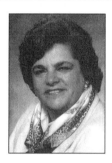

"There are some good managed care plans out there, but as the opportunity to make a buck increases, a number are cutting here and there and coming up woefully short of acceptable standards for care."

— Dr. Nancy Dickey,
president,
American Medical Association

nications and electric utilities: Should the government impose reforms or allow the free market to sort things out and give consumers all of the necessary protections?

The question packs added punch in the case of health care because many Americans believe access to emergency care, experimental treatments and medical specialists already is restricted and will get worse in the future. What's unclear is whether proposed patient-protection regulations will improve access to the health system or intensify the pressure to cut costs and ration care.

In essence, the whole point of managed care is rationing. Insurers promote the health services and providers they believe are the most cost-effective and limit access to those that aren't. The managed care industry says passing laws that would guarantee clients a choice of doctors, more power in selecting treatments and expand the right to sue their plans would drive up costs and raise premiums, ultimately leaving more Americans uninsured. [10]

"In the end, real working people are going to pay either directly or indirectly for whatever Congress mandates," AAHP President Ignagni says. "The fundamental question is whether patient-protection legislative proposals are really in the patients' interests."

Ignagni and others point to the experience of the late 1980s and early '90s, when the increased use of diagnostic tests, new drugs and technologies and more physician visits combined to sharply drive up the nation's health-care costs. Insurers raised the cost of coverage, and employers passed on the increases to workers. Many young and low-income workers opted out of their health plans entirely rather than ante up. Some businesses made the decision for them by dropping coverage altogether.

The number of uninsured Americans has been a growing concern for policy-makers. EBRI estimates that

Industry Warns About New Regulation

The managed care industry says increased government regulation will drive up employers' premiums or reduce the value of benefits that plans offer members. Some believe this will ultimately lead to more health-care rationing.

Possible Effects If Employers' Premiums Rise 10 Percent

- Increased employer contributions (1999-2003): **$116.7 billion**
- Increased employer contributions per covered worker (1999-2003): **$1,593**
- Decrease in number of insured individuals in 1999: **3.2 million**
- Total potential wage loss (1999-2003): **$122.8 billion**
- Wages lost per covered household (1999-2003): **$1,869**

Source: Barents Group, April 21, 1998

about 43 million people currently have no health coverage.[11] Federal law allows workers to purchase insurance if they leave a group plan without having another plan to join. But policy experts say insurers commonly screen applicants for "pre-existing conditions" and charge them many times the normal price if something is found. As a result, affordable insurance is only available to a handful with a clean bill of health.

Reform-minded lawmakers say regulation is needed now precisely so market power will be shifted back in consumers' direction. With consumer complaints on the rise, the politicians argue that new patients'-rights laws would help tens of millions of managed care participants who currently don't have any legal protections because of the nation's patchwork sys-

tem of regulating health care. These lawmakers say patients should be active participants in their care and treatment, and have access to a fair process to resolve differences with their insurers and doctors.

Under the current regulatory scheme, states are the primary regulators of employer-based health insurance. Some 15 states have enacted health-care consumer protections. According to a recent U.S. General Accounting Office survey, they range from improved access to emergency services and specialists to prohibitions on "gag rules" that some contend prevent doctors from discussing treatments that won't be covered by insurance.[12]

But the federal Employee Retirement Income Security Act of 1974 pre-empts state laws for the approxi-

mately 48 million people enrolled in self-insured group health plans (plans typically sponsored by large companies in which the employer, rather than an outside insurance company, assumes the financial risk). The ERISA exemption protects these plans from member lawsuits and requirements that they open their networks to a broader selection of health-care providers.

"Even where states have acted to deal with particular problems, too often the action fails to provide the full protection patients need," Sen. Kennedy says.

While lawmakers appear to agree on broad principles for overhauling managed care, they remain divided along partisan lines on specifics. Republicans, favoring an approach that keeps regulation to a minimum, have offered a proposal in the Senate that would extend protections to the 48 million Americans in self-insured plans. The GOP plan is spearheaded by Sen. James M. Jeffords, R-Vt., chairman of the Senate Health, Education, Labor and Pensions Committee.

Democrats, though, say there are at least 113 million Americans in managed care who need federal protection because of the hit-or-miss nature of state regulations. They include state employees and workers who buy health insurance independently.[13]

"Enormous differences exist today in the protections that are afforded to people based on the accidental happenstance of a consumer's state of residence, and the payer and form of that consumer's health plan," says Ronald Pollack, executive director of the liberal-leaning advocacy group Families USA.

Regardless of whether regulations are passed, few experts predict health-care rationing will go away. Instead, they say, decisions about painful cuts will gradually shift from insurers to health-care professionals, employers and the workers themselves. Some corporations confronted with premium increases may elect to forgo buying health coverage for workers and instead give their employees vouchers or lump-sum payments. The workers will then have to decide what is the most appropriate coverage they can buy for that amount. Similarly, insurers who face higher costs may increase deductibles and copayments, forcing plan members to decide if they want to pay more for certain procedures.

"You can't avoid the reality of rationing, it just will shift from sector to sector," says Mark Hall, professor of law and public health at Wake Forest University and author of the 1997 book *Making Medical Spending Decisions.*

Health-care economist Fronstin predicts current labor conditions may prevent consumers from shouldering too much of the burden. With skilled labor in demand, he thinks companies will go out of their way to avoid passing along premium increases, cutting administrative costs and taking other steps to keep workers happy.

"As long as there's a tight labor market, employers will be very reluctant to do anything to create more job openings," Fronstin says. "But if there's a recession, costs will be shifted, and you could end up with many more people uninsured."

Should physicians and hospitals be subject to performance ratings or guidelines?

Cleveland Health Quality Choice was one of the first communitywide efforts in the nation to measure the quality of local health care. But come July, the nonprofit health program will

shut its doors permanently, a victim of the topsy-turvy health-care market.

Launched in 1989 by a group of businesses alarmed by spiraling medical costs, the program issued semiannual report cards on how 27 northern Ohio hospitals cared for patients suffering from serious conditions like heart attacks and strokes. The businesses anticipated using the results as guides to buying health coverage for their workers. Plan administrators even took the unusual step of releasing the report cards to the public,

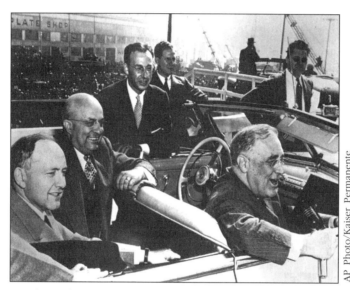

Industrialist Henry J. Kaiser, second from left, visits the Kaiser shipyard in Portland, Ore., in 1942, with President Franklin D. Roosevelt. In 1945, Kaiser opened enrollment in his company's prepaid health-care system to the public.

AP Photo/Kaiser Permanente

hoping the evaluations would show that simply choosing the cheapest health-care providers was, in fact, not always cost-effective in the long run.

But problems soon developed. Hospitals complained that the plan didn't always allow for differences in the severity of patients' illnesses and even accused each other of falsifying results. A spate of hospital mergers changed the nature of health-care contracting, forcing purchasers to decide whether to contract with all or none of the hospitals in a group and reducing the need for individual

hospital performance ratings.

In January, the Cleveland Clinic and the eight hospitals in its system — which reluctantly participated in the program in the first place, largely to avoid losing insurance contracts — decided the approximately $2 million annual cost of compiling the data wasn't worth the effort and dropped out of the program, effectively dooming it.

"We focused on the quality of health care when everybody else was focused on cost," says Dr. Dwain Harper, the program's director. "When something like this fails, it's the community that loses."

The Cleveland Health Quality Choice plan's experience illustrates the dilemmas surrounding health-care quality standards. While advocates say such measures are needed to protect and inform consumers in an increasingly complicated marketplace, it's difficult to agree on precisely what to measure, how the measurements should be compared and whether the results should be used internally or released to the public.

Many believe some type of agreed-upon standards are necessary because health care in the United States varies widely from region to region, rendering traditional medical guidelines for specific procedures inadequate. Dartmouth Medical School researchers have documented how fewer than three out of every 200 breast cancer patients in Rapid City, S.D., received breast-conserving surgery instead of mastectomies, while in suburban Elyria, Ohio, 96 out of 200 did. The two procedures are deemed about equally effective. In gerontological care, spending for hospital treatments during the last six months of life is nearly twice as much in retiree-rich Greater Miami ($14,212 per person) as in Minneapolis ($7,246), the Dartmouth researchers found. [14]

Another argument for standards is that not everyone agrees on what is generally accepted care. A recent study in the AMA's *Archives of Internal Medicine* found more than 47 percent of 1,710 patients who had recurrent heart attacks between 1986 and 1995 had not received aspirin, beta-blockers and lipid-lowering drugs to control cholesterol after the first attack. Doctors in recent years have increasingly turned to the medications to reduce the risk of cardiovascular death. [15]

Doctors and hospitals are traditionally reluctant to endorse a single treatment as the most effective, arguing that medical cases are almost always too complicated to merit such a black-and-white approach. However, managed care companies and big employers increasingly have used their market power to impose statistical guidelines, which they say accurately point caregivers in the right direction.

In the early 1990s, a group of employers and HMOs developed the Health Plan Employer Data and Information Set (HEDIS), a now widely accepted standard that measures how frequently people in health plans receive more than 40 basic tests and services. While groundbreaking, the quality reports have been criticized as being heavily weighted toward primary-care — such as cancer screening and cholesterol tests — and inadequate for measuring how seriously ill people are treated:

More recently, the health-care community has embraced "outcomes research," a more complicated type of assessment that systematically tracks a patient's clinical treatment and responses to the treatment. This involves the use of still-evolving statistical measurements to account for differences between patients. An effective grading system could, for instance, track the success rate of coronary by-pass surgeries while recognizing that certain teaching or research hospitals in a community see more complex heart cases.

To date, there is no single accepted standard for measuring quality of care. The AMA recently launched an accreditation program aimed at evaluating physicians' clinical performance and patient-care results. The program, which would release results to the public, is viewed skeptically by some as an attempt by doctors to set standards for each other instead of leaving the task to regulators or insurers. [16]

"Our opponents like to portray us as arbitrary, having little regard for outcomes research," says AMA President Dickey, defending the effort. "It's really a question of determining the best medical practices and digging beneath the political rhetoric."

Managed care also is incorporating new quality reviews as part of the industry's accreditation process. The National Committee for Quality Assurance (NCQA), a watchdog agency set up by the managed care industry to police health plans, announced in March that, starting in July 2000, it will begin requiring accredited plans to submit to outside reviews by specialists if they deny patients access to certain care or procedures. The move is designed to fight perceptions that managed care makes decisions based on cost considerations instead of what's best for the patient. It also could blunt proposed congressional legislation that would make it easier for patients to sue their health plans if certain coverage is denied. [17]

"A health plan that does well under Accreditation 2000 [the new review process] puts its members first," says NCQA President Margaret O'Kane.

Meanwhile, large employers in several cities are teaming up to launch independent programs similar to Cleveland Health Quality Choice. In Dayton, Ohio, a coalition of businesses that assumes financial risk for insuring 70,000 employees plans to issue a community report card on area hospitals within two years. In Texas, doctors and hospitals in Dallas and Fort Worth are working with large employers in the area to develop a report card for health-care consumers based on benchmarks such as recovery times and complication rates from procedures.

"This information is not available today in our marketplace," Sue Nelson, manager of health promotions and benefits for Dallas-based Texas Instruments Inc., recently told the *Dallas Morning News*. "If you were to go out and seek medical care, we believe you should know answers to the key questions." ∎

BACKGROUND

Cost Concerns

After resoundingly rejecting President Clinton's 1993 plan for government-run health care, Americans appeared content to let for-profit managed care companies figure out how to balance medical costs with quality of care. The industry's failure to do so has created turmoil throughout the health-care system and new fears about the availability of care to millions of patients and employers.

Managed care companies absorbed more than $800 million in losses over the past two years, prompting a wave of mergers and consolidations. In December, Aetna Inc. purchased Prudential Health

Chronology

1880s-1920s
The concept of modern health care evolves with the advent of group practices, health insurance and community rating.

1883
William Mayo and his son, William James, open the Mayo Clinic in Rochester, Minn., becoming the first medical group practice.

1911
The Equitable Life Assurance Society of America writes the first group coverage employee life insurance policy. Interest from big employers leads to expansion of employee benefits, including "'medical catastrophe coverage," the first fee-for-service indemnity plans.

1929
Baylor University contracts with its hospital to provide care for the university's faculty for a flat rate per person. This "community rating" system becomes the predecessor of Blue Cross health plans.

---·---

1940s-1950s
Large-scale major medical plans evolve out of wartime industry.

1941-1945
A shortage of skilled workers and a wartime freeze on wages and corporate profits lead companies to expand employee health benefits. Collective bargaining and favorable court decisions help unions win generous health benefits that are standardized into fee-for-service medical plans.

1945
Industrialist Henry J. Kaiser provides health-care coverage and services on a prepaid basis for his shipyard workers in Oakland, Calif., and Vancouver, Wash., then opens the plan to the public. The plan evolves into Kaiser Permanente, the first managed care organization, now serving about 9 million clients.

1950
More than 100 rural health plans exist, and about 20 HMOs are in operation. The St. Louis branch of the Teamsters, the Appalachian United Mine Workers and the Detroit United Auto Workers have prepaid group coverage.

1959
The Federal Employee Health Benefit Program is formed.

---·---

1960s-1980s
The advent of government-financed health systems leads to greater demand for medical services, driving up health-care spending.

1965
Medicare is enacted. The tax-payer-financed system provides the elderly and disabled with access to short-term medical services. At enactment, slightly half of those age 65 and older have hospital insurance.

1988
Allied-Signal Corp. cancels the health-care arrangements of 80,000 employees and dependents and transfers them into the HMO plans of Cigna Corp. Cigna agrees to cap Allied-Signal's health-care costs for three years. The trend of employers channeling workers into managed care accelerates.

---·---

1990s
Managed care organizations hold down health-care inflation but encounter public backlash.

1991-1997
Increases in HMO premiums among firms with more than 200 employees slow from 12.1 percent to 2 percent.

1993
The Clinton administration proposes the National Health Security Act, designed to provide all Americans with health insurance. Spearheaded by first lady Hillary Rodham Clinton, the plan is defeated by a coalition of business interests, the medical lobby and Republicans.

1996
Fifty million Americans now receive health care through employer-sponsored HMOs, up from 15 million in 1985. Another 50 million are in preferred-provider organizations (PPOs).

1997
A proposed "Patients' Bill of Rights" is issued by Clinton's Advisory Commission on Consumer Protection and Quality in the Health Care Industry.

1999
Enrollment in managed care plans continues to surge despite complaints about service. Congressional Democrats and Republicans offer differing versions of health-care consumer bills.

Care — the latest in a series of acquisitions that has essentially concentrated power around six big insurers: Aetna, Cigna, United Healthcare, Foundation Health Systems, Pacificare and Wellpoint Health Networks. [18]

These combined companies wield enormous power in some cities, giving them the ability to dictate prices and lock dissenting doctors and hospitals out of their networks. In some areas, insurers have used so-called "all-or-nothing" contracts to pressure doctors to participate in their lowest-paying health plans. The practice has sparked several nasty disputes; 400 Texas doctors in Arlington and Fort Worth left Aetna last year and refused to see the insurer's patients. [19]

Despite the intense pressure to cut costs, a growing number of observers question how much more efficiency the industry can squeeze out of the health-care market. Health plans recently have experienced problems keeping control of rising drug costs and the demand for expensive medical technologies. One industry survey last year found the number of drug prescriptions filled per 1,000 HMO members rose 7 percent over 1997 figures. And with the majority of workers now in some form of managed care, insurers can't rely as much on the one-time savings from switching people over from traditional indemnity plans. [20]

Princeton University economist Reinhardt blames managed care's woes on timing and economic conditions. Reinhardt says it was easier to cut costs and force health-care rationing on employers and workers during the recession of the late 1980s and early '90s, when employees were worried about losing their jobs. Now, the economy is strong, labor markets are tight and employers must offer generous fringe benefits to attract skilled workers. As a result, health

plans are under pressure to be more flexible. Increasingly, HMOs and their gatekeeper systems are giving way to less restrictive point-of-service contracts and "preferred provider" networks, which allow patients to obtain care from outside the managed care network.

"Boom times in the economy have eroded the power of selective contracting and, thereby, clipped the wings of managed care," Reinhardt wrote in a 1998 essay, "The Managed Care Industry in Perspective." He says the industry increasingly is powerless to impose market discipline and is "slouching once again to something resembling . . . warmed-over, fee-for-service indemnity insurance." [21]

That hasn't stopped health-care consumers from worrying about the future — and harboring suspicions about their plans. The spate of HMO "horror stories" over the past two years has fueled the perception that many people are receiving substandard care, even though managed care executives contend they sometimes are being blamed for medical accidents that could happen in any health-care system. Doctors also are reminding patients about the freedom they have lost in procuring health care and raising their anxiety over further rationing. Public opinion is so brittle that Helen Hunt's tirade against her HMO in the 1998 movie "As Good As It Gets" drew standing ovations in some theaters.

Meanwhile, employers are concerned about managed care mergers limiting the choice of available health plans and raising premiums. In Philadelphia, the Aetna-Prudential merger has given the combined company a projected 39 percent share of the health-care market. Aetna and a large Blue Cross company, Keystone Health Plan East, together control more than four out of every five members of Philadelphia-area managed care networks.

"A marketplace this large should not be subject to a near monopoly," Alan Hillman, director of the University of Pennsylvania Health Policy Center, told The New York Times in January, soon after the merger was announced. Hillman says the financial demise of either big provider would leave one health plan in charge of care for a large percentage of the working population.

Search for Solutions

Big business, consumers and health professionals are all appealing to Congress for legislative remedies. But lawmakers remain divided over how to respond to the various concerns.

Republicans, in keeping with their generally anti-regulatory leanings, prefer market-based solutions. One option broached by Rep. Bill Thomas, R-Calif., influential chairman of the House Ways and Means Subcommittee on Health, House Majority Leader Dick Armey, R-Texas, and others would shift health care away from the current employer-based system to one based on tax credits. [22] Most of the proposals would offer a refundable tax credit to individuals who buy health insurance. In theory, this would give consumers more control over how much coverage they want to buy and spur managed care companies to compete on price and service, not on how they can limit benefits in ways hidden to most consumers.

It wouldn't be the first time the federal tax code is used to shape social policy — proposals already abound to use tax credits for education and long-term care. But critics say the approach ignores the fact that high-risk individuals with pre-existing conditions probably won't be able to find affordable, comprehensive policies unless the government forces

Employers Now Make Many Choice Decisions

The Clinton administration's 1993 health-care reform proposal foundered in large part because many Americans didn't want the government to decide what medical care they receive. Instead, the task is falling to the nation's large employers, who increasingly are channeling employees and their dependents into managed care and, in the process, defining the health-care marketplace.

The practice dates to 1988, when Allied-Signal Corp. canceled the health-care plans of 80,000 employees and their dependents and transferred them into Cigna Corp.'s HMO plans.[1] In return, Cigna gave the company a discounted price and agreed to cap Allied-Signal's health-care costs for three years. The move saved the company millions of dollars and soon had corporate executives across the country chanting the managed care mantra.

Yet studies show that employees often have little choice in selecting what managed care coverage they receive. A 1998 survey of 21,000 employers conducted by the RAND Corp. and the Research Triangle Institute found that only 17 percent of workers employed by private companies were offered a choice among plans. Only one-third of the businesses with 100 or more employees allowed workers to select from a variety of plans. The survey also found that only one-quarter of the large businesses gave employees anything beyond basic plan descriptions.

Paul Ginsburg, president of the Center for Studying Health System Change, says despite the fact that most workers weren't given a choice of health plans, they did have more choice of physicians than in the past. That's because employers, responding to worker concerns, expanded hospital and physician networks within the managed care framework.

"It's important to recognize that employers have responded to consumer demands for choice," Ginsburg says.

The situation is less optimistic for smaller businesses, who have less clout negotiating health coverage and are more sensitive to premium increases. Some — particularly in retail trade, agriculture and resources — have stopped offering health coverage at all, or only give their employees limited choice.

Choice is important because experts say workers are sensitive to small changes in the cost of premiums. One 1997 study in the *Journal of Health Economics* documented how 26 percent of health-plan members switched to a cheaper plan when the monthly premium for their own plan rose by $10. The sensitivity primarily benefits HMOs, whose premiums usually are slightly lower than indemnity insurers and preferred provider organizations that offer more choice.

Some lawmakers and public-policy experts have suggested reforming health insurance so it is no longer employer-based. They note that by switching from one managed care company to another, a big company can force thousands of workers and their families to leave their personal physicians. Reform advocates also contend that most big employers aren't concerned with the quality of care, just the cost, and lack the means to measure how well their workers are being cared for. A number have suggested using tax credits to allow workers to buy their own health coverage.

Employers say they want to continue to sponsor health plans, noting they now provide coverage for 150 million workers and their families and finance one-third of all health-care spending in the United States. But they fear new federal mandates on managed care will drive up the cost of insurance at a time when tight labor markets dictate they must offer generous benefits to retain workers.

"The marketplace is responding to the needs and desires of consumers," Marcia Comstock, a health-care policy fellow at the U.S. Chamber of Commerce, testified at a U.S. Senate hearing in March. "Mandating today's favored practices or services runs counter to ... quality improvements and drives up costs unnecessarily."[2]

---

[1] For background, see Thomas Bodenheimer and Kip Sullivan, "How Large Employers Are Shaping the Health-Care Marketplace," *The New England Journal of Medicine*, Vol. 338, No. 14 (April 2, 1998), pp. 1003-1007.

[2] Comstock testimony before Senate Committee on Health, Education, Labor and Pensions, March 11, 1999.

insurers to cover them. The size of subsidies for low-income families and the working poor also would have to be substantial to cover the full cost of coverage.

Some critics, such as Rep. Pete Stark, D-Calif., ranking Democrat on the Ways and Means Health panel, believe employers will use the availability of the credits as an excuse to stop providing health coverage that would be preferable to anything that could be bought with the credits. Others believe Congress should instead address underlying problems in the insurance industry, like the lack of standards for what health procedures should be covered.

"None of the tax-credit proposals adequately addresses the need for reform in the [insurance] market. In the absence of such reform, tax-credit proposals could seriously erode health coverage for individuals and families with substantial pre-existing conditions," the advocacy group Consumers Union recently declared.

With the 2000 campaign season looming and odds stacked against substantial reforms, GOP leaders are

How States Are Regulating Managed Care

Here are some of the most common types of patient-protection legislation and the states where they are in force:

Prevent health plans from penalizing doctors who discuss options not covered by the plan or inform patients about grievance or appeal rights:

California, Colorado, Connecticut, Florida, Kentucky, Maryland, Massachusetts, Minnesota, New Jersey, New York, Ohio, Oregon, Pennsylvania, Texas, Vermont.

Protect enrollees if a health insurer denies coverage for emergency services because enrollee didn't seek prior approval:

California, Colorado, Connecticut, Florida, Kentucky, Maryland, Minnesota, New Jersey, New York, Ohio, Oregon, Pennsylvania, Texas, Vermont.

Allow women in health plans to designate obstetricians and gynecologists as their primary-care physicians:

California, Connecticut, Kentucky, Maryland, Minnesota, New Jersey, New York, Oregon, Pennsylvania, Texas, Vermont.

Force managed care firms to provide easier access to medical specialists:

California, Colorado, Connecticut, Florida, Minnesota, New Jersey, New York, Ohio, Oregon, Pennsylvania, Texas, Vermont.

Require managed care firms to list prescription drugs they normally cover, and/or disclose providers for obtaining drugs not on the list:

California, Connecticut, Florida, Kentucky, Minnesota, New York, Oregon, Pennsylvania, Texas, Vermont.

Source: "Managed Care: State Approaches on Selected Patient Protections," March 11, 1999, U.S. General Accounting Office

publican congressional leaders this year are allowing committees with jurisdiction over health care to draft and approve managed care legislation — a process that will give Democrats more input and could result in a degree of bipartisanship. Last year, the Republican managed care bill was written outside the committee process by a GOP health-care task force that didn't solicit Democratic input. The task force produced a bill that narrowly passed the House by a vote of 216-210, mostly along party lines, and drew a veto threat from Clinton, who said it didn't provide enough patient protections.

"I'm encouraged by the consensus that has emerged on the core elements of a Patients' Bill of Rights," Sen. Jeffords says. "I believe we have an obligation to act responsibly, without unduly raising the cost of health coverage or upsetting the existing balance between state and federal regulation of health coverage." ∎

likely to offer more modest, piecemeal proposals. But they are expected to clash with the goals of President Clinton and congressional Democrats, who believe Republicans won't go far enough in giving patients the protection they need. The differences were evident at last month's 13-hour markup of the Senate Republicans' patients'-protection bill, when Democrats on the Senate Health, Education, Labor and Pensions Committee offered 18 amendments that were all defeated by party-line votes. The bill — which relies on market-based solutions but has been criticized for covering just the 48 million Americans in self-insured health plans — was fi-

nally approved by a 10-8 vote, with all Republicans voting for it and all Democrats opposing it.

Democrats want any reforms to apply to all Americans with private insurance, and they continue to press for provisions that would make it easier for patients to sue managed care providers for denial of treatments. Republicans oppose such measures, saying they would drive up health-care costs, increase the number of frivolous lawsuits and prompt employers to scale back the health benefits they now offer.

Despite such tensions, some observers believe it's still possible for lawmakers to arrive at a bipartisan solution. Re-

CURRENT SITUATION

"Managed Competition"

For most of the 1990s, employers embraced managed care as a way

Uninsured Americans Now at 43 Million

Managed care gets credit for controlling medical costs and offering a private-sector solution to the nation's health-care woes. But a number of studies suggest Americans who are unable to get into its health plans are finding it increasingly difficult to obtain essential medical services.

The number of uninsured Americans has risen from 37 million in 1992 to approximately 43 million today. Health-care economists blame increasingly expensive premiums, cutbacks in employer coverage and other cost pressures stemming from the changing medical environment. And experts caution the traditional safety net of charity care is eroding as doctors and hospitals struggle with shifting reimbursement policies and limits on federal aid.

"Many people don't focus on the uninsured because they're busy gauging the opinions of people who are already in health plans, who, for the most part, are satisfied because they're healthy," says Paul Fronstin, health-care economist for the Employee Benefit Research Institute. "The fact is the problems with the uninsured are getting worse, and something needs to be done."

The uninsured are usually defined as those people who don't have health coverage through employer-based plans, Medicare or Medicaid. An estimated 30 million are members of low-income working families who can't afford to buy coverage but also aren't poor enough to qualify for Medicaid, the federal-state health program for the indigent. Most people in this group are less likely to receive basic care and tend to delay seeking treatment until they get seriously ill, sometimes requiring emergency-room visits.

Many health-care providers provide charity care to these people knowing they won't get compensated — an American Medical Association study estimates that doctors provide about $11 billion worth of free or discounted care annually. Some have tried to shift the cost to their insured patients. But with managed care tightening payments to doctors, hospitals and clinics, recouping the losses is more difficult, leading some practitioners to abandon the practice altogether. [1]

A recent study sponsored by the Washington-based Center for Studying Health System Change illustrates the problem. The study of 12,000 physicians, published in March in the *Journal of the American Medical Association*, found that doctors whose income depends the most on HMOs and other managed care organizations devote, on average, 40 percent less time to charity care as doctors with little involvement in managed care. [2]

In addition, doctors who practice in regions with a large number of managed care plans spent less time providing charity care, regardless of how many managed care patients they saw in their own practice. The survey found more than 77 percent of respondents said they still provide at least 10 hours of care to uninsured patients each week.

An earlier study by the center found that, in states where Medicaid programs rely heavily on managed care, uninsured people were less likely to have a primary-care physician or have visited a doctor or clinic for regular care in the past year.

Managed care companies respond that employers and state governments, not health insurers, are to blame for the added pressure on health care's bottom line. Both the American Association of Health Plans and the Health Insurance Association of America contend the managed care industry has improved the quality of care by keeping medical inflation down, thus making health insurance more affordable. AAHP President Karen Ignagni cites industry studies showing that even a 1 percent increase in premiums can result in 300,000 more people losing health coverage.

Federal officials and health-plan administrators are taking some efforts to widen access to care. Congress in 1997 approved a $24 billion, five-year program to provide coverage for the nation's approximately 11 million uninsured, non-Medicaid-eligible children. Similarly, HMO giant Kaiser Permanente has earmarked money to treat uninsured children and asked doctors to work in clinics that cater to at-risk, uninsured patients. [3]

Peter Cunningham, author of the two Center for Studying Health System Change studies, says lawmakers should get more involved. He suggests providing direct funding to care for the uninsured or compensating health-care providers for the charity care they deliver by creating a pool of money financed by federal and private sources.

"The research suggests that the holes in the safety net may be widening," Cunningham says.

---

[1] See Amy Goldstein, "Physicians Cutting Back Charity Work," *The Washington Post*, April 5, 1999, p. A1.

[2] See Peter Cunningham et al., "Managed Care and Physicians' Provision of Charity Care," *Journal of the American Medical Association*, Vol. 281 (March 24/31, 1999), pp. 1087-1092.

[3] Goldstein, *op. cit.*

---

of keeping costs in line. But many privately believed they could do an even better job containing health-care inflation if they banded together to collectively purchase health insur-ance. With premiums on the rise, more and more are.

Last year, nine Chicago-area businesses — including Ford Motor Co., Bank of America and Navistar Inter-national Transportation — negotiated 1999 premiums with local HMOs at rates that were just 4 percent above last year's level. That's less than half of what most employers are expecting to pay this year. After five years of little or no premium growth, three-quarters of American businesses expect health insurance rates to rise an average of 9 percent this year, according to the benefits consulting firm William Mercer.

"We saw the HMO market in Chicago merging, and costs were going up, so we felt by coming together we could expand our leverage," Larry Boress, executive director of the alliance — the Chicago Business Group on Health — told the *Chicago Tribune.* [23]

Group purchasing is built around what health-care experts call the concept of "managed competition." The companies jointly solicit proposals for health coverage and evaluate the resulting bids to obtain competitive rates and certain performance guarantees. In the process, they bypass insurance companies who traditionally act as middlemen and impose their own restrictions on care. The added clout allowed the Chicago-area companies to require the HMOs to provide employees with preventive medical services, such as mammograms, or participate in wellness programs.

But joint purchasing isn't always easy. Thomas Bodenheimer, a family and community medicine specialist at the University of California at San Francisco School of Medicine, says it can be difficult to get participating companies to agree on a standard set of benefits so that all involved are essentially buying the same insurance product. The companies also have to abide by the joint negotiating process and agree not to bargain on the side for even cheaper insurance from managed care providers. [24]

Purchasing groups have been used in a number of different ways across the country with varying success. One of the oldest is the Cleveland-based Council of Smaller Enterprises, which began as a joint-purchasing program

for small businesses in the late 1970s and today offers insurance to 13,000 companies with 200,000 employees and dependents. Organization officials say the group's leverage in negotiating rates has pushed insurance costs in northern Ohio down 20 percent below the national average.

A more recent example is the Pacific Business Group on Health, formed in the early 1990s by Wells Fargo, Bank of America and other large San Francisco-area employers. The coalition, which now includes 33 companies and more than 3 million members, negotiates premiums with managed care companies and ties 2 percent of the premium to performance. If the organizations don't provide appropriate preventive care, as defined by the coalition, they must pay back the amount. This summer, the coalition will try to expand its system to include smaller businesses, which tend to experience higher rate increases because they have less negotiating power.

An arguably more dramatic variation on the theme is found in Minneapolis and St. Paul, Minn., where a 29-company coalition, the Buyers Health Care Action Group, for the past two years has contracted directly with groups of hospitals and physicians, essentially designing its own care systems. Bodenheimer says the coalition — which includes corporate giants 3M, General Mills and Honey-well — succeeded in creating a price war among health-care providers, driving down premiums 8.5 percent below what they would have been had the companies contracted through HMOs. But, he adds, the alliance adopted a complicated system for reimbursing the health professionals, preventing some of the savings from being translated immediately into expanded medical services. [25]

The Clinton administration and many local governments believe

joint purchasing could be the way of the future, particularly for small businesses that currently are experiencing premium increases of 10-13 percent this year. Clinton has proposed a tax credit for small businesses with fewer than 25 workers that establish purchasing alliances, also known as "health marts." Clinton proposed a similar incentive for purchasing pools in his 1993 health plan. Several localities, among them New York City, also have launched their own pilot programs with business groups to form new purchasing alliances. [26]

Drop in Care Denials

Health insurers say they aren't concerned about direct contracting and other collaborative efforts driving them out of business. Managed care executives contend only the largest corporations have the financial means to independently process claims, deal with customer complaints and offer workers a choice of several health-care options. "It's going to be difficult for all but the largest groups of employers to do it," says HIAA's Kahn, predicting some alliances may eventually contract with health plans for claims processing and other administrative functions.

If managed care companies are not fazed about the potential shift in power, new data suggest they appear to be making a concerted effort to be more accommodating to patients. Health-care statistics collected by several states over the past two years indicate health plans actually are not denying much care despite the well-publicized horror stories about HMOs cutting off access to medical treatments.

New York, New Jersey and Connecticut, among others, have begar to require managed care plans tc

At Issue:

Should legislators shift responsibility for interpreting "medical necessity" from insurers to health-care providers?

RICHARD F. CORLIN, M.D.
Speaker, American Medical Association House of Delegates

FROM A STATEMENT TO THE SENATE COMMITTEE ON HEALTH, EDUCATION, LABOR AND PENSIONS, MARCH 2, 1999.

*t*here is currently no issue more pressing than the question of who determines the "medical necessity" of patient care. . . . Consider, for instance, how integral the determination of medical necessity is for sound internal and, especially, external appeals programs. . . . [R]egardless of how sound and effective the actual appeals procedures may be, if the "medical necessity" standard that is being applied in both the internal and external appeals is arbitrarily dictated by the plan administrator or plan documents, the patient will never be guaranteed a fair, objective evaluation of the appropriate level of covered treatment. . . .

Information-disclosure requirements can also be adversely influenced by how "medical necessity" is determined and by whom. For instance, many plans in their information-disclosure statements indicate that the plan will provide coverage for all "medically necessary" treatment. As a result, patients and prospective enrollees believe that they are covered for all medical treatment which is clinically appropriate. . . . When the patient suffers an illness, however, plans that have arbitrarily defined the term "medical necessity" can deny coverage for a wide range of accepted treatments that do not fall within their own arbitrary definition of medically necessary treatment. . . .

Frequently, a patient's right to have access to specialty care hinges on whether the plan decides that it is not medically necessary based on an arbitrary definition of "medical necessity" crafted by the plan. . . . In such a case, upon appeal, if further constrained to use only the plan's "medical necessity" definition, the final outcome would deny needed patient care. Under appeals regulations currently in effect, a patient can be "slow walked" through an appeals process, while awaiting referral to an appropriate specialist. . . .

Reviews of managed care contracts last year revealed that language imposing "lowest cost" criteria had been included in many contracts' definitions of medical necessity. Health plans' concern about their profits remains the driving force behind these definitions, which emphasize cost and resource utilization over quality and clinical effectiveness. To say the least, this is alarming both to patients and to physicians. . . . The AMA believes that "medical necessity" or "medical appropriateness" decisions are ultimately medical decisions and must continue to be treated as such. Permitting health plans to decide "medical necessity" according to financial or cost considerations creates a dangerous precedent.

HEALTH INSURANCE ASSOCIATION OF AMERICA

FROM "MEDICAL NECESSITY AND HEALTH PLAN CONTRACTS," MARCH 1999.

*t*he question is provoked by legislation that has been proposed on Capitol Hill and in many states. At first blush, such legislation, which would place determinations of "medical necessity" solely into the hands of treating physicians, seems innocuous, even reasonable: Why shouldn't treating physicians define what is medically necessary? But, in fact, this proposed change — which would have a detrimental effect on health care in America — reflects the widespread public confusion about "medical necessity" as a boundary of health coverage and "medical necessity" as a clinical determination by a treating physician.

The "medical necessity" provisions in currently proposed federal legislation represent a radical rewriting by public officials of the contract between insurers and health plans and their customers. When the provider, rather than the health plan or insurer, interprets the scope of coverage under the contract, health plans and fiduciaries cannot guarantee to the insured that health-care dollars are being spent fairly and equitably on medical treatments that are safe, proven and effective. Indeed, such legislation could give some providers incentives to overtreat patients to enhance their incomes. Under such a regime, who can doubt that insurers' denials of payment or determinations of non-coverage would be regularly challenged?

In effect, the proposed "medical necessity" provisions represent an attempt to turn back the clock. Such proposals would do more than simply return the health-care system to the unconstrained fee-for-service system of payment that was responsible for the double-digit inflation in health-care costs of the 1970s and 1980s. It would undermine efforts by all types of health-plan delivery models, from HMOs through PPOs and fee-for-service coverage. Even in the earlier era of fee-for-service medical coverage, insurers reviewed claims to ensure that the services already delivered had in fact been medically necessary.

Far from protecting patients, passage of such legislation would be deeply inimical to the interests of health-care consumers, driving up the cost of medical care and possibly even placing patients in harm's way. The legislation would needlessly raise costs for plans, thereby promoting premium increases and reducing the affordability of health insurance. In the long run, such legislation threatens to diminish the availability of coverage and increase the number of the uninsured.

Glossary for a New Millennium

The advent of managed care has created a new lexicon. Here are some of the more commonly used health-care terms:

Managed Care — A catchall term that refers to a wide variety of health-care organizations, including health maintenance organizations (HMOs) and preferred provider organizations (PPOs), which control costs by monitoring how member doctors and hospitals treat patients, and by limiting access to specialists and certain expensive procedures.

Fee-for-Service — The traditional system of paying doctors for services rendered, as opposed to by salary or a fixed amount.

Third-Party Payer — The insurer, employer, government or other party that mediates between doctors and patients and negotiates fees for medical services. This is the opposite of when patients make payments out-of-pocket directly to a doctor or other health-care provider.

Utilization Review — A system used by many health insurers and health-care providers to monitor doctors' diagnoses, treatment and billing practices. The reviews are designed to lower costs by discouraging unnecessary treatment but have been criticized for interfering with physicians' decisions.

Medicare — The government-financed health-care system that provides the elderly and disabled with access to short-term medical services. Funded by payroll deductions and general revenues, the plan covers acute illnesses but doesn't cover prescription drugs or routine hearing, vision and dental care.

Health Maintenance Organization (HMO) — A health-care plan that provides health services for members who prepay a premium that generally covers a range of health services with limited co-payments.

Preferred Provider Organization (PPO) — A health-care provider who furnishes services on a negotiated fee schedule. Enrollees are offered a financial incentive to use doctors on the preferred list and must pay a deductible and co-payment to use out-of-network physicians.

Point-of-Service Plan — A managed care plan that combines features of prepaid and fee-for-service insurance. Enrollees decides whether to use network or non-network providers when care is needed, and are usually charged large co-payments for choosing the latter.

Managed Competition — One approach to health-care reform in which health plans compete to serve the needs of enrollees. Typically, enrollees are offered a choice of plans during an open season.

Community Rating — The practice of setting premium rates based on the cost experience of a managed care plan's entire membership, instead of a particular employer group.

Capitation — A health insurance payment mechanism in which health-care providers are paid a fixed amount of money each month per insured person to cover services over a period of time.

Cost Shifting — A situation in which a health-care provider compensates for decreased revenue from one payer, say an uninsured person, by increasing charges to another.

Source: George Halvorson, *Strong Medicine*, 1993.

report incidents of care denials and how they were resolved. While the information is still incomplete, it suggests health plan administrators now appear reluctant to second-guess physicians, possibly fearing lawsuits or political backlash. [27]

The records show HMOs primarily denied access to medical specialists who weren't part of their network, or refused to pay for treatments the plans decided weren't essential for a patient's recovery. Also denied were experimental procedures, such as bone-marrow transplants. But the relative numbers were low: the six largest managed-care firms in New York have averaged about 2.5 appeals per 1,000 patients. In New Jersey, the state last year recorded just 69 appeals from some 2.5 million enrollees in managed care plans.

The figures bear out managed care executives' contention that the amount of denials and the appeals they generate is overstated. But the low numbers concern some health-care experts, who say plan administrators are abdicating their responsibility to control health costs, likely in response to the political pressures. There is "an urgent need for managed care to second-guess decisions by physicians [that] subject patients to needlessly risky surgery and needlessly costly tests," Alain Enthoven, a health economist and one of the academicians who coined the concept of managed care in the 1980s, proclaimed recently in *The New York Times*. [28]

OUTLOOK

Rx for Medicare?

While Congress and the Clinton administration ponder ways to rein in managed care, lawmakers simultaneously are looking at ways the industry can help solve the financial squeeze surrounding the federal Medicare program.

Medicare provides subsidized health insurance to 39 million elderly or disabled Americans. But with costs rising faster than revenues, the $207 billion-a-year system is projected to go broke in about 2008, when the first of 77 million "baby boomers" born between 1946 and 1964 begin retiring. One solution would be to introduce some form of managed competition by having the government offer incentives for private managed care plans to compete against traditional health insurers, which pay fixed rates for specific medical services. This could be accomplished by giving the elderly health-care vouchers with which they could shop for the most appropriate coverage. Because recipients are presumably more sensitive to price and quality than government bureaucrats, this system — called "premium support" — would, in theory, deliver more benefits and better care at a lower price. [29]

But the recent experience of a federal commission charged with finding a solution to Medicare's woes shows how politically difficult it is to introduce such reforms — and more broadly raises questions about whether it's at all possible to overhaul the American health system. The 17-member commission, after a year of study, in March came up one vote short of the 11 needed to endorse formal recommendations to Congress or President Clinton. Members were divided over a plan offered by panel co-chairman Sen. John B. Breaux, D-La., that would have given seniors a fixed amount of money to buy private health insurance. Opponents, particularly more liberal Democrats appointed by President Clinton, said it wouldn't necessarily save money and questioned whether it would undermine a 1960s Great Society pact to protect the nation's sick and needy.

Breaux has indicated he may take another stab by introducing legislation in the Senate. Clinton, meanwhile, has offered his own solution, proposing to divert nearly $700 billion of government surpluses over the next 15 years to shore up Medicare.

Managed care reform and Medicare reform are separate but closely related issues. Len Nichols, a health-care economist at the Urban Institute in Washington, estimates federal and local governments buy health care for approximately 27 percent of Americans through Medicare and Medicaid. Annual spending for these beneficiaries amounts to nearly 40 percent of all health services delivered — worth more than $500 billion. With a flood of current workers set to retire early in the next century and health-care costs on the rise, policy-makers know they have to control the program's costs. They can't without changing the fundamental way health care is delivered and paid for — likely through some kind of managed care legislation. But the system is so complex — and the current pace of medical breakthroughs so fast — that government regulators can't keep up.

The federal government already has tried to link managed care to Medicare. In 1997, lawmakers created Medicare+Choice, a program that created more health insurance options for seniors by making it easier for private managed care plans to enter the Medicare market. About 17 percent of all Medicare beneficiaries have since switched to HMOs, and many like their willingness to pay for preventive services and prescription drugs that currently aren't covered under traditional Medicare coverage.

The federal government has set up pilot programs in several cities to see whether Medicare costs could be reduced if HMOs had to bid for senior-citizen patients. But patient and health-care professionals' concerns that benefits would also be cut led to the scuttling of the programs in Baltimore and Denver. Implementation of a program in Phoenix, where 40 percent of area seniors are enrolled in Medicare HMOs, has been delayed.

Plan administrators also complain the government's reimbursement policies haven't adequately kept up with rising costs. In response, many managed care plans unexpectedly dropped out of Medicare or scaled back their service areas over the past two years, leaving approximately 500,000 seniors stranded. Most had to go back to conventional Medicare coverage.

"It is absolutely impossible to micromanage health care in the 21st century," Breaux said, after his panel deadlocked on the latest Medicare debate.

That assessment is shared by many experts, who caution there is no "magic bullet" to answering the larger question of how to improve health-care quality and keep costs down. Indeed, most say any practical solution will require politically unpalatable sacrifices from beneficiaries, health-care providers and insurers.

"We can no longer start our public debate with the false but comforting assumption that our social abundance can support social safety nets and minimum entitlements to everyone in society," University of Chicago legal scholar Richard A. Epstein writes in his 1997 book *Mortal Peril: Our*

Inalienable Right to Health Care?

AAHP's Ignagni puts it equally bluntly: "Republicans and Democrats both want to do something. The question is what is it, and can each side get beneath the political debate and truly assess the costs and benefits?" ∎

Notes

[1] For background, see Kenneth Jost, "Patients' Rights," *The CQ Researcher*, Feb. 6, 1998, pp. 97-120, and Sarah Glazer, "Managed Care," *The CQ Researcher*, April 12, 1996, pp. 313-336.
[2] See Katherine Levit et al., "National Health Expenditures in 1997: More Slow Growth," *Health Affairs*, November/December 1998, pp. 99-110.
[3] See Milt Freudenheim, "Group Sues to Halt Kaiser Permanente Ads," *The New York Times*, March 18, 1999, p. C7.
[4] See Julie Marquis, "HMO Case Renews Debate on Patients' Rights," *Los Angeles Times*, Jan. 22, 1999, p. A3.
[5] See Karen Foerstel, "Health Care Forces Fight To Frame the Debate," *CQ Weekly*, April 3, 1999, pp. 799-801.
[6] See Michael Conlan, "It's Up, Down: Medicaid Covers Viagra, But Insurers Cite Safety Concerns," *Drug Topics*, July 20, 1998, p. 18.
[7] See S. Rosenbaum, et al., "Who Should Determine When Health Care Is Medically Necessary?" *The New England Journal of Medicine*, Vol. 340, No. 3 (Jan. 21, 1999), pp. 229-232.
[8] See Dahlia Remler et al., "What Do Managed Care Firms Do to Affect Care?" *Inquiry*, Vol. 34 (fall 1997), pp. 196-204
[9] See "Fraud: The Hidden Cost of Health Care," Health Insurance Association of America, 1996.
[10] See Ellyn Spragins, "Making HMOs Play Fair," *Newsweek*, May 4, 1998, p. 88.
[11] For background, see "Sources of Health Insurance and Characteristics of the Uninsured," Employee Benefit Research Institute Issue Brief No. 204, December 1998.
[12] See U.S. General Accounting Office, "Managed Care: State Approaches on Selected Patient Protections," March 1999.
[13] See Karen Foerstel, "Debate on Managed Care Legislation Diverges Along Familiar Lines," *CQ Weekly*, March 20, 1999, pp. 701-702.
[14] See "The Dartmouth Atlas of Health Care 1998," *American Hospital Publishing*, 1998.
[15] See Danny McCormick et al., "Use of Aspirin, Beta-Blockers and Lipid-Lowering Medications Before Recurrent Acute Myocardial Infarction: Missed Opportunities for Prevention?" *Archives of Internal Medicine*, 159:561-567 (March 22, 1999).
[16] See Judith Graham, "Physician Performance Initiatives Gain Ground," *1999 Comparative Performance Data Sourcebook*, Faulkner & Gray Inc.
[17] See "NCQA To Require Independent Appeals," A.M. Best Co./BestWire, March 16, 1999.
[18] See Milt Freudenheim, "Concern Rising About Mergers in Health Plans," *The New York Times*, Jan. 13, 1999, p. A1.
[19] See Peter Kilborn, "400 Doctors in Dallas Break Contracts with Aetna's HMO," *The New York Times*, Oct. 20, 1998.
[20] See Michael Casey, "HMOs Tally Up Costs and Raise Their Rates," *Medical Industry Today*, Feb. 2, 1999.
[21] For background, see Stuart Altman and Uwe Reinhardt, "Strategic Choices for a Changing Health System," *Health Administration Press*, 1996.
[22] See Mary Agnes Carey, "Managed Care Overhaul Shows New Signs of Life," *CQ Weekly*, Jan. 16, 1999, pp. 129-134.
[23] See Bruce Japsen, "Employers Pool Muscle," *Chicago Tribune*, Dec. 24, 1998, p. B1.
[24] For background, see Thomas Bodenheimer and Kip Sullivan, "How Large Employers Are Shaping the Health Care Marketplace," *The New England Journal of Medicine*, Vol. 338, No. 14 (April 2, 1998), pp. 1003-1007.
[25] *Ibid.*
[26] See Jennifer Steinhauer, "Health Insurance Costs Rise, Hitting Small Business Hard," *The New York Times*, Jan. 19, 1999, p. A1.
[27] See Michael Weinstein, "Managed Care's Other Problem: It's Not What You Think," *The New York Times*, Feb. 28, 1999, p. C1.
[28] Quoted in *Ibid.*
[29] See Robert Pear, "Politically and Technically Complex, Medicare Defies a Sweeping Redesign," *The New York Times*, March 18, 1999, p. A23 and "Medicare Reform Promises, Promises," *The Economist*, March 27, 1999, pp. 29-30.

Bibliography

Selected Sources Used

Books

Altman, Stuart, and Uwe Reinhardt, eds., *Strategic Choices for a Changing Health-Care System*, Association for Health Services Research, 1996.
Two prominent health-care scholars outline policy and management issues, including health-care spending, rationing and reorganization of the delivery system.

Anders, George, *Health Against Wealth*, Houghton Mifflin, 1996.
A *Wall Street Journal* reporter documents how the HMO system can turn against patients confronting medical emergencies and serious diseases.

Epstein, Richard, *Mortal Peril: Our Inalienable Right to Health Care?* Addison-Wesley, 1997.
A University of Chicago legal scholar argues that a hands-off approach to regulating health care will guarantee greater access to quality medical care for more people.

Halvorson, George, *Strong Medicine*, Random House, 1993.
America's health system focuses on procedures, not outcomes, creating massive waste, a managed care executive contends.

Articles

Cunningham, Peter, et. al., "Managed Care and Physicians' Provision of Charity Care," *Journal of the American Medical Association*, Vol. 281 (March 24/31, 1999), pp. 1087-1092.
Health-system changes may be affecting the ability of doctors to provide care with little or no compensation from patients who are uninsured and underinsured and may result in decreased access to physicians for uninsured patients, researchers say.

Lewis, Diane, "Doctors Join Union to Fight Ills from HMOs," *The Boston Globe*, March 2, 1999, p. A1.
In an attempt to regain clout lost to HMOs, 15,000 doctors have joined a new alliance formed by the AFL-CIO and promised to fight managed care by spending $1 million over the next year to bring discontented physicians into their fold.

McLaughlin, Catherine, and Paul Ginsburg, "Competition, Quality of Care and the Role of the Consumer,"
The Milbank Quarterly, No. 4, Vol. 76 (December 1998), p. 737.
Two health-policy experts argue there is little evidence of any relationship between competition and the quality of medical care.

Millenson, Michael, "What Doctors Don't Know: Problems With the Health-Care System," *The Washington Monthly*, December 1998, No. 12, Vol. 30, p. 8.
A journalist-turned consultant argues that physician autonomy in making health-care decisions isn't always a good thing.

Rosenbaum, Sara, et al., "Who Should Determine When Health-Care is Medically Necessary," *The New England Journal of Medicine*, Vol. 340, pp. 229-232 (Jan. 21, 1999).
The authors argue that physicians, not insurers, should be responsible for deciding what care patients receive.

Samuelson, Robert, "Myth of the Managed Care Monster," *The Washington Post*, July 29, 1998, p. A21.
The economics columnist argues that, if Americans can get whatever health care they — or their doctors —want, then society will ultimately be worse off.

Reports

"Medical Necessity and Health-Plan Contracts," Health Insurance Association of America, March 1999.
A health-insurance industry analysis of proposed congressional patients'-rights legislation outlines how new regulations would mean higher costs and lower-quality care.

"Sources of Health Insurance and Characteristics of the Uninsured," Employee Benefit Research Institute, Issue Brief No. 204, December 1998.
A nonpartisan group provides comprehensive summary data on the insured and uninsured populations in the nation and in each state and discusses the characteristics most closely related to individuals' health-insurance status.

Nichols, Len, "Health-Care Quality: At What Cost?" No. 13 of the series "The Future of the Public Sector," The Urban Institute, May 1998.
As Medicare and Medicaid adopt cost-control techniques used in managed care, the author argues that the uninsured will find it even more difficult to afford medical treatment.

8 Medical Mistakes

SARAH GLAZER

Karl Shipman's fall from a ladder in 1997 should have ended in straightforward treatment for his broken wrist.

But after the 64-year-old internist's accident, almost everything that could have gone wrong did, according to his daughter Debra Malone, a nurse. First, Shipman's doctors misdiagnosed as back strain an infection in his wrist that had spread to his spine.

When his condition worsened, Shipman went to the intensive-care unit of Presbyterian-St. Luke's Medical Center, the Denver hospital where he had practiced for 35 years. There, according to Malone, a nurse who lacked intensive-care training and an intern just out of medical school failed to recognize his worsening condition. By the next morning, when a physician trained in critical care came on duty, Shipman was suffering from shock, respiratory failure and cardiovascular collapse. He died 18 days later. [1]

Shipman's case illustrates how flaws in the American system of medical care — the most technologically advanced medical system in the world — often combine with human mistakes to cause death and injury. In fact, more people die each year from medical mistakes in American hospitals than are killed in car crashes or by breast cancer or AIDS. (See table, p. 144.)

Experts have known that medical errors are widespread for more than a decade. But the problem has received a new dose of attention from the public and Congress following a recent report from the prestigious Institute of Medicine (IOM) confirming the extent of the phenomenon

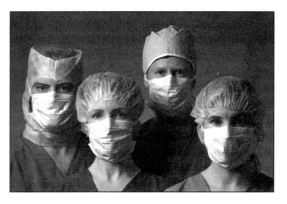

and urging reforms.[2] And on Feb. 22, President Clinton added his voice to the call for mandatory reporting of errors. (See "At Issue," p. 151.)

Shipman's case also illustrates how a hospital's refusal to admit mistakes often puts it in an adversarial position with patients and their families and blocks improvements. A blue-ribbon panel appointed by the IOM argues that the failure to acknowledge and analyze mistakes deprives hospitals of important information that could help prevent similar mistakes in the future.

The antagonism that such an attitude creates among patients' families was painfully clear last December, when Malone told a congressional committee investigating medical mistakes about her father's death.

"The pain of our loss is compounded by the knowledge that his death was probably preventable," she said. "What became even more upsetting was the stonewalling, defensive posture the hospital took when I attempted to address these issues with them. The risk-management office assured me that they had reviewed the case and found nothing wrong with the care my father received." [3]

Yet federal and state health officials probing Shipman's death found deficiencies in eight areas, especially the hospital's failure to assure that all its nurses were competent. Even then, the hospital issued an official statement con-

From *The CQ Researcher,* February 25, 2000.

tending, "the care and treatment provided was appropriate." [4]

The stand taken by Presbyterian-St. Luke's is all too common, some in the profession say. "The culture of this is that hit-and-run is OK if you don't get caught. If the patients don't sue you, you've gotten off," says Steve S. Kraman, chief of staff at the Veterans Affairs Medical Center in Lexington, Ky. The facility is one of the few hospitals in the nation that informs patients and their families if they are victims of medical error and offers to compensate them. (See story, p. 146.)

Kraman says hospitals fear that admitting mistakes will spark a double-whammy: Patients will file malpractice suits, and malpractice insurers will drop the hospital from coverage. In addition to suits, medical experts say individual doctors and nurses who are honest with patients face the prospect of being ostracized by their colleagues or fired.

The solution is to create an atmosphere in hospitals that fosters less blame, not more, according to the IOM report. "We have punitive environments in our hospitals," says IOM committee member Lucian Leape, an adjunct professor at the Harvard School of Public Health. "If something goes wrong in a hospital, the assumption is frequently that somebody screwed up, and they should be made to pay. Punishing the person turns out not to be very effective at preventing someone else from doing the same thing later. It's a system that's been used for the last hundred years, and it's gotten us where we are today — which is an incredibly unsafe system."

The IOM points to the aviation industry as its model for safety reform, noting that pilots can report errors anonymously to the National Aeronautics and Space Administra-

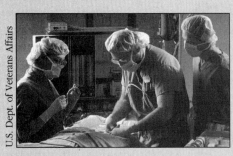

U.S. Dept. of Veterans Affairs

When Doctors Are Disciplined

Doctors in the United States committed more than 14,000 offenses for which disciplinary action was taken by a state medical board in 1995 or 1996. More than one-third of the offenses were for substandard care or resulted in a criminal conviction.

OFFENSE	NUMBER	PERCENT
Criminal conviction	2,545	18.1%
Substandard care, incompetence or negligence	2,531	18.0
Misprescribing or overprescribing drugs	1,632	11.6
Substance abuse	1,566	11.1
Professional misconduct	1,576	11.2
Noncompliance with a board order	953	6.8
Noncompliance with a professional rule	1,233	8.8
Practicing without a license	477	3.4
Practicing without a controlled-substance license	55	0.4
Providing false information to medical board	384	2.7
Sexual abuse of or sexual misconduct with a patient	425	3.0
Physical or mental impairment	365	2.6

Note: Percentages do not add to 100 because only major categories of offenses are listed.
Source: Public Citizen Health Research Group, "16,638 Questionable Doctors," 1998

tion (NASA). "The way aviation got so safe was to recognize that you didn't keep planes from crashing by punishing pilots but by redesigning the planes and the procedures and experience," says Leape, co-author of a landmark 1991 study of the high medical-error rate in New York state. "We have to take that approach in health care."

For example, simply having a doctor specially trained in critical care on duty at Presbyterian-St. Luke's' intensive care unit might have saved Shipman's life. Research suggests this step alone could reduce patient deaths by 10 percent, according to Leapfrog, a group of leading U.S. employers who are launching an effort to steer their workers to hospitals with safer practices.

But a blame-free atmosphere alone won't satisfy consumer advocates. Many consider it an outrage that prospective patients can't find out which hospitals or doctors have the best — and worst — performance records.

"The No. 1 reason these mistakes occur is because hospitals are not accountable," says Charles B. Inlander, president of the People's Medical Society, a consumers' group in Allentown, Pa. "There's no public disclosure of these mistakes. Not a single hospital in the country publicly reports its drug errors to any authority," nor its rate of hospital-

produced infections from improperly sterilized equipment. "There's not a hospital that publicly releases the names of doctors whose privileges they've suspended or revoked, which is usually done for ineptitude or negligence."

The dilemma faced by policymakers is how to balance the public's right to know with the creation of a blame-free, mistake-admitting culture. Consumers and large employers want to know hospitals' error rates so they can put market pressure on hospitals and doctors to improve patient safety. But the American Medical Association (AMA) and the American Hospital Association (AHA) counter that disclosure would only foster fear of lawsuits among doctors and nurses, making them even more secretive. And that would undermine the long-term public goal of finding out what causes errors and how to prevent them, the health industry lobbies contend.

As state and federal lawmakers, the Clinton administration and medical professionals contemplate legislation dealing with medical mistakes, here are some of the questions they are asking:

Should hospitals be required to report their medical errors?

In diluted form, potassium chloride is commonly used as an additive to intravenous solutions to replace potassium in critically ill patients. The solution is never supposed to be injected full strength. Yet each year, fatal accidents occur when hospital staffers mistakenly inject full-strength potassium chloride into severely ill patients. [5]

After Massachusetts hospitals reported several such incidents to the Massachusetts Board of Registration in Medicine, the board recommended that hospitals only stock their patient-care units with diluted potassium chloride prepared by the hospital pharmacy.

IOM panel member Leape points to Massachusetts as a model of how a state can learn from its mistakes. Hospitals there have been required to report unexpected deaths and major complications of treatment to the board since 1987, along with preventive steps they are taking.

By examining approximately 500 reports a year, the state board has identified problems ranging from chemotherapy overdoses to infections caused by certain types of endoscopic equipment used to visualize the interior of organs. It has followed up with safety alerts and guidelines to hospitals. [6]

"Most people feel this has been effective in getting hospitals to take responsibility and to make changes," Leape says. Expanding the system nationwide, he believes, "would make it possible to collect data and aggregate it and learn from it. It would make it easier for parties that have facilities in more than one state [to correct mistakes] and it would make it easier to get together and inform consumers."

Taking a cue from the aviation industry, where pilots' identities are destroyed within 72 hours after they report an error to NASA, the IOM report recommended that hospitals encourage a similar approach. [7] Near-misses — errors not resulting in serious harm — should be reported on a voluntary basis, the IOM recommends, with the information confidential and

protected by law from public scrutiny. To encourage information-sharing nationwide, the panel recommended that Congress create a Center for Patient

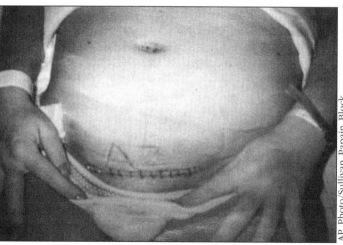

Allan Zarkin (top), a New York obstetrician, cut his initials into a patient's abdomen with a scalpel after performing a Caesarean section on her last year. It was months before his license was suspended. He faces assault charges and a $5 million lawsuit.

Safety within the federal government to track such patient safety reports, research the cause of mistakes and disseminate information on ways to prevent errors.

But, some panel members observe, deaths or serious injuries from medical errors are more akin to the devastation from a plane crash, where passengers die, and the public expects to learn findings of the investigation. For mistakes that hurt people, the panel made its most controversial recommendation — creation of a nationwide mandatory reporting system to collect such information.

About one-third of the states now require hospitals to report treatment-related deaths and injuries to state health departments. [8] State agencies would continue to be the primary collectors of that information under the recommendation. However, the panel wants to extend the system to all states and to make reporting standards uniform so the information could be shared among hospitals and state agencies.

The recommendation has strong support from consumer groups, which have been pushing for stronger reporting systems at the state level. But the AMA opposes mandatory reporting, arguing that it could open hospitals and doctors to malpractice litigation.

"If the fear of litigation continues to pervade efforts to improve patient safety and quality, our transformation into a culture of safety on behalf of our patients may never be fully realized," Nancy W. Dickey, immediate past

Three Mistakes — Three Victims

Willie King's wrong leg was amputated in 1995. Surgeon Rolando Sanchez said he realized he was removing the wrong leg after he had started cutting through the muscle of the 51-year-old diabetic, a retired equipment operator, at University Community Hospital in Tampa. Two months later, the hospital was stripped of its accreditation needed to receive Medicare and Medicaid funds. After the incident attracted national headlines, the state of Florida beefed up enforcement of its program requiring hospitals to report mistakes. Sanchez's license was suspended for six months The state Board of Medicine noted King's other leg probably would have been amputated anyway. King sued, and the hospital settled the lawsuit for $900,000. Five months later, Sanchez was accused of amputating a woman's toe without her consent, and his license was again suspended for six months. In July 1998 the state rescinded Sanchez's license for putting a catheter into a major vein of the wrong patient. He was permitted to resume his medical practice in April 1999.

❑ **Ben Kolb**, 7, died on Dec. 13, 1995, after going into the hospital for an operation to remove a benign tumor from inside his ear. A lab investigating the case later discovered that the anesthetic syringe had been filled mistakenly with topical adrenaline, a medication that is never supposed to be injected. The death spurred changes at Martine Memorial Medical Center in Stuart, Fla., which took the unusual step of informing Ben's family that his death was due to a mistake. A special filtering device is now used to transfer medications directly to a syringe and must occur under the observation of two nurses.

❑ **Betsy Lehman**, 39, a health columnist for *The Boston Globe*, died on Dec. 3, 1994, of a chemotherapy overdose at Dana-Farber Cancer Institute, where she was being treated for breast cancer. Lehman's physician mistakenly misread the dose, leading to fatal heart damage. The mistake was not discovered until February 1995, when hospital clerks were doing a routine review of records. The case made front-page headlines in the *Globe* on March 23, 1995.

president of the AMA, told the Senate Committee on Health Education, Labor and Pensions on Jan. 25.

The AHA, often an ally of the AMA, has not joined it in opposing mandatory disclosure, although it shares the AMA's concerns about liability. "The reporting systems that are in place now are inadequate," says AHA Senior Vice President Richard Wade. There is too great a fear of retribution among doctors and other hospital staff to report honestly to state agencies or hospital administrators under current systems, he says.

"You need to create a set of protections so you make it safe for people to report," Wade says. "The traditional systems for error reporting have been search and destroy. As the IOM said, this should not be about blame-fixing and finding the guilty party and firing them."

The failure of existing systems to protect patients' safety has led to the unfair singling out of nurses as scapegoats, when the real problem was a systemic failure within the hospital, according to the American Nurses Association, which supports mandatory reporting. The group points to the case of three registered nurses in Colorado who were charged with criminally negligent homicide after a medication error resulted in the death of an infant in 1996. After a physician had ordered a single, intramuscular dose of penicillin, a hospital pharmacist mistakenly sent up a much larger dose. The neonatal nurse changed the medication to intravenous to avoid sticking the child repeatedly with such a large dose. Two of the three nurses pleaded guilty and received two years' probation and 24 hours of public service. The third nurse was acquitted.

Contending that state mandatory-reporting systems have not demonstrated that they can reduce medical errors, the AMA argues against instituting mandatory reporting on a national level. IOM panel members concede they have no hard proof of the effectiveness of reporting because there have been no studies at the state level. In the two states with the most extensive reporting systems — Florida and New York — consumer advocates and state officials say inaccurate and sometimes dishonest reporting have been problems.

In Florida, which has the country's oldest and most comprehensive reporting system, hospitals reported some 5,091 patient injuries in 1998. But Ray McEachern, president of the Association for Responsible Medicine in Tampa, Fla., says Florida hospitals are "scofflaws" when it comes to the reporting system because virtually nobody reports their mistakes or errors accurately. And he says the state government is "aiding and abetting the cover-up by hiding the identity of the wrongdoers."

McEachern founded the patients-rights group in 1993 after a doctor's mistake left his wife, Pat, partially paralyzed. For the first 10 years the law was in effect, the state made no attempt to enforce it, McEachern contends. The number of errors reported doubled statewide in 1996, the year after the state began conducting on-site audits at hospitals.

Anna Polk, who directs the risk-management program that enforces the law for the Florida Agency for

Health Care Administration, concurs that Florida hospitals don't report their errors accurately, but she adds, "It's not simply Florida, it's anywhere." Hospital administrators learn of only 5 to 10 percent of the errors occurring at their own institutions, according to studies cited by Polk. She attributes Florida's under-reporting in part to a culture of silence and a fear among hospital staff that retribution from colleagues could destroy their careers.

"There can be very serious reprisals for nurses or other professionals for reporting. You just don't tell on each other. That's part of the traditional taboo that's been in place forever," Polk says. "Some doctors have told me they've suffered a loss of referrals" after discussing another doctor's mistakes in hospital meetings.

Consumers like McEachern say the solution is to strengthen Florida's reporting system, not do away with it. The state needs a tough system of verification backed up by stiff fines and criminal penalties for doctors or hospitals that fail to report errors honestly, he argues.

In New York state, where treatment-related injuries are reported more extensively than anywhere in the country — at a rate of 15,000 to 20,000 a year — the system has been plagued by underreporting, critics say, and is now in its third redesign.

"Having a collection system doesn't reduce errors; you have to act on it," says Blair Horner, legislative director of the New York Public Interest Research Group (NYPIRG), a consumers' organization.

"In New York, there's no evidence that there's been an aggressive effort to reduce errors in health-care settings."

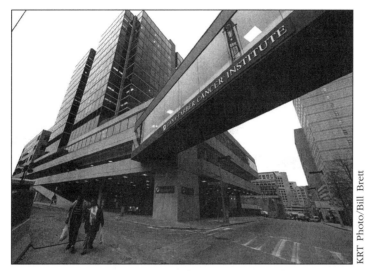

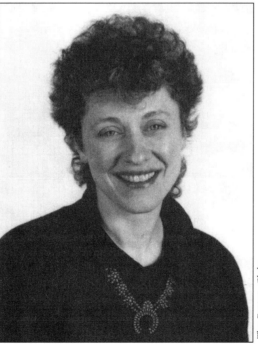

Betsy Lehman, a Boston Globe *health columnist, died in 1994 at the Dana-Farber Cancer Institute (top) when her doctor mistakenly quadrupled her chemotherapy dosage. A clerk discovered the error three months later.*

New York's reporting system was already in place in 1991 when Harvard researchers reported that close to 7,000 patients had died in one year from negligence in New York hospitals — more than died in murders or car crashes combined in New York City, according to Horner. [9] Yet even those startling statistics "never triggered any kind of patient-safety program," Horner observes. "No one has argued the number has changed."

The bizarre case of physician Allan Zarkin has highlighted further flaws in the New York system. Last year, after performing a Cesarean, Zarkin carved his initials into the patient's abdomen. Zarkin continued to practice in New York City for four months after the incident before his license was suspended. According to state officials, the hospital did not file the mandatory report on the incident to the state bureau of hospitals. Zarkin has not denied the charge, but his lawyers say he suffers from Pick's disease, an Alzheimer's-like degeneration of the brain's frontal lobe. [10]

"Zarkin's like the poster child of what can go wrong. The hospital didn't even report the incident to the state Health Department in a way that would have allowed the health commissioner to yank his license through an emergency proceeding," Horner says. "It was a classic failure of the system to protect the public. Zarkin is the most outrageous example of what happens in hospitals every day."

Horner sees the IOM report as an opportunity to push the New York state legislature to strengthen and expand its reporting program, improve the disciplinary system and create whistleblower protection for hospital workers who see mistakes or miscreant behavior. "I doubt [Zarkin] was in there by himself," Horner says. "Why didn't someone stop him? It's not that other physicians don't see what's going on. They chose not to report it."

But IOM panel member Donald M. Berwick says the public perception that most errors are caused by people like Zarkin is inaccurate. A major finding of the IOM report is that most safety problems pervade even the best organizations. "So we're not going to solve the problem by firing some docs or closing some hospitals," says Berwick, president of the Institute for Healthcare Improvement, a private organization in Boston that trains hospital staff in safer practices.

However, Berwick warns, an environment of mandated reporting and reprisal would be "pretty toxic to real improvement. Mandatory reporting will improve trust and a sense in the public that we're not hiding things," and that's the main reason the panel recommended it, he says. "But the main route to safety is through voluntary reporting and deep study about why the hazards exist."

Should reports of medical errors be made public?

Crane operator Mark Baas of Allentown, Pa., was scheduled to undergo open-heart surgery when he stumbled across a booklet that may have saved his life. It listed the bypass success rates of surgeons and hospitals throughout Pennsylvania, and to Baas' surprise ranked both his hospital and his surgeon with a minus sign. The symbol meant that more patients died there than would be expected given their risk of death before surgery. Baas also noticed that a nearby hospital rated a diamond for its surgical program, indicating its

mortality rate was within the expected range. The booklet also gave a "plus" rating to one of the hospital's doctors, signifying that he performed better than expected. Baas had his operation at the second, diamond-rated facility without incident. [11]

The booklet Baas consulted was published by the Pennsylvania Health Care Cost Containment Council, an independent state agency created in 1986 to help labor unions and businesses throughout the state find cost-effective health care. The council has reported on mortality rates, average length of hospital stays and the cost of up to 60 common medical procedures.

Some consumer advocates and major employers want similar information about the medical-error rates at hospitals that they are about to patronize. "By law, we get more information about funeral homes, bank loans and refrigerators than we do about a hospital or a doctor," says Inlander of the People's Medical Society. He argues that Pennsylvania's system for reporting mortality rates and complications from surgery — known as performance outcomes — should be the model for reporting medical errors. He points to studies showing market pressures have forced hospitals to improve and become safer.

Under the Pennsylvania system, hospitals with poor ratings have tended to lose market share at first. But in subsequent years they improved the most if they were under competitive pressures from nearby hospitals with better ratings, researchers at the University of Pittsburgh and Carnegie Mellon University concluded. Between 1992 and 1997, when ratings for coronary bypass surgery were reported annually, the state's overall death rate from the procedure dropped 26 percent, according to Joe Martin, communications director of the cost-containment council.

The IOM's proposal that hospitals be required to report their mistakes to government agencies has led many observers to assume that such reports would be available to the public in much the same form that Baas found. However, the IOM report is vague on the question of whether mandatory reports of serious harm would be available to the general public in a form that clearly identified individual doctors or hospitals.

Currently, even states that require reporting of mistakes do not disclose hospitals' or doctors' error rates. In Florida, state law forbids the agency that collects data to reveal the number of mistakes reported by an individual hospital. In New York, the state is not legally barred from releasing the number of adverse events reported by an individual hospital, but it has never done so. In most states, consumer information has been limited to the total number of adverse events reported statewide, and is sometimes broken out by type of accident.

Consumer advocates argue that members of the public should know a hospital's error rate so that they can make wise choices before receiving patient care. The IOM report has given new impetus to consumer groups in New York to lobby for making more information about hospitals and doctors accessible to consumers.

"I think the only way to get institutions to act is to make the information publicly available," says NYPIRG's Horner. His group is lobbying to beef up New York's reporting system with aggressive auditing and penalties for not reporting. As for hospital report cards on error rates, "Once we know the data is valid," he says, "then it should be reported."

Authors of the IOM report stress that the most important contribution of a national reporting system in their view would be the ability to standardize the collection of errors across

Preventing Mistakes the Modern Way

New York's Montefiore Medical Center has turned to high technology to reduce mistakes from a major source of problems. The big facility in the Bronx requires all prescriptions to be entered on a computer.

If a patient is allergic to the prescribed medication, the word "Allergy" pops up on the screen in red letters — and the computer describes how the patient may react to the incorrect drug. And if a drug is prescribed that could interact with one the patient is already taking, the computer flashes "Interaction" and warns that blood tests should be monitored to avoid a dangerous complication.

Instead of pulling out a paper chart to check a patient's prescribed medication, nurses at the hospital check a hand-held computer clamped onto their rolling equipment table. Doctors at Montefiore can write prescriptions on their home computers, at their office or on a wireless hand-held computer in the patient's room. Not only that, if one of their patients walks into any of Montefiore's 35 outpatient centers, the medical staff can pull up his most recent prescriptions and entire medical history.

Montefiore is among only 1 percent of U.S. hospitals that require all drug and patient orders to be entered directly into a computer.

Yet about 20 percent of hospitals have the technological capacity to do so, according to Arnold Milstein of the Leapfrog Group. The group of leading employers, including General Motors, is using its market power to encourage more hospitals to adopt the system. A study at Brigham and Women's Hospital in Boston found that direct computer entry by doctors reduced the rate of serious medication errors by more than half. [1]

If such a system had been in place at Boston's Dana-Farber Cancer Institute in December 1994, it could have prevented the mistaken chemotherapy dose that killed 39-year-old *Boston Globe* reporter Betsy Lehman, some experts believe. Dana-Farber's computer system was set to go into operation a few months after Lehman died. [2]

Perhaps the most obvious problem the system corrects is doctors' notoriously illegible handwriting. "A lot of mistakes go with paper order entry," says Robert Lynn, a kidney specialist at Montefiore. "I've had orders not followed because people can't read my handwriting."

The system also avoids the kinds of mistakes that used to arise if there was a discrepancy between the prescription sent to the pharmacy and the paper order the nurse was consulting. "Now everyone's looking at the same screen," nurse Christine Imperio says, because the doctor's order arrives simultaneously at the computers in the pharmacy and nurse's station. The warning signals in the program make it "harder to order the wrong dose," she adds.

Not surprisingly, the system has glitches. Lynn complains that it takes longer to enter batches of orders than to scribble them on a piece of paper. The red-letter "Interaction" warning comes up so frequently in the program, he says, that hospital staffs tend to ignore it.

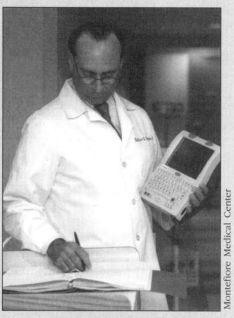

Dr. Matthew A. Berger of Montefiore Medical Center, New York City, uses a hand-held computer to write prescriptions.

Matthew A. Berger, medical director of Montefiore's clinical information system, says the system permits a large hospital like Montefiore to track how long it takes a patient to receive a test or an antibiotic from the time it is ordered and to improve its overall procedures. Moreover, hospital staff cannot erase orders to cover up mistakes, a well-recognized problem for state regulators overseeing hospitals. [3]

"You wouldn't run a big bank or a business without an inventory-control system. That's why a big hospital is willing to put up $10-$20 million for this," Berger says. Training staff on the system is costly, he says, requiring two weeks of initial training followed by two weeks of follow-up help.

Cost is the main reason the system has not been more widely adopted, according to Richard Wade, a spokesman for the American Hospital Association. "More than 40 percent of hospitals are in some kind of financial difficulty," he says. "One-third to one-half of our hospitals couldn't think of anything that expensive today." For rural hospitals, he adds, "It may not be the most effective use of the money in a 20-bed hospital."

---

[1] David W. Bates et al., "Effect of Computerized Physician Order Entry and a Team Intervention on Prevention of Serious Medication Errors," *Journal of the American Medical Association*, Oct. 21, 1998, pp. 1311-1316.

[2] Michael L. Millenson, *Demanding Medical Excellence* (1997), p. 91.

[3] Robert Gray Palmer, "Altered and 'lost' medical records," *Trial*, May 1999, pp. 31-36.

The High Toll of Medical Mistakes

Between 44,000 and 98,000 people die each year because of mistakes in medical treatment in hospitals, according to two recent studies. Medical errors ranked eighth among the top causes of death in the United States in 1997, even when the lower estimate is used.

Heart disease	727,000
Cancer	540,000
Stroke	160,000
Lung disease	109,000
Accidents	96,000
Pneumonia and flu	86,000
Diabetes	63,000
Medical errors	44,000
Breast cancer	42,000
Suicide	31,000
Kidney disease	25,000
Homicide	20,000
AIDS	17,000

Sources: Centers for Disease Control and Prevention; Institute of Medicine

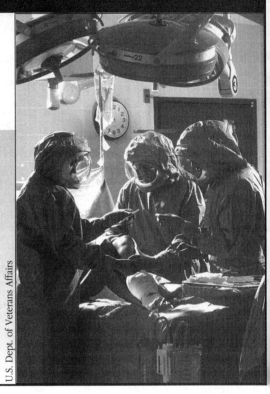

U.S. Dept. of Veterans Affairs

state lines. That way the medical profession could learn what kinds of practices across the nation are causing errors and could help hospitals learn how to prevent them by sharing that information.

Most state laws consider the information in internal hospital reviews of physicians' competency as privileged and unavailable to patients or the public. But a recent investigation by the *Philadelphia Inquirer* of records at the Medical College of Pennsylvania Hospital opened during a bankruptcy proceeding revealed hundreds of cases of patients killed or injured by medical errors. Neither the patients nor their families, however, had been informed. In one case, doctors operated on the wrong side of a patient's chest; he died three months later. The family learned of the mistake from the Inquirer. [12]

The IOM panel wrestled with the conflict between providing a non-punitive atmosphere, where doctors feel free to report mistakes, and the public's right to know, several panel members say. "We have to balance the very real need for accountability with the reality that reporting is often punishment — and often unjustified," says Leape, who opposes identifying doctors involved in mistakes. "Our feeling is we should hold the institutions responsible," he says, "and that's where the reporting level ought to be."

Lowell S. Levin, a professor emeritus of public health at Yale University, believes hospital errors should be visible. "After all, these are mainly public institutions," he says. "If not publicly owned, they're publicly supported. And as taxpayers and citizens we're entitled to full disclosure of all that goes on within the walls of these institutions."

Powerful groups with very different interests in the availability of such information are primed to clash over how much should be made public. In response to the IOM report, a group of leading employers, including General Motors Corp., has launched an effort to steer its employees to hospitals with the lowest rates of error-caused death or serious injury. The Leapfrog Group is a steering committee of The Business Roundtable in Washington, D.C., which represents 100 of America's leading corporations, employing approximately 10 million Americans.

The error rates reported by the IOM "imply that every hour one of our member-company enrollees suffers an avoidable death and five suffer an avoidable disability due to hospital errors," said Leapfrog member Arnold Milstein, medical director of the Pacific Business Group on Health. [13]

Milstein says he would like to see hospital-by-hospital reporting of deaths and serious injuries publicized. Leapfrog is developing purchasing standards to guide companies in choosing health-care providers with the best quality and safety records.

According to Milstein, the group wants to send hospitals and health plans a blunt message: "Depending on your performance, we'll encourage our people to use you, discourage our people from using you, we'll exclude you or we'll vary how much we pay you."

The AMA and AHA insist such information should remain confidential because it could open the medical profession to lawsuits and also could give the public a misleading picture of which hospitals are most dangerous. Both organizations caution that hospitals that report the highest death and injury rates may be those with sicker populations or ones that perform more difficult surgeries.

"Whatever we do has to have a degree of honesty with the public where it's useful information and it's not something that frightens the public and unfairly paints a picture of what may be happening," says the AHA's Wade.

A mandatory reporting system is unlikely to provide a reliable report card along the lines the business groups are hoping for, some experts believe. "To try to say, based on the number of error reports you get through mandatory reporting, that you will show that one hospital is better than another is wishful thinking and will do a great disservice," Leape cautions. "It will penalize those hospitals that are honest and report their errors and let the ones that cheat get away with it."

Whether or not statistics are published for each hospital, doctors and hospitals fear malpractice lawyers would engage in a feeding frenzy to try to subpoena any information collected by state health departments as part of pretrial discovery. Any approach to improving patient safety, the AMA has testified, should include "federally guaranteed legislative protection from discovery for all aspects of information gathered to improve patient safety." [14]

But does the risk of a lawsuit justify withholding the information, particularly from a patient who has been seriously injured? "Should the injured party have a right to know? Our answer is yes," says the IOM panel's Berwick. " The committee's view is that there is a moral obligation to reveal that. Right now, hospitals would object to even that. Although they might say it's ethical to tell them, they'd say it's unrealistic to tell them because of the malpractice climate."

Some legal experts agree that public release of hospital errors could influence litigation. "If five people come to your law office Thursday and ask if you'll take their cases, and one of them says he was injured in a hospital with pretty bad numbers to begin with, that might seem like a better target of opportunity," says Thomas W. Mayo, an associate professor of law at Southern Methodist University who specializes in health care.

But Mayo doubts that publicizing such information would initiate a flood of lawsuits. He points to the federal government's former practice of reporting mortality levels at hospitals providing Medicare. For several years, those reports were published annually in local newspapers. They came in for harsh criticism from hospitals for failing to adjust the statistics according to the relative sickness of each hospital's population. Even so, "The sky didn't fall in with those numbers being reported every year," Mayo says, in terms of malpractice claims against hospitals with comparatively worse data.

Only a tiny percentage of injured patients ever file malpractice suits, and of those a very small percentage wins, experts agree. [15] Under lobbying pressure from the medical profession, several states have passed tort-reform laws placing caps on damages a patient can win in a medical malpractice suit or placing other hurdles to filing. Those laws have dampened lawyers' interest in bringing such cases to court. "Across the board, malpractice suits are down, especially in states with historically high rates of malpractice filings — Florida, New York, Texas, California — because of tort-reform measures," Mayo observes.

In Pennsylvania, individual physician ratings have not led to a single lawsuit, according to Martin of the cost-containment council. New York publicizes mortality rates for coronary-artery bypass surgeries for each surgeon and each hospital. The publicity has not spurred malpractice suits in New York, according to the designer of the system, Edward Hannan, chairman of the Department of Health Policy Management at the State University of New York at Albany.

Some experts remain skeptical that confidentiality protection will make much difference in encouraging honest reporting of errors. In Florida, for example, although state law makes hospital reports of errors confidential, hospitals still underreport, Polk notes.

Is the current system of disciplining doctors working?

To consumer advocate Horner, prospective patients in New York have to act like James Bond to find out if any complaints have been filed against the doctor they're considering using. Like virtually all the states, New York won't release information on pending complaints — only those that have resulted in final action. [16] Even then, many consumers don't know where to find the information, Horner says. In some states, the state board can take years to reach a decision on a complaint while the doctor is still practicing — two-and-a-half years on average in Virginia, for example. [17]

But conscientious consumers in New York would have to work even

When Honesty Is the Cheapest Policy

Kentucky farmer Claudie Holbrook, 67, died of a blood clot in his lung in 1997 because he had been getting the wrong formulation of blood-thinning medicine for several months.

But the Veterans Affairs Medical Center in Lexington, Ky., didn't try to cover up the Army veteran's death. Hospital officials informed the family that the hospital's medication error was responsible. The hospital's attorney also explained that the family could file a lawsuit against the hospital, offered to help fill out the paperwork and proposed a monetary settlement as an alternative. [1] Even more surprising, Holbrook's family decided not to sue.

Contradicting the conventional wisdom among hospitals that admitting errors is an invitation to lawsuits, the big hospital has discovered it can limit the costs associated with malpractice suits by reporting mistakes to patients or their families as soon as possible and offering reasonable compensation. In a study comparing the Kentucky hospital with 35 similar veterans' hospitals from 1990 to 1996, the Kentucky hospital paid less than all but seven other facilities. In five of the hospital's 88 malpractice claims for hospital errors involving death or injury during that period, the patients probably would not have learned of the mistake if the hospital had not told them, according to the study's lead author, Steve S. Kraman, the facility's chief of staff. [2]

Holbrook's family received an indication that Holbrook had been getting the wrong medication about a week before he went into the hospital with the fatal blood clot.

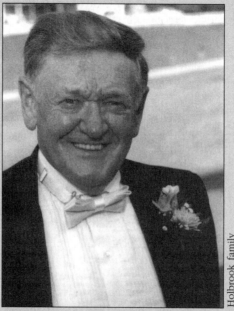

After an error killed Claudie Holbrook in 1997, the Veterans Affairs Medical Center in Lexington, Ky., admitted responsibility and offered to compensate his family.

Holbrook family

A supervisor for the home-nursing agency that was monitoring Holbrook's blood told the family he had the wrong medication. The hospital's pharmacy mistakenly had supplied Holbrook with a blood thinner that was one-tenth the strength needed to combat his blood-clotting disorder, according to Kraman. The mistake apparently came about because the pharmacy was not accustomed to sending the high-concentration version home with a patient, Kraman says.

Holbrook's daughter Sandy Reynolds, the main family member responsible for injecting her father with the blood-thinner twice a day over a 13-month period, remembers being wracked with guilt, anger and questions about his medication as she drove her father to the hospital one final time that morning in February 1997. In two previous visits to the hospital, she says, the medical staff found her father's blood at dangerous levels of viscosity but still didn't catch the medication mistake. If the hospital had not later admitted its mistake, the Kentucky business-woman says, "I would have been madder than hell and I would have sued them."

Instead, the hospital's attorney and a hospital nurse visited the family several weeks after Holbrook's death and, in Reynolds' words, admitted "they were responsible for my dad's death." It was an emotional scene, and Reynolds broke down crying. "The people that came out and dealt with us were very friendly and caring, and patted and hugged and cried a little bit. It appeared as if they were truly sorry," Reynolds recalls.

One of the reasons the family decided not to sue was that the compensation the hospital offered was similar to

harder to uncover a doctor's malpractice history. That's because they would have to travel to every courthouse in the state where a suit has been filed. The state collects that information but doesn't make it available.

Horner's group has been lobbying the state's legislature to pass a bill

known as "Lisa's Law," in memory of Lisa Smart, a 30-year-old woman who died in 1997 during routine gynecological surgery at Beth Israel Medical Center in Manhattan. An assisting surgeon was on probation with the state at the time. The bill would expand the information currently available on the state Health

Department's Web site by including a doctor's malpractice history, educational background and any dismissal from a hospital staff.

Lisa's Law is modeled after a Massachusetts law that makes a doctor's malpractice history publicly available on a comparative basis with other doctors in the same

the amount their attorney told them to expect from a lawsuit, Reynolds says. The settlement of $50,000 was modest, Reynolds concedes. But she said that next to an apology, the most important thing to her was the hospital's commitment to make sure that kind of mistake never happened again. "If we can get one pharmacist to check the zeros, one doctor to think twice, then Dad didn't die without a purpose," she says.

In response to Holbrook's death, the hospital has made several changes. It has placed the high-concentration blood-thinner in a different section of the pharmacy from the low-dose version to avoid mix-ups, according to Kraman. It has placed more pharmacists on duty during the pharmacy's busiest time of day. Now no patient leaves the hospital without an individual consultation with the pharmacist in a private booth on how to use prescribed medicine. And University of Kentucky faculty are teaching the case to medical students as an example of how medical errors can happen.

What most injured patients and their families want are an apology and a promise that the problem will be fixed to prevent future errors, Kraman has found. "Sometime if they get the first two, they don't want monetary compensation. They've resisted occasionally, and we've had to talk people into accepting it," Kraman says. The hospital has only been forced to pay malpractice judgments twice in the 13 years since initiating its tell-and-pay approach.

The hospital initiated its rather radical policy in 1987 after losing two malpractice judgments totaling more than $1.5 million. A policy advising veterans' hospitals to inform patients of their rights to file claims for hospital-caused injuries has been buried in the policy manual of the Department of Veterans Affairs (VA) since 1995. But hospital attorney Ginny Hamm says Lexington is the first in the system to carry out the policy aggressively. Partly in response to the publication of Kraman's article last December, the VA is considering a new policy of actively informing patients of error-caused injuries, according to VA spokesman Terry Jemison. "In recent months we've become much more committed to a corporate atmosphere of reporting errors" at all VA hospitals, Jemison says.

The Kentucky hospital's experience seems to confirm several studies finding that almost all medical malpractice cases involve a breakdown in the physician-patient relationship. Almost half of newborn-related injury lawsuits in Florida were motivated by a suspicion of a cover-up or a desire for revenge, one study found.[3]

In an accompanying editorial, Albert W. Wu of Johns Hopkins University School of Medicine, in Baltimore, Md., called the Lexington center's approach "the rare solution that is both ethically correct and cost-effective." But Wu also raised some questions about how well the VA's experience would transfer to non-federal hospitals. The VA's patients consist mainly of "older men of limited means, a group that may have finite expectations and a low level of litigiousness," Wu noted. In the Veterans Affairs system, patients can also qualify for compensation without a finding of negligence if their injuries are "service connected."[4]

Hospitals that are privately insured would probably have to persuade their insurance companies that a policy of open disclosure would cost them less in liability and litigation costs than the usual policy of keeping mum, Kraman concedes. But he's convinced that "one lawsuit with a cover-up" could cost 10 times more than the value of the case. "If you make errors and hide in the bushes hoping no one will sue you, it will be impossible for [an injured patient's] lawyers to ignore that," Kraman says. "If you identify the errors and fairly compensate the patients, then there's nothing for the lawyers to do."

---

[1] Under the Federal Tort Claims Act, a veteran can sue a VA hospital for compensatory damages. The United States government is not liable for punitive damages. However, federal judges have wide discretion on awarding damages and some judgments have been in the millions of dollars. In order for the Lexington VA hospital to offer a payment to an injured patient, the patient must first file a claim under the Tort Claims Act and the hospital must offer to settle it before it reaches court.

[2] Steve S. Kraman and Ginny Hamm, "Risk Management: Extreme Honesty May Be the Best Policy," Annals of Internal Medicine, Dec. 21, 1999, pp. 963-967.

[3] Cited in Albert W. Wu, "Handling Hospital Errors: Is Disclosure the Best Defense?" Annals of Internal Medicine, Dec. 21, 1999, pp. 970-972.

[4] Ibid., p. 971.

---

specialty.[18] The Medical Society of New York strongly opposes posting doctors' malpractice histories, contending that the data can be misleading because some specialties have higher rates of malpractice suits, as do doctors who take on high-risk cases. The society also argues that there could be internal politics behind a doctor's dismissal from a hospital.[19]

The issue has taken on greater urgency in New York because of the Zarkin case. At the time that he cut his initials in a patient's abdomen, the Department of Health had already received at least two patient complaints about the doctor, one well over a year old. But neither the abused patient nor a clinic director who hired Zarkin after the incident could have known that, because health officials were not permitted to say he was being investigated until his license was officially suspended.[20]

Consumer advocates have long argued that the self-policing approach of state medical boards is inadequate for disciplining negligent doctors, in large part because doctors form the majority of every medical board in the country. "It's the foxes guarding the chicken coops because the boards are predominantly physicians," Inlander says. "They are not protecting the public; they are protecting the industry."

The number of doctors disciplined is very low compared with those thought to be negligent or substandard. In 1985, *The New England Journal of Medicine* concluded that 5 percent of the nation's doctors "ought not to be practicing." But that year less than one-half of 1 percent were disciplined. [21] According to the Public Citizen Health Research Group, only 2,731 doctors nationwide were subject to serious discipline in 1996. By contrast, the consumers' group estimates that some 80,000 patients are killed and 234,000 injured as a result of negligence in hospitals. [22] The group's director, Dr. Sidney Wolfe, calls that a "worrisome discrepancy."

Furthermore, consumers argue, disciplinary action is too soft. Only 32 percent of the physicians disciplined for substandard care, incompetence or negligence in 1996 had to stop practicing, even temporarily, according to the Health Research Group. [23]

Wide discrepancies among states' rates of discipline seem to reflect how tough a state's board is on doctors, rather than the quality of its professionals. "People who live in a state with poor doctor discipline such as Massachusetts are at risk of being injured or killed by doctors who would have been thrown out of the practice of medicine in states that are more aggressive like Vermont," Wolfe asserts.

Dr. James Winn, executive vice president of the Federation of State Medical Boards, disputes these criticisms. He says it is not clear what portion of negligence incidents each year is caused by doctors, as opposed to nurses and other hospital professionals. Winn also disagrees that the boards are soft on doctors.

"Medical boards come into play when there is a pattern of care that is obviously substandard," Winn says. "I've seen no medical boards giving out a weak slap on the wrist for those kind of doctors."

But Winn believes the boards are hobbled by insufficient reporting of bad doctors. Citing the 1991 Harvard study in New York, Winn notes that only a tiny percent of the state's 7,000 deaths and 877 disability cases caused by negligence resulted in lawsuits. "If it didn't result in a lawsuit, I can guarantee it didn't get reported to the medical board," Winn says. "You can't turn around and say the medical board is doing a weak job because they're not disciplining people they don't even know about."

Currently, the federation believes hospitals are not reporting all cases of negligence to state medical boards, according to Winn, although he says he's not sure how widespread underreporting is. Under a 1986 law establishing a National Practitioner Data Bank, hospitals must report to the data bank and to their state medical boards whenever they deny hospital privileges to a doctor for more than 30 days. Hospitals are required to consult the data bank before hiring a doctor to find out whether the doctor has ever lost hospital privileges, had his license suspended in another state or been the subject of malpractice suits. But hospitals are often reluctant to suspend privileges for fear the doctor will sue them, Winn says.

"We are aware of situations where lawyers for the [disciplined] physician and lawyers for the hospital board create a settlement of a problem [of substandard care] where the

doctor just moves to another locality or state so that they avoid any reporting requirement," Winn says. "So the incident doesn't get reported; the guy just gets out of town."

One of the data bank's main purposes was to keep doctors whose licenses had been lifted by one state from jumping to another state to practice, unbeknown to a state board or hospital. However, under pressure from doctors, Congress closed the only national repository on doctors' disciplinary records to the public. This remains a sore point with consumers.

"Here you are gathering all the information about the lousy things doctors do, and it's closed to the public because the AMA moaned, groaned and donated," Inlander says. "It turns out to be one of the most anti-consumer pieces of legislation ever passed." ∎

BACKGROUND

Common Malady

The plague of medical mistakes in modern American medicine is actually old news. In *Demanding Medical Excellence*, author and health consultant Michael L. Millenson quotes a doctor as early as 1955 describing accidents produced by well-intentioned therapy as "one of the commonest conditions" in a hospital. But Millenson argues that doctors tended to view such accidents as the inevitable cost of practicing increasingly complex modern medicine. [24]

In the 1970s, a sudden surge in malpractice premiums raised the question of whether the cause was improved lawyering or declining doctoring. A large-scale study backed

Chronology

1950s *Some doctors acknowledge that well-intentioned physicians are injuring patients in hospitals, but the medical profession takes no active steps to combat mistakes.*

1955
Journal of the American Medical Association publishes article by David Barr calling accidents from medical treatment one of the "commonest" conditions in hospitals.

———— • ————

1970s *Malpractice insurance premiums skyrocket, raising questions about how much litigation stems from faulty medical care.*

1978
Study of California hospitals backed by California Medical Association finds medical treatment is killing more Americans per year than in the entire Vietnam War.

———— • ————

1990s *Widely publicized cases of patients killed or hurt by hospital mistakes and new studies finding widespread errors raise public awareness of medical mistakes.*

1991
Harvard study of New York hospitals is published in *New England Journal of Medicine* finding substantial number of patients die from medical errors

— 98,000 each year nationwide in today's terms.

1992
Harvard study is corroborated by study of Colorado and Utah hospital patients who die from errors — or 44,000 Americans each year.

1993
Ray McEachern founds a patients'-rights group, the Association for Responsible Medicine in Tampa, Fla., after a doctor's mistake leaves his wife, Pat, partially paralyzed.

February 1995
Willie King, a retired equipment operator, has the wrong leg amputated at a Tampa hospital.

March 1995
Boston Globe reports that health columnist Betsy Lehman died from a chemotherapy overdose because of a hospital staff error.

December 1995
Seven-year-old Ben Kolb enters Stuart, Fla., hospital for minor ear operation and dies after being injected with the wrong medication.

1996
The number of medical errors reported at Florida hospitals doubles a year after the state began conducting on-site audits at hospitals.

September 1999
Philadelphia Inquirer series reports hundreds injured and 66 killed by errors at a Philadelphia hospital after records are opened in bankruptcy proceedings.

Nov. 29, 1999
Institute of Medicine issues report urging the nation to cut the death and injury rate from medical errors.

———— • ————

2000 *Members of Congress and administration officials study ways to implement Institute of Medicine proposals to reduce errors.*

Jan. 25, 2000
Senate Appropriations Subcommittee on Labor holds hearings on medical errors.

Jan. 26, 2000
Senate Committee on Health, Education, Labor and Pensions holds first of a series of hearings on medical mistakes.

Feb. 8, 2000
Sens. Arlen Specter, R-Pa., and Tom Harkin, D-Iowa, introduce legislation encouraging states to report hospital errors. The bill would give grants to states to collect information on medical errors and to pass it on to the federal Agency for Healthcare Research and Quality. Responding to concerns of the American Medical Association and the American Hospital Association, all information collected by the federal government would be barred from use in pretrial discovery or Freedom of Information Act inquiries.

Feb. 22, 2000
President Clinton calls for mandatory reporting of medical errors.

by the California Medical Association sampled over 20,000 medical charts from 23 California hospitals in 1974. It concluded that one patient in 20 was harmed by treatment. On a nationwide basis, the California study suggested hospital care produced 121,000 deaths every year. [25]

If that statistic was right, it meant that medical treatment was killing twice as many Americans in a single year as died in the Vietnam War.

The 1991 Harvard study, which reviewed 30,000 of New York's 1984 hospital discharges, reported figures similar to the California findings. Extrapolated on a nationwide basis to current-day figures — the more than 33 million admissions to U.S. hospitals in 1997 — the Harvard study suggests that as many as 98,000 patients die each year from medical errors. [26] This figure has been widely quoted as the upper end of the range reported by the IOM study.

Disability or prolonged hospitalization caused by medical management occurred in 3.7 percent of the hospitalizations, the New York study found. The proportion of such "adverse events" attributable to errors and therefore preventable was 58 percent. Twenty-eight percent of the "adverse events" were linked to negligence. Of those, almost 14 percent resulted in death, and almost 3 percent caused permanent, disabling injuries. Drug complications were the most common adverse event, followed by wound infections and technical complications. [27]

The Harvard findings have since been corroborated by a study of hospital discharges in Colorado and Utah in 1992. Extrapolation to current nationwide hospital admissions led the IOM to its lower-range estimate that at least 44,000 Americans die in hospitals each year as a result of preventable medical errors. [28]

Although the Harvard findings have been widely quoted since the IOM report came out last year, at the time of their publication in 1991, the headlines announcing the study "changed nothing at all," Millenson writes. The following year, a study of Harvard's own hospitals found injuries from preventable drug errors were "common." [29]

Perhaps more effective in shaking up public complacency about hospital treatment was a *Boston Globe* report in March 1995 that a young health columnist for the newspaper, Betsy Lehman, had died of a chemotherapy overdose. Lehman's death at Boston's Dana-Farber Cancer Institute had been due to a rather simple mistake: Her physician believed that the figure showing the total dose of the chemotherapy drug over a four-day period was the amount to be given each day for four days. [30]

Even more horrifying, the error was only discovered three months later by Dana-Farber clerks — not clinicians — during a routine review of the records. [31]

A series in the *Philadelphia Inquirer* in September of last year also shook up health-industry observers. The newspaper's search of medical records at the Medical College of Pennsylvania hospital found that hundreds of patients had been seriously injured and at least 66 had died after medical mistakes from 1988 to 1989. The paper discovered that its numbers mirrored estimates by Harvard's Leape that 1 million patients nationwide are injured each year by errors. [32]

The series also highlighted the fact that patients are rarely informed of mistakes. In a 1991 study, researchers at the University of California found only 24 percent of medical residents told patients or their families of mistakes. [33]

It's not clear whether medical errors are on the rise, but some observers fear the problem may be growing as more drugs are prescribed, technology becomes more complex and untrained staff are put in jobs beyond their competency. From 1983 to 1993, medication errors produced a twofold increase in inpatient deaths and an eightfold increase in outpatient deaths, according to the IOM. [34]

Starting in the 1990s, hospitals searching for ways to cut overhead actually had cleaning and maintenance staff handle some tasks once performed by nurses, giving them minimal training to operate or interpret results from complex machinery, says Mary Foley, president of the American Nurses Association.

"You do wonder whether we are back to the way it is in the Middle East, where you need a family 'sitter' to sit there and make sure everything is handled correctly," Foley says. "Someone terribly ill is the last person who can look up and say, 'Is that the right antibiotic?'" ∎

CURRENT SITUATION

Harsh Criticism

The existing system of hospital regulation has come in for harsh criticism from consumers' groups. Most of the mud slinging has been aimed at the main body charged with inspecting and accrediting hospitals, the Joint Commission for Accreditation of Healthcare Organizations.

"The joint commission is essentially a wholly owned subsidiary of the hospitals," says Public Citizen's Wolfe, noting that hospitals pay the commission to inspect them. "It does a lousy job. It should be abolished."

At Issue:

Should hospitals be required to report deaths and serious injuries resulting from their medical mistakes?

BILL CLINTON
President of the United States

FROM STATEMENT DELIVERED AT THE WHITE HOUSE, FEB. 22, 2000

Last December, I directed our . . . health-care quality task force to analyze the [Institute of Medicine] study [and] to report back with recommendations about how we can follow the suggestions they made to protect patients and promote safety. This morning I received the task force report, and I am proud to accept all its recommendations.

Our goal is to . . . reduce preventable medical errors by 50 percent within five years. Today I announce our national action plan to reach that goal. . . .

First . . . I propose the creation of a new center for quality improvement and patient safety. My budget includes $20 million to support the center, which will invest in research, develop national goals, issue an annual report on the state of patient safety and translate findings into better practices and policies.

Second, we will ensure that each and every one of the 6,000 hospitals participating in Medicare has patient-safety programs in place to prevent medical errors, including medication mistakes. . . .

Third, as we seek to make sure that the right systems are in place, we need to make sure they are working. Today I am releasing our plan for a nationwide state-based system of reporting medical errors, to be phased-in over time. This will include mandatory reporting of preventable medical errors that cause death or serious injury and voluntary reporting of other medical mistakes. . . .

We also wanted to replace what some call a culture of silence with a culture of safety — an environment that encourages others to talk about errors, what caused them and how to stop them in the first place. So we'll support legislation that protects provider and patient confidentiality, but that does not undermine individual rights to remedies when they have, in fact, been harmed. . . .

Finally, I'm . . . calling on the Food and Drug Administration to develop new standards to help prevent medical errors caused by drugs that sound similar or packaging that looks similar. In addition, we'll develop new label standards that highlight common drug interactions and dosage errors.

Taken together, these actions represent the most significant effort our nation has ever made to reduce medical errors. It's a balance, a common-sense approach based on prevention, not punishment, on problem solving, not blame-placing.

NANCY W. DICKEY, M.D.
Immediate past president, American Medical Association

STATEMENT, FEB. 22, 2000

The AMA supports President Clinton's goal of reducing health-system errors and improving patient safety, and we agree with many of his proposals.

However, we are concerned that the proposal for mandatory reporting will not improve patient safety and may, in fact, have the perverse result of driving errors underground. Effective aviation safety programs have taught us that a culture of safety is created by avoiding a culture of blame. The same principle holds true for the health system.

The AMA and the medical-specialty societies have been pioneers in the effort to reduce health-system errors. Based on our work, we agree with many of the president's proposals for steps that the private sector and government can take to improve patient safety.

We support the president's call for increased funds to research errors and disseminate the findings to improve health care. We also concur with the proposal to modify pharmaceutical packaging and marketing practices to reduce medication errors. Prompt action is needed on many consensus areas for improving patient safety.

However, the AMA is opposed to the expansion of mandatory reporting of medical errors. There is no evidence to show that mandatory reporting improves patient safety. Before we expand data collection activities, we need to analyze existing state systems to determine the most effective use of finite resources.

The AMA appreciates President Clinton's statement of support for protecting the confidentiality of peer-review activities.

But we are concerned that the protections do not go far enough to promote the type of information sharing that would help create a culture of safety where all members of the health system can learn from and prevent errors.

About 70 percent of the organization's funding comes from the fees it collects for inspections, but that's not much different from an accounting firm whose clients pay it by the audit, responds commission President Dennis S. O'Leary.

In Wolfe's view, the IOM's call for a nationwide, mandatory-reporting system for medical errors is a "an indirect slap at the joint commission because if they were doing their job, they would get these data and make them public."

Over the past three years, less than 1 percent of the 5,000 hospitals the organization inspects have failed to receive accreditation. The commission's efforts to get hospitals to report serious injuries or deaths from errors are equally unimpressive. Over a five-year period, the organization received fewer than 500 reports from the 5,000 hospitals it inspects, fewer than would be expected from one large hospital, critics say.

"These are pathetically small numbers," O'Leary agrees. "We are a classic example of why voluntary reporting doesn't work." Hospitals "are afraid to report in the absence of confidentiality protections, because they think it will create a feast for trial lawyers."

The AHA's Wade confirms that hospitals became increasingly mistrustful of the joint commission once states used the organization as a proxy for state licensure, and the federal government tied conditions for participating in Medicare to accreditation. "The hospitals say they're paying the joint commission to be a consultant," Wade says. "They ask 'Are you a performance-improvement consultant or the cop from Washington, D.C.?'"

Both organizations say the solution to honest reporting is providing federal guarantees of confidentiality so hospital staff won't be afraid to report errors. O'Leary adds that he thinks it is just a matter of time before mandatory reporting goes into effect.

Like an Army base that gets a new coat of paint just before inspection, hospitals spend months getting ready for the joint commission's regular, announced inspections every three years. That may be one reason the commission rarely flunks a hospital for accreditation, critics charge. Even for "surprise" inspections, hospitals are routinely given at least 24 hours' notice. In the wake of the IOM report and an extremely critical report from the inspector general of the Department of Health and Human Services (HHS) last year, the commission has announced that it will start making surprise inspections without prior notice this year.

Doctors' Offices

While most estimates of medical errors focus on hospitals, injurious mistakes could be occurring at an even higher rate in doctors' offices, some consumer advocates believe. "The worst place to have anything done is the doctor's office," Inlander says. "No one is monitoring them."

In recent years, patients have been undergoing a growing range of elective surgeries, from laser eye surgery to knee operations, in doctors' offices and other types of outpatient clinics. Such facilities are rarely subject to state requirements for reporting error-related injuries. Most don't have to undergo any kind of licensing inspection. As a result, there's little hard data about what happens.

Nevertheless, some recent reports are disturbing. The death rate for liposuction, the popular cosmetic surgery performed mainly in doctors' offices and clinics, is 20 to 60 times higher than the death rate for all operations performed in hospitals, according to a recent study. In liposuction, fat is sucked out of the thighs, bellies and other parts of the body, usually by plastic surgeons. More than 170,000 people undergo the procedure each year. The study published in *Plastic and Reconstructive Surgery*, found that for every 5,000 liposuction procedures from 1994 to 1998, one patient died. [35]

Harvard's Leape calls that death rate "pretty scary." The IOM panel has recommended that mandatory reporting of medical errors should be required initially of hospitals but eventually should be expanded to walk-in settings as well. Leape says the few studies of major procedures performed outside hospitals suggest "their risk of errors and injuries is about the same as in the hospital, and possibly even worse. ◼

OUTLOOK

Doctors vs. Consumers?

As Congress begins drafting legislation aimed at tackling medical errors, the interests of hospitals and doctors already are colliding with those of consumers and employers. On Feb. 8, the first major bill — the Medical Error Reduction Act of 2000 — was introduced by Sens. Arlen Specter, R-Pa., and Tom Harkin, D-Iowa. It would keep all medical information collected by the federal government confidential. The bill would give grants to states to collect information on medical errors and to pass it on to the federal Agency for Healthcare Research and Quality. Responding to concerns of the AMA and AHA, all information collected by the federal government would be barred from use in pretrial discovery or from inquiries under the Freedom of Information Act.

Clinton's Medical-Error Initiative

On Feb. 22, President Clinton announced he was endorsing virtually every recommendation of the Institute of Medicine, including its goal of reducing preventable medical errors by 50 percent within five years. The president's initiative included:

❑ Support for a nationwide system of mandatory reporting for hospitals, phased in over three years. The president is urging state health agencies to require that hospitals report any errors causing death or serious injury, with hospitals publicly identified.

❑ Encouraging the development of voluntary reporting of errors that do not harm patients.

❑ Support for legislation that protects hospital analyses of medical errors and the identity of doctors from legal discovery for malpractice suits. But the president said patients or their family members should have access to information about an error that caused them serious injury or death.

❑ Regulations requiring the more than 6,000 hospitals participating in Medicare to carry out programs to reduce errors, such as computerized drug prescribing by doctors.

❑ New standards to be developed by the Food and Drug Administration to help prevent medical errors caused by drug names.

❑ Creation of a new Center for Quality Improvement and Patient Safety.

❑ The use of computerized order entry for drugs at all Veterans Affairs hospitals this year.

❑ A mandatory error-reporting system in the 500 military hospitals and clinics system serving over 8 million patients.

Such "closed-to-the-public" provisions make Inlander suspicious of efforts to create a national collection system. "The only other time the feds did anything like this was when they created the National Practitioner Data Bank — and it's closed to the public," he observes. Consumers should have access to individual hospitals' error rates, Inlander says, because "That's the only thing that's going to help me [as a consumer]. I'm the one that has to go in there."

To answer some of the questions raised about the relative merits of public disclosure and mandatory vs. voluntary reporting, Specter and Harkin have proposed demonstration projects at 15 hospitals throughout the nation. One-third of the facilities would have to inform HHS of any medical errors; one-third would also inform the patient and/or his family; and the rest would only inform HHS of errors on a voluntary basis.

On Feb. 22, President Clinton called for a nationwide system of reporting medical errors, similar to the system used by airlines to report aviation safety hazards. Rather than trying to impose a federal requirement now, he is pressuring the states to adopt mandatory reporting require-

ments within three years. Clinton endorsed virtually all of the recommendations made in November by the Institute of Medicine. [36]

Previous statements by administration officials had worried some lawmakers about the administration's commitment to mandatory reporting. [37] Several administration officials recently said they were not convinced of the effectiveness of mandatory reporting or were concerned that disclosing hospitals' and doctors' names could inhibit reporting. [38] However, the president sided with consumers in proposing that hospitals be publicly identified when reporting mistakes that cause harm.

Sens. Joseph I. Lieberman, D-Conn., and Charles E. Grassley, R-Iowa, are drafting legislation that may require hospitals to report all medical mistakes as a condition of receiving Medicaid and Medicare funds. And Sen. Edward M. Kennedy, D-Mass, is developing legislation to encourage reporting of medical mistakes along the lines of the IOM report. [39]

No matter what the government does, big-business leaders say they are committed to putting economic pressure on hospitals to become safer. The Leapfrog business group

will urge employers to reward hospitals that take at least three steps shown to save lives:

• requiring doctors to enter prescriptions on a computer;

• issuing report cards showing mortality and complication rates for surgical procedures, as Pennsylvania does; and

• keeping specially trained personnel on duty in intensive-care units.

The attention to medical errors also has given publicity to new technologies that could help prevent mistakes, such as putting bar-coded wrist bands on patients to identify them and packaging medication with bar-coded labels. [40]

For its part, the IOM has proposed a raft of practical solutions, from periodically re-examining doctors and nurses to stocking only diluted solutions of dangerous drugs on patient wards. Taken together, the IOM says the steps it is proposing could help the nation reduce medical errors by at least 50 percent over the next five years. As evidence, it points to the aggressive, successful efforts to build a safe aviation system.

Meanwhile, the IOM appears to have achieved its immediate goal: "to break [the] cycle of inaction." [41]

Notes

[1] Testimony of Debra Malone, Hearing on Medical Mistakes, Dec. 13, 1999, U.S. Senate Appropriations Subcommittee on Labor, Health and Human Services, Education and Related Agencies, transcript by Federal Document Clearing House, pp. 21-23.

[2] Linda T. Kohn et al., eds., "To Err is Human: Building a Safer Health System, Committee on Quality of Health Care in America," Institute of Medicine, National Academy Press (1999).

[3] Malone, *op. cit.*, p. 21.

[4] Ann Schrader, "Officials Find Hospital Errors Led to '97 Death; Presbyterian-St. Luke's Cited in 8 Areas," *Denver Post*, April 14, 1999, p. B-01.

[5] Kohn, et al., *op. cit.*, p. 167.

[6] The program is described in Lucian L. Leape et al., "Promoting Patient Safety by Preventing Medical Error," *Journal of the American Medical Association*, Oct. 28, 1998, pp. 1444-1447.

[7] Kohn et al., *op. cit.*, p. 109.

[8] Sixteen states and the District of Columbia have a law requiring hospitals to report unexpected patient deaths or serious injuries from medical treatment, according to a March 1999 phone survey conducted by the Joint Commission on Accreditation of Healthcare Organizations: Alabama, Alaska, District of Columbia, Florida, Idaho, Iowa, Louisiana, Massachusetts, Minnesota, Nevada, New Jersey, New York, Pennsylvania, Tennessee, Texas, Washington and Wisconsin. According to the Institute of Medicine, additional states with mandatory reporting systems include California, Colorado, Kansas, Mississippi, Rhode Island and South Dakota.

[9] Troyen A. Brennan et al. "Incidence of Adverse Events and Negligence in Hospitalized Patients," *New England Journal of Medicine*, Feb. 7, 1991, p. 373. The study estimated 6,895 deaths from negligent care in New York in 1984.

[10] Jennifer Steinhauer and Edward Wong, "How Doctor Got Work after Carving into Patient," *The New York Times*, Jan. 27, 2000, pp. B1, B5.

[11] This incident is described in Michael L. Millenson, *Demanding Medical Excellence* (1997), pp. 208-209.

[12] Andrea Gerlin, "Mum is often the word when caregivers stumble," *Philadelphia Inquirer*, Sept 14, 1999.

[13] Statement by Arnold Milstein, MD, Medical Director, Pacific Business Group on Health on Behalf of The Business Roundtable before the Senate Committee on Health, Education, Labor and Pensions, Jan. 25, 2000.

[14] "Statement of the American Medical Association to the Senate Committee on Health, Education, Labor and Pensions, by Nancy W. Dickey, M.D., immediate past president. Re: Preventing Health System Errors," Jan. 25, 2000, p. 3.

[15] For example, a study of a Chicago hospital found that almost 18 percent of patients had a serious adverse event related to inappropriate care but only 1 percent of them filed a claim for compensation. Cited in Albert W. Wu, "Handling Hospital Errors: Is Disclosure the Best Defense?" *Annals of Internal Medicine*, Dec. 21, 1999, pp. 970-971.

[16] According to the Federation of State Medical Boards, Kentucky is the only state where complaints against a doctor are a matter of public record prior to investigation and action by the state medical board.

[17] Kohn et al., *op. cit.*, p. 123.

[18] Other states that provide data on malpractice claims include California, Florida, Idaho and Tennessee, according to Public Citizen's Health Research Group. California, Florida, Idaho and Massachusetts report disciplinary actions taken by hospitals against physicians on the state medical boards' Web sites.

[19] Jennifer Steinhauer, "Albany Bill Would Help Patients Learn Doctors' Discipline Records," *The New York Times*, Dec. 27, 1999, p. 1.

[20] Steinhauer and Wong, *op. cit.*

[21] Millenson, *op. cit.*, p. 70.

[22] Public Citizen's Health Research Group, "15,638 Questionable Doctors — 1998 Edition."

[23] *Ibid.*

[24] Millenson, *op. cit.*, p. 56.

[25] *Ibid.*, p. 58-59.

[26] Kohn et al., *op. cit.*, p. 1.

[27] *Ibid.*, p. 25.

[28] *Ibid.*, p. 26.

[29] Millenson, *op. cit.*, p. 63.

[30] *Ibid.*, p. 52, 54.

[31] *Ibid.*, p. 52

[32] Andrea Gerlin, "Health Care's Deadly Secret: Accidents Routinely Happen," *Philadelphia Inquirer*, Sept. 12, 1999.

[33] Cited in Gerlin, "Mum is the Word," *op cit.*

[34] Kohn et al., p. 28.

[35] Cited in Robert Davis, "Liposuction death rate 'unacceptable,'" *USA Today*, Jan. 18, 2000, p. 1A.

[36] "Moving Fast on Patient Safety," (editorial), *The New York Times*, Dec. 8, 1999, p. 22.

[37] U.S. Senate press release, "Senators Push Federal Agencies to Move More Aggressively on Medical Errors in Major Programs: Lieberman, Grassley, Kerrey, Nickles send letters demanding reports from HHS, DOD, OPM and VA on action plans," Feb. 8, 2000.

[38] Robert Pear, "U.S. Health Officials Reject Plan to Report Medical Mistakes," *The New York Times*, Jan. 24, 2000, p. 14.

[39] See Mary Agnes Carey and Rebecca Adams, "Deadly Medical Mistakes: Congress Urged to Go Slow in Weighing Legislative Fix," *CQ Weekly*, Jan. 29, 2000, p. 188.

[40] See Milt Freudenheim, "Corrective Medicine: New Technology Helps Health Care Avoid Mistakes," *The New York Times*, Feb. 3, 2000, pp. C1, C26.

[41] Kohn et al., *op. cit.*, p. 3.

FOR MORE INFORMATION

Agency for Healthcare Research and Quality, 2101 Jefferson St., Suite 501, Rockville, Md. 20852; (301) 594-1364; www.ahcpr.gov. This recently renamed arm of the Department of Health and Human Services supports research to improve quality and decrease errors in health care.

Institute of Medicine, 2101 Constitution Ave. N.W., Washington, D.C. 20418; (202) 334-2000; www.nationalacademies.org. This arm of the National Academy of Sciences published "To Err is Human," an influential report on medical errors.

National Patient Safety Foundation at the AMA, 515 North State St., 8th Floor, Chicago, Ill. 60610; (312) 464-4848; www.npsf.org. This American Medical Association group studies why errors occur in health care.

People's Medical Society, 462 Walnut St., Allentown, Pa. 18102; (610) 770-1670; www.peoplesmed.org. This national consumer organization aims to make the health-care system more responsive to consumers.

Bibliography

Selected Sources Used

Books

Inlander, Charles B., and Ed Weiner, *Take this Book to the Hospital With You*, St. Martin's Paperbacks, 1997.
Published by the People's Medical Society, this book offers tips on protecting oneself in the hospital and has a section on hospital-caused injuries.

Millenson, Michael L., *Demanding Medical Excellence: Doctors and Accountability in the Information Age*, University of Chicago Press, 1997.
This well-written book by a former *Chicago Tribune* journalist contains chapters on the growing understanding of medical errors and on efforts by Salt Lake City's LDS hospital to prevent mistakes.

Articles

Brennan, Troyen A. et al., "Incidence of Adverse Events and Negligence in Hospitalized Patients: Results of the Harvard Medical Practice Study I," *The New England Journal of Medicine*, Feb. 7, 1991, pp. 370-376.
This landmark study of New York hospital patients established the basis for today's estimate that 98,000 patients nationwide die annually from medical errors.

Freudenheim, Milt, "Corrective Medicine: New Technology Helps Health Care Avoid Mistakes," *The New York Times*, Feb. 3, 2000, p. C1.
This article discusses high-tech measures being taken by hospitals to combat mistakes.

Gerlin, Andrea, "Health Care's Deadly Secret: Accidents Routinely Happen," *The Philadelphia Inquirer*, Sept. 12, 1999; Part I of a four-part series. The entire series can be accessed at http://health.philly.com/specials/mistakes/hosp12.asp.
The *Inquirer*'s series on "Medical Mistakes" was touched off when bankruptcy proceedings opened the records of the Medical College of Pennsylvania, revealing that errors had injured hundreds of patients.

Kilborn, Peter T., "Ambitious Effort to Cut Mistakes in U.S. Hospitals," *The New York Times*, Dec. 26, 1999, p. 1A.
Reactions to an Institute of Medicine report on medical errors — from business groups, the hospital accrediting agency and members of Congress — constitute "the most ambitious effort ever to confront mistakes in the nation's hospitals," the author concludes.

Kraman, Steve S., and Ginny Hamm, "Risk Management: Extreme Honesty May be the Best Policy," *Annals of Internal Medicine*, Dec. 21, 1999, pp. 963-967.
In Lexington, Ky., the Veterans Affairs hospital's unusual policy of informing patients when they are the victims of medical mistakes appears to control malpractice costs.

Pear, Robert, "U.S. Health Officials Reject Plan to Report Medical Mistakes," *The New York Times*, Jan. 24, 2000, p. 14.
Some federal health officials express doubts about the value of a mandatory reporting system for medical errors as the administration conducts a review of the Institute of Medicine's proposals.

Shapiro, Joseph P., "Doctoring a Sickly System," *U.S. News & World Report*, Dec. 13, 1999, p. 60.
The Veterans Affairs hospital system is becoming a model for quality improvement, the article says, such as scanning bar-coded wristbands on patients to check against medication mistakes.

Reports and Studies

Demian, Larry et al., Survey of Doctor Disciplinary Information on State Medical Board Web Sites, Public Citizen Health Research Group, Feb. 2, 2000, www.citizen.org/hrg/publications/1506.htm.
This report by a consumer group found that 10 states provide no information on their Web sites.

Kohn, Linda T. et al., eds., To Err Is Human: Building a Safer System, Institute of Medicine, National Academy Press, 1999.
This report by an IOM blue-ribbon panel gained widespread media attention for pointing out that more people die in hospitals than car crashes. It proposes mandatory reporting of hospital medical errors.

Office of the Medical Inspector, Veterans Health Administration, Department of Veterans Affairs, Special Report: VA Patient Safety Event Registry: First Nineteen Months of Reported Cases Summary and Analysis; June 1997 through December 1998, July 15, 1998.
The VA's first systematic attempt to require reports of medical mistakes from VA hospitals documented almost 3,000 incidents of medical errors and adverse events from medical treatment.

Public Citizen Health Research Group, 16,638 Questionable Doctors, March 1998, www.citizen.org/hrg/qdsite/PUBLICATIONS.
This report rates states according to the toughness of disciplinary measure they take against doctors whose competence is under question.

9 Embryo Research

ADRIEL BETTELHEIM

Last fall, teams of scientists working separately at the University of Wisconsin and Johns Hopkins University made a groundbreaking discovery — and kicked up a tempest.

The researchers isolated from human embryos and fetuses a primitive variety of cells that are capable of developing into virtually every kind of tissue in the body. The so-called stem cells could provide valuable tools for curing ailments such as Parkinson's disease and diabetes, if scientists can learn how to train them to grow into a desired healthy body part.

"These findings . . . bring medical research to the edge of a new frontier that is extraordinarily promising," National Institutes of Health (NIH) Director Harold Varmus said, echoing the optimism that swept the scientific community. "It is not too unrealistic to say that this research has the potential to revolutionize the practice of medicine and improve the quality and length of life."

But while the findings generated headlines and drew comparisons to landmark moments in 20th-century science, they also reignited a simmering legal and ethical debate over embryo research. Scientists, theologians, politicians and government officials have sparred in recent months over whether a 1995 federal ban on funding research on embryos should apply to stem cells. Congress and the NIH are attempting to devise new guidelines in light of the developments. But officials first must arrive at a consensus on such thorny philosophical questions as when life begins, and whether an embryo has the same moral status as a person.

"It's a watershed issue that cuts

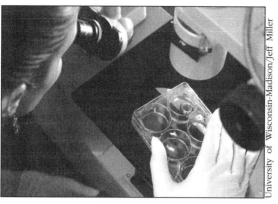

University of Wisconsin-Madison/Jeff Miller

deeply into the future of the biomedical community," says Ronald M. Green, chairman of the Ethics Institute at Dartmouth College. "Science is forcing us to rethink our ethical, moral and religious considerations, but all the recent developments make it difficult to draw lines in the sand."

Human stem cells are hardly the first scientific discovery in recent years to challenge people's beliefs in this way. The advent of recombinant DNA technology in the 1970s led to developments allowing scientists to clone sheep and other mammals, raising the very real but unsettling prospect that human beings also could be replicated. [1]

Around the same time, scientists developed a deeper understanding of how DNA carries chemical messages, allowing them to identify specific human genes linked to diseases, and, possibly, certain types of behavior. That has raised questions about how much of our existence is predetermined, and whether science should be allowed to intervene via techniques such as gene therapy. [2]

The stem cell discovery could potentially have even more profound meaning, because it offers a glimpse at human life in its simplest form. The microscopic clumps of cells are found in the interior of days-old embryos before they develop rudimentary nervous systems and are capable of achieving something resembling awareness.

When isolated in culture dishes, the cells — through a still-unknown mechanism — can grow into specific body parts, such as brain cells or heart muscle. They also can replicate indefinitely in the laboratory, providing a potentially endless source of replacement tissue. Scientists have watched with amazement as some of the cells spontaneously evolve into tiny bundles of beating heart muscle, clumps of nerves or even hair and teeth. [3]

However, scientists don't yet know how to make a stem cell "committed" to becoming a particular body part. And they still aren't sure whether the spare body parts they create won't be rejected by the patient's immune system — a problem that frequently arises in organ transplants.

Some of the stem cells were extracted from spare embryos created in fertility clinics that were deemed unsuitable for implantation in the womb. Others came from the gonads of aborted fetuses. Because of uncertainties over whether the existing funding ban applies to stem cells, the University of Wisconsin and Johns Hopkins scientists relied on private funding for their work, including financing from Geron Corp., a Menlo Park, Calif., biotechnology firm with a strong interest in anti-aging products.

Most scientists believe the stem cells are biologically closer to other types of cells — say, blood cells — than to a complete embryo. They argue the government should fund research into how the cells can be coaxed into becoming a specific type of tissue, pointing to the wide-ranging health benefits that could follow. With this knowledge, researchers say they could perform tasks like creating new bone and cartilage cells for patients suffering from osteoporosis

From *The CQ Researcher,*
December 17, 2000.

or arthritis, or nerve cells for stroke victims or people with spinal cord injuries.

"The world would be better off if public funding were available, because it would allow the best biomedical scientists in academia to enter the field," says James A. Thomson, the University of Wisconsin biologist who first isolated the human stem cells and used them to grow heart tissues. "Although a great deal of basic research needs to be done before these cells can lead to human therapies, I believe in the long run they will revolutionize many aspects of transplantation medicine."

However, anti-abortion groups and many Catholic theologians oppose using taxpayer money to fund the work, arguing the scientists are destroying life to advance their research. The critics, who believe that life begins at conception, contend the stem cells, however primitive, are distinct entities that have the same moral status as humans. They criticize the researchers for playing up the biological qualities of the stem cells while paying less attention to the methods that extract them from embryos. And they worry that advances in cloning will soon lead scientists to create embryos specifically so they can extract their stem cells.

"These embryos are far beyond conception; fertilization has taken place and we have a genetically unique individual," says C. Ben Mitchell, senior fellow at the Center for Bioethics and Human Dignity, a nonprofit group in Bannockburn, Ill., that is leading the fight against federal funding. "Giving an embryo a different moral status based on the time of gestation is simply an act of arbitrariness. There's no scientific evidence to point to a specific time when the moral status moves higher."

Public figures and advocacy groups are already joining the debate. Groups advocating for victims

of various diseases have mounted a major lobbying push in favor of federal funding, even going as far as recruiting the help of conservative Sen. Strom Thurmond, R-S.C., an abortion foe whose daughter suffers from juvenile diabetes, and 33 U.S. Nobel Prize winners.

Opponents, including the National Conference of Catholic Bishops, have issued strongly worded position papers supporting the ban, saying any researcher who understands the origin of the stem cells is "morally complicit" in their destruction. Those coming out against federal funding include no less than 70 members of Congress and former Surgeon General C. Everett Koop.

Lawmakers considering what to do must first consider the 1995 ban, authored by Rep. Jay Dickey, R-Ark. that prohibits spending federal money on any biomedical research involving human embryos outside the womb. [4] The ban, which didn't contemplate the extraction of stem cells, has been attached for the past four years as a rider to the annual bills that fund NIH.

Congress could elect to expand the ban so it explicitly mentions stem cell research. Lawmakers also could take the more dramatic step of extending the ban to privately funded research — a move that experts say would almost certainly would trigger legal challenges because it could infringe on individuals' reproductive rights. Congress also could elect to simply let the ban stand and defer to NIH on the issue of stem cell research — a move that appears increasingly likely given the sharp philosophical divide over the issue.

NIH in December released draft guidelines recommending the funding of stem cell research based on a legal opinion by Harriet Rabb, general counsel of the U.S. Department of Health and Human Services (HHS). [5] The opinion states that stem

cells "do not have the capacity to develop into a human being, even if transferred to the uterus." As a result, Rabb wrote, destruction of the cells during the course of research wouldn't constitute the destruction of an embryo. President Clinton's National Bioethics Advisory Commission and the American Association for the Advancement of Science (AAAS) have similarly endorsed federally funded stem cell research.

To get around the issue of the current funding ban, NIH said it would not use federal funds to create embryos for research but would support studies that use embryos developed by private sources. Moving with caution, the agency is seeking public comment on the draft guidelines and has assembled an oversight panel to review grant proposals.

"The ethical and social issues associated with stem cell research are complex and controversial and require thoughtful discourse in public fora to reach resolution," Varmus says.

But critics say the NIH's preliminary decision reflects a concerted effort to defy the funding ban and present a new definition of an embryo. "The researcher's temptation is to think that if something technically can be done it ethically should be done," Richard Doerflinger, associate director for policy development for the National Conference of Catholic Bishops, told a Senate Appropriations subcommittee hearing on stem cell research last December. "A civilized society will appreciate the possibilities opened up by research, but will insist that scientific progress must not come at the expense of human dignity." [6]

Geron is watching the debate closely. It wants to learn how to convert a patient's ordinary cells into stem cells that then can be used for transplantation and self-repair. The company announced in May that i

At the Beginnings of Life

The isolation of human embryonic stem cells, shown below, represents a landmark in biomedical research and offers the highest-resolution view yet into early human development. Controversy arises because stem cells are isolated from aborted fetuses or early-stage embryos.

Culturing Human Embryonic Stem Cells

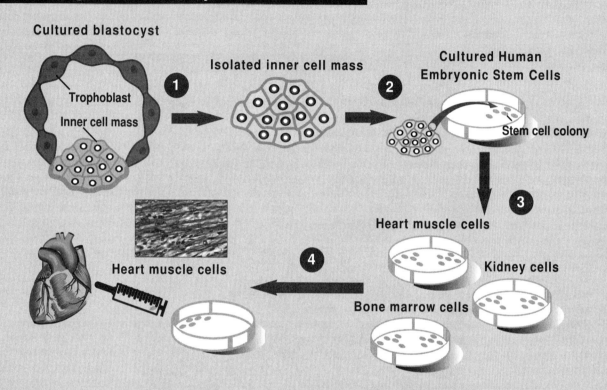

Cultured blastocyst — Trophoblast — Inner cell mass — **1** — Isolated inner cell mass — **2** — Cultured Human Embryonic Stem Cells — Stem cell colony — **3** — Heart muscle cells — Kidney cells — Bone marrow cells — **4** — Heart muscle cells

1 Scientists isolate the inner cell mass from a microscopic five-day-old embryo, or blastocyst.

2 The cells are placed in a tissue culture dish and mixed with growth factors that allow them to mature into stem cells.

3 When the growth factor is removed, the stem cells differentiate into specific cell types. University of Wisconsin researchers used stem cells to grow heart tissues while scientists at Johns Hopkins University coaxed them into becoming nerve cells.

4 Other body parts could be grown in this way and used to treat assorted ailments, such as heart disease.

Source: University of Wisconsin–Madison

---

ormed a $20 million research alliance with the Roslin Institute of Scotland, which first focused worldwide attention on cloning in 1997 by creating Dolly, a cloned sheep. But Geron has denied it is interested in creating cloned human embryos.

Geron's involvement has made some observers uneasy because it operates entirely outside the scope of the funding ban and, by extension, without any federal oversight. Dartmouth ethics expert Green, among others, believes federal funding of stem cell research would ensure that other companies entered the field, and that NIH or some other federal authority would oversee the scope of the work.

"You would have a serious ethical issue if some company, not necessarily Geron, were deliberately creating embryos only to dismember them, and reaping huge financial benefits," Green says.

Geron says it convened its own ethics panel for advice on how to proceed, adding it understands the moral questions and general unease swirling around stem cell research.

"We are sensitive to the ethical issues surrounding our respective technologies," Geron President and Chief Executive Officer Thomas Okarma said in announcing the alliance with the Roslin Institute. "Both our organizations have been and remain committed to pursuing these technologies in an open and responsible manner."

As scientists, ethics experts, religious leaders and government officials continue to debate stem cell research and what it means for broader experiments involving human embryos, here are some questions they are asking:

Is the use of stem cells from embryos morally or ethically wrong?

The isolation of human stem cells created tensions between two of the modern world's most important ethical commitments: curing disease and protecting human life. For many, resolving the issue hinges on draw-

ing a series of careful distinctions about the source and nature of the stem cells.

The Johns Hopkins researchers' technique of extracting stem cells from aborted fetuses has stirred up slightly less controversy because the research didn't affect the ultimate fate of the embryos. Notwithstanding the separate and incendiary national

The human embryonic stem cells isolated at the University of Wisconsin–Madison randomly differentiated into a variety of cell types: (A) gut, (B) neural, (C) bone marrow, (D) cartilage, (E) muscle and (F) kidney.

debate over abortion, using stem cells from already-dead fetuses has been likened to the well-established medical practice of obtaining donor tissue from cadavers. Many experts additionally believe this research would currently qualify for federal funding because of the wording of the congressional ban on embryo research.[7]

The University of Wisconsin team's

use of spare embryos from fertility clinics is much more controversial. About 16,000 embryos are created in clinics each year, the majority of which are deemed unsuitable for transplantation in the mothers' wombs. They typically are stored in liquid nitrogen and eventually discarded. However, using them to obtain stem cells involves the direct destruction of the embryos — an act that is expressly singled out in the congressional funding ban.

President Clinton's 17-member National Bioethics Advisory Commission believes the federal government should fund researchers using these two extraction techniques because a ban would conflict with the ethical goals of medicine — namely healing, prevention of disease and research. But the panel draws a distinction between the use of existing embryonic tissue and the hypothetical creation of a "research embryo" strictly so it can be used as a source of stem cells. The ethics panel says "there is no compelling reason" to generate an embryo for purposes other than creating a child, and recommends against using taxpayer funding for research using embryos produced for research purposes.[8]

Harold Shapiro, president of Princeton University and chairman of the ethics panel, says coming to some moral agreement on issues of birth and death is difficult because science is constantly evolving and testing individuals' beliefs. The result, he says, is anxiety about the future direction of technology and, in some cases, a temptation to "stop" science

"We need new sources of reflection to enrich the ongoing ethical debates," Shapiro said. The "nervousness, ethical malaise, anxiety or even foreboding reflect, I believe, a shared understanding that humankind's destiny will not be decided in full in the laboratory or at the genetic level, where we have a lot more confidence in our ability to find solutions." [9]

Some theologians parse the ethical question differently, drawing distinctions not between the source of the embryos but between whether they exist inside or outside of the womb. Four leading theologians took this tack in October, when they wrote to Congress contending that human stem cell research can be conducted ethically and in harmony with religious principles.

"According to our religious beliefs, all human life must be protected," the theologians wrote. "However, they also indicate that there is a significant difference between an embryo suspended in liquid nitrogen that will never be implanted inside a womb, and an unborn child who is already in the womb." The group added that religious teachings stressing compassion for the sick further justify federal funding of the research.*

Theologians also are re-evaluating the question of precisely when life begins, postulating that such a thing as a "pre-embryo" may exist. Following this line of thinking, it may be permissible to extract stem cells before the embryo reaches some critical developmental milestone in which it becomes a distinct entity — for instance, the point at which it is capable of dividing in two to form twins.

The letter was signed by Margaret Farley, a Roman Catholic nun and professor of Christian ethics at Yale University Divinity School; Nancy Duff, a Presbyterian theologian and associate professor at the Princeton Theological Seminary; Rabbi Elliott Dorff, professor of philosophy at the University of Judaism in Los Angeles; and Abdulaziz Sachedina, an Islamic scholar at the University of Virginia.

However, opponents of stem cell research contend such distinctions are designed to achieve political compromises and don't address the broader ethical issues surrounding experiments on human subjects. The critics say society must rigorously apply those principles or face the prospect of treating people as things.

"Members of the human species who cannot give informed consent should not be the subjects of an experiment unless they personally may benefit from it, or the experiment carries no significant risk to harming them," says the National Conference of Catholic Bishops' Doerflinger. He notes that U.S. law already allows for such considerations, permitting states to pass statutes prohibiting harmful experiments on human embryos, despite prohibitions on restricting access to abortions.

The Center for Bioethics and Human Dignity rejects using compassion for the sick as justification for conducting stem cell research, saying the Bible teaches that people are not free to pursue good ends through immoral or unethical means.

"We must not sacrifice one class of human beings to benefit another," says the center's Mitchell, citing as an example the use of data from Nazi medical experiments on concentration camp inmates to gain insights into human physiology.

Both groups believe the correct ethical approach would be to find alternate sources for stem cells. Indeed, lab techniques have been identified that could stimulate growth and specialization of stem cells extracted from adult tissues, bone marrow or umbilical-cord blood. However, scientists say those stem cells aren't biologically equivalent to the ones found in embryos and are less capable of evolving into the desired tissue.

Experts believe the debate over ethics will continue but that new scientific discoveries will gradually make the potential applications of stem cell research overshadow the moral reservations. Arthur Caplan, director of the Center for Bioethics at the University of Pennsylvania, predicts patient-advocacy and disease-related interest groups will besiege undecided lawmakers with evidence that stem cell research can create such medical miracles as virus-free blood or help repair spinal-cord damage until the politicians give in. "That lobby, I think, will overwhelm moral reservations," Caplan said. [10]

Should stem cell research be eligible for federal funding?

To patient-advocacy groups, Michelle Puczynski is a living argument for federal funding of stem cell research. The 15-year-old from Toledo, Ohio, was 13 months old when she was diagnosed with juvenile diabetes. Since then, she has taken 16,500 injections of insulin simply to survive. The advocates, who invited Puczynski to a Washington news conference in May, say the government should bankroll research into how stem cells can be grown into insulin-producing pancreatic cells. Such cells could then be injected into Michelle's body to begin reversing the debilitating condition.

"Events in the lab are overcoming the fear of the unknown," says Daniel Perry, executive director of the Alliance for Aging Research and head of Patients' Cure, a Washington-based coalition of 35 patient organizations advocating federal funding. "This debate needs to include the voices of people who face tragic and catastrophic illnesses — conditions that potentially could be relieved."

But Congress has been leery about giving its blessing to new varieties of developmental biology. The 105th Congress took up a measure to ban a process known as somatic cell nuclear transfer that could be used to

Stem Cells' Unlimited Potential

Researchers believe that human embryonic stem cells can be grown into a variety of body parts, enabling them to fight many common afflictions.

Cells Derivable From Stem Cells	Target Diseases
Insulin-producing cells	Diabetes
Nerve cells	Stroke, Parkinson's disease, Alzheimer's disease, Spinal cord injury
Heart muscle cells	Heart attacks, Congestive heart failure
Liver cells	Hepatitis, Cirrhosis
Blood cells	Cancer, Immunodeficiencies
Bone cells	Osteoporosis
Cartilage cells	Osteoarthritis
Eye cells	Macular degeneration
Skin cells	Burns, Wound healing
Skeletal muscle cells	Muscular dystrophy

Source: Geron Corp.

create a human embryo. The process involves replacing the nucleus of an egg cell with another cell that wouldn't multiply if left in its original state. The remaining part of the egg cell can "program" the new nucleus to multiply. Scientists believe the process could help them clone cells that could treat cancer, heart disease and other conditions, but lawmakers expressed serious concerns about creating carbon copies of living or dead people. The Senate finally voted against taking up the bill because it was too broadly written. [11]

Defenders of stem cell research

this year tried to insert a measure in a Senate spending bill that would have permitted government-supported research on spare stem cells donated by couples who went through in-vitro fertilization. But the provision was stripped out by Sen. Arlen Specter, R-Pa., chairman of the Senate Appropriations subcommittee that controls NIH's budget, who said the issue should be decided outside the budget process. Specter and Senate Majority Leader Trent Lott, R-Miss., indicated they will introduce legislation in February to define the conditions for federally supported stem cell research. [12]

The 1995 congressional funding bars the use of federal money for research in which embryos are "destroyed, discarded or knowingly subjected to risk, injury or death" but doesn't specifically mention stem cells. One key question surrounding the ban and its effect on the current research is whether stem cells can develop into embryos on their own and, thus, should fall under the funding ban. The answer appears to be "maybe."

Scientists at the University of Toronto in 1993 grew entire mice out of stem cells. But the scientists first wrapped the stem cells in an envelope of genetically modified cells that couldn't grow into part of the fetus but helped the stem cells attach to the wall of the female mouse's uterus. Without this kind of artificial protection, many scientists believe the stem cells alone aren't capable of evolving into a person. [13]

"Embryonic stem cells on their own can't make certain embryonic tissues, they can't form an embryo and we aren't cloning here," says John Gearhardt, director of the division of developmental genetics at the Johns Hopkins School of Medicine. He is the scientist who coaxed stem cells isolated from the gonads of aborted fetuses into becoming nerve cells.

But Gearhardt points out there are

different kinds of stem cells. He believes the ones he and the University of Wisconsin's Thomson isolated are "pluripotent" stem cells, meaning they are capable of becoming a wide array of human tissues but cannot become cells of the placenta or other tissues needed for implantation in the womb.

However, the scientists can't be sure. That is because very early in development, an embryo is also believed to possess "totipotent" stem cells that can form every kind of cell in the body. The researchers can't test whether the cells they isolated are totipotent because it would involve injecting the stem cells into another embryo to create a test environment to determine whether the cells retain all of their developmental powers. That would conflict with virtually all accepted ethical guidelines.

Rep. Dickey, the author of the congressional funding ban, says that such uncertainties are precisely why the ban should be applied to stem cells. He says scientists should study stem cells in animals and in less controversial adult cells without getting involved in politically volatile embryo research. He adds NIH's preliminary indications that it will fund stem cell research are a deliberate attempt to flout the law.

"Any NIH action to initiate funding of such research would violate both the letter and spirit of the federal law banning federal support for research in which human embryos are harmed or destroyed," Dickey wrote Secretary of Health and Human Services Donna E. Shalala in May.

Dickey has numerous allies. Sen. Sam Brownback, R-Kan., calls the

research "immoral, illegal and unnecessary," adding, "there are better, more promising avenues to follow in order to continue our fight against some of the diseases with which we are battling." Brownback issued a highly critical position paper on stem cell research this summer that was endorsed by Catholic and Protestant anti-abortion leaders.

Despite the passionate feelings, political realities are thwarting the critics from enacting legislation. Dickey in September indicated he would draft an amendment to NIH's

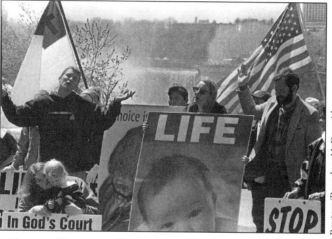

The use of human embryonic stem cells in medical research is rekindling the debate over whether fetuses should be considered human beings. Above, abortion foes from Operation Rescue protest at an abortion clinic in Niagara Falls, N.Y., last April.

fiscal 2000 spending bill that would have extended the ban to stem cells. But he was talked out of the move by House Majority Whip Tom DeLay, R-Texas, who was seeking to eliminate controversial amendments in an effort to speed up the budget process. The fight will likely continue during the next Congress.

"Congress is crossing a moral Rubicon, and the people fighting the abortion wars see [stem cell research] as a kind of proxy for the fight over when does life begin," says the Alliance for Aging Research's Perry. "We're taking a middle-of-the-road

approach and hoping NIH will release its guidelines soon so we can develop a funding policy through an honest, thorough and open process."

Are the potential benefits of stem cell research being oversold?

A hiker suffers a serious heart attack in a remote part of a national park. By the time he reaches a hospital, only one-third of his heart is still working. Eager to return to active life, he provides doctors with a sample of his skin cells, which are then injected into specially prepared, donated human eggs. The eggs are grown in a lab for a week, developing into early-stage embryos that yield stem cells that are a perfect genetic match for the patient. Doctors grow the stem cells into heart-muscle cells, inject them into the patient and watch as the new cells begin to replace old damaged ones. Before long, the patient is restored to health.

This hypothetical scenario — outlined recently in *Scientific American* magazine by Roger Pedersen, a stem cell researcher at the University of California at San Francisco — illustrates the tremendous potential for therapeutic cures arising from stem cell research. If it were possible to control how stem cells differentiate into body parts, Pederson writes, the resulting cells could potentially help repair damage from Parkinson's disease, diabetes and other debilitating conditions that result from the death or damage of one or several cell types. [14]

But observers caution there are huge scientific hurdles ahead, and that significant health benefits from the current research may not be seen for decades, if ever. In particular, some worry that researchers — under pressure to produce and deliver results for politicians, potential investors and the public — may bc hyping the field's potential before they even know whether stem cell-based transplantation works in humans.

"I hate to be the skunk at the garden party, but the probability of success simply isn't guaranteed," says Charles Jennings, editor of *Nature Neuroscience*, a scientific journal. "The brain, for example, has a hundred-billion neurons in an incredibly complicated array, firing 10 to 100 actions every second. You just can't expect to go patch up the holes in it with cellular putty-filler."

Jennings and others question whether stem cell researchers are moving too quickly toward human clinical trials without fully understanding the underlying science and possible risks. Without knowing precisely what kind of brain cells govern certain neurological functions, for example, the skeptics say it will be difficult to pinpoint a cure for Parkinson's disease — a progressive disorder characterized by the loss of dopamine-producing neurons in the brain. It also will be hard to recruit patients for trials on potential therapies. To test the efficacy, scientists will need one group that receives transplanted cells and another control group that receives a placebo. But skeptics question how many people will be willing to volunteer to have holes drilled into their heads or needles injected into their brains, on the chance they may receive an unproven treatment.

"Neural transplantation is quite risky," Jennings says. "And once the new cells are implanted, it's difficult to monitor physiological changes because you can't just decide to biopsy that part of the brain. It raises major concerns."

Some patient advocates have elected to remain silent on stem cell research until the outcome of experiments and the political debate become clearer. The American Cancer Society last summer pulled out of the Patients' Cure coalition, reportedly over internal policy disagreements. The organization also had received a letter from Cardinal William Keeler of Baltimore asking the cancer society to reconsider its membership. Officials denied that pressure from the Roman Catholic Church influenced their decision, saying they were conducting their own analysis of the issue and at some point in the future would issue a policy statement. [15]

Even some lawmakers generally sympathetic to scientific causes are openly expressing reservations about endorsing a major government role in stem cell work. Specter describes the issue as "fuzzy" — intriguing because of the medical potential but also fraught with troubling legal and moral implications. "I don't think you can rush to judgment on it," he says. "This is obviously on the cutting edge."

Most scientists acknowledge there are concerns but defend pushing forward, saying stem cell research is doing more than just promising future cures. It also is offering insights into events that can't be studied directly in the human embryo. The University of Wisconsin team, for example, has observed how stem cells differentiate into the three primary "germ lines" in the body, and subsequently into arrays of tissue cells, including cartilage, bone, muscle and neural and gut cells. Understanding these steps will yield new insights into birth defects, infertility and miscarriage, according to Thomson. And testing how specific, differentiated cells respond to certain drugs will allow researchers to sort out which medications are helpful or harmful. [16]

"We're not just a bunch of cow-

boys looking to stick strange cells into the heads of people," says Ronald McKay, a leading stem cell researcher and chief of the laboratory of molecular biology at the National Institute of Neurological Disorders and Stroke in Bethesda, Md. "This work has appeal to many different segments of the scientific community because stem cells give us a tool to look at very complex cellular functions."

Many researchers in the field are now focusing on chemicals that can act as growth factors and stimulate stem cells to produce specific kinds of cells. Researchers at Washington University School of Medicine in St. Louis, for example, found that the vitamin A derivative retinoic acid seems to stimulate a set of genes in stem cells to make them produce neurons while inhibiting genes that trigger other types of cell formation. [17]

Gearhardt of Johns Hopkins and other prominent researchers take pains to note that stem cell work is not a new, hype-driven branch of science but builds on more than a half-century of pioneering work in developmental biology. Viewed in this context, he says it is reasonable to expect careful, steady progress, but no breathtaking applications overnight.

"Our work is simply an extension of work that's gone on for decades," Gearhardt says. "We're taking discoveries that go back to the 1930s and '40s and just applying them to humans." ∎

BACKGROUND

Early Breakthroughs

S cientific breakthroughs like the discovery of penicillin and the

Chronology

1960s *Biologists studying mice begin to postulate how "master cells" existing in embryos can create different kinds of tissue. However, they can't isolate the cells. Meanwhile, other types of fetal research yield a vaccine against measles and improved treatment of blood diseases.*

1970s *Embryo research accelerates and becomes a public issue.*

1973
The U.S. Supreme Court recognizes the constitutional right to abortion in *Roe v. Wade.*

1975
The U.S. Department of Health and Human Services (HHS) bars research on live fetuses but allows studies on dead fetuses or their tissues if permitted by state law.

1980s *Scientists continue their studies and begin transplanting fetal tissue. Anti-abortion groups oppose the use of biological materials from aborted fetuses.*

1981
Researchers in England and the United States derive stem cells from mouse embryos at an early stage. This allows them to begin developing cultures in laboratories to prompt the stem cells to form certain tissues.

1988
Scientists at the University of Colorado perform the first fetal tissue transplant on a patient with Parkinson's disease. HHS imposes a moratorium on federal funding of fetal tissue transplant research.

1990s *New discoveries offer a detailed view of early human development — and fan controversies.*

1993
Scientists at the University of Toronto announce they grew an entire mouse from individual stem cells extracted from mouse embryos. The experiment proves stem cells can grow into an entire healthy organism. President Clinton, in one of his first acts as president, removes prohibitions on fetal tissue research.

1994
A panel of experts convened by the National Institutes of Health (NIH) concludes that public funds should be spent on embryo research, as long as the embryos in question were not created strictly for research purposes. President Clinton soon after announces that his administration will forbid taxpayer funding for research with human embryos, regardless of their source.

1995
Congress incorporates language in the spending bill that funds NIH forbidding taxpayer funding for research with human embryos, regardless of their source.

The ban is included in subsequent annual spending bills. University of Wisconsin researchers isolate the stem cells of a monkey and discover unique properties inherent to primates.

November 1998
Scientists at the University of Wisconsin and Johns Hopkins University announce that they isolated human embryonic stem cells for the first time.

Jan. 19, 1999
NIH Director Harold Varmus announces the federal government can pay for some stem cell research, as long as publicly funded researchers don't grow the cells themselves.

May 4, 1999
Geron Corp., in Menlo Park, Calif., forms an alliance with the Roslin Institute of Scotland to blend stem cell research with the cloning technology that produced Dolly the sheep in 1997.

June 28, 1999
The National Bioethics Advisory Commission recommends that federally funded scientists be allowed to extract stem cells from human embryos, as well as conduct research on embryos derived by others.

Aug. 18, 1999
The American Association for the Advancement of Science endorses private and public research on stem cells, citing the potential medical benefits to individuals.

polio vaccine have long given Americans hope that other still common afflictions such as cancer, heart disease and mental illness could be stopped, too. In fact, progress has come painfully slow. Consider that when President Richard M. Nixon signed the National Cancer Act in 1971, marking the official declaration of war on the disease, many scientists believed they were within a decade of curing or controlling the disease. Nearly 30 years later, scientists are still learning the basic underpinnings of the disease and how to prevent specific cancers. [18]

It is precisely because of this incremental nature of scientific research that the isolation of human embryonic stem cells is both a watershed event and only the latest development in nearly a half-century of research into human tissue growth and transplantation. It may take many more decades — if ever — before the knowledge is harnessed into practical therapies that allow the body to replicate parts of itself.

The idea of a "master cell" that could prompt many kinds of tissue growth began to gain currency in the 1960s, when scientists noticed that cancerous cells in mice could form several different types of tissue. The discovery had limited research applications, however, and scientists for nearly two decades were unable to create non-cancerous, self-renewing stem cells from mouse embryos.

In 1981, researchers at the University of Cambridge in England and the University of California at San Francisco were able to derive stem cells from mouse embryos at an early, 100-cell stage. This allowed scientists to begin tinkering with cultures that could allow the cells to multiply. They also were able to combine mouse stem cells with separate embryos, giving rise to a genetically hybrid mouse. But the researchers soon

learned there were major differences in developmental biology between mice and humans, leading to research on higher mammals.

In 1995, the University of Wisconsin's Thomson isolated the stem cells of a monkey. The work was notable because Thomson soon noticed unusual characteristics as he closely examined the behavior of stem cells. For instance, he found that primate stem cells quickly differentiated into various tissues unless they were grown in tissue culture dishes along with a special type of mouse cell called a "feeder cell" that prevents them from specializing. Scientists don't yet understand how the feeder cells work — a hurdle that will have to be overcome if they are ever to generate enough tissue for commercial purposes. [19]

Thomson subsequently applied his primate stem cell extraction technology to spare embryos from fertility clinics, which enabled him to perform the first successful extraction of human stem cells in February 1998. Around the same time, Johns Hopkins' Gearhardt also isolated and cultured human stem cells. Gearhardt's work arose out of two decades of research on how genetic errors give rise to Down's syndrome, a condition that occurs when one of an embryo's chromosomes copies itself once too often.

"It feels great [to be first], but it's just the beginning," Thomson says. "Up until this point, we've had no way to study questions about human development during the early weeks so we can see all of the critical decisions being made in the body plan. This gives us a nice source of material to study."

The University of Wisconsin and Johns Hopkins each patented the respective extraction techniques the scientists used and then licensed them to Geron. The biotech company believes it could be on the cusp of a

financial bonanza if the stem cells can be harnessed to provide anti-aging products. But company President Okarma acknowledges this will involve much more research, including developing a much better understanding of human development. [20]

Unanswered Questions

One big question is why are stem cells so active in embryos but hardly in evidence after birth? Each of the body's cells carry the organism's unique genetic code imprinted in DNA and, theoretically, could use it to create replacement tissue during adulthood. But other than regenerating skin cells and occasionally mending some bone fractures, the human body outside of the womb typically does not take advantage of this option. In contrast, salamanders and certain other animals can regrow tails and limbs. [21]

Another focus is the cellular mechanism that shuts off stem cell division, which centers on the portion of a chromosome called a telomere. Cells are born with a length of telomere that gets shorter each time a cell divides. Conventional human cells divide about 50 times, then die of old age — a driving factor in the broader phenomenon of human aging. However, Geron scientists have perfected a way of building telomeres back up with an enzyme called telomerase. Scientists using the enzyme have been able to make stem cells divide 200 times or more, creating healthy cells that could increase the life span. But it's still unclear whether they can make enough cells to save a patient suffering from the late stages of conditions such as Alzheimer's disease or cirrhosis of the liver.

Longer term, stem cell research could be used to replace a human

Religious Views Vary on Stem Cell Research

Stem cell research, and the broader issue of using fetal tissue for biomedical purposes, has prompted a broad spectrum of religious views. The following sampling is culled from a one-day workshop organized by the National Bioethics Advisory Commission last May at Georgetown University. [1]

■ **Catholicism** — Roman Catholics view human life as a continuous progression from single-cell embryos to death, according to Edmund D. Pellegrino, director of the Center for Clinical Bioethics at Georgetown University Medical Center. Catholics therefore object to extracting stem cells from aborted fetuses or spare embryos from fertility clinics, believing that those who do are destroying the equivalent of a human being. They also are highly skeptical about designating just those embryos that are past a certain stage of development as human beings, viewing the practice as arbitrary.

A differing view is offered by Margaret Farley, a Catholic nun and professor of Christian ethics at Yale University Divinity School. Farley believes a case can be made for stem cell research and raises the possibility that embryos in their earliest stages of development may not constitute an individual human entity. She believes the break point may be when the embryo develops the first signs of a nervous system and can begin to respond to its surroundings, usually around 14 days after conception.

■ **Judaism** — Jewish law doesn't bestow legal status on embryos outside the womb. Moreover, it doesn't recognize fetuses as a human beings until they emerge from the uterus, regarding them during the first 40 days of gestation "as if they were simply water," according to Rabbi Elliot Dorff, professor of philosophy at the University of Judaism in Los Angeles. Therefore, current stem cell research is permissible, and even in keeping with the Jewish tradition of accepting both natural and artificial means to overcome illness. Judaism still prohibits abortions except when absolutely necessary, but it wouldn't frown on using stem cells extracted from a fetus to save other people's lives if the abortion were performed for sufficient reason.

■ **Islam** — Islamic law doesn't provide a universally accepted definition of "embryo" or define specifically when the fetus becomes a moral-legal being, according to Abdulaziz Sachedina, professor of Islam in the department of religious studies at the University of Virginia. A majority of Shiite and Sunni scholars divide pregnancies into two stages by the end of the fourth month, when they believe ensoulment takes place. Therefore, Sachedina says, research using stem cells from early-stage embryos is an act of faith in God, so long as the purpose is to improve human health.

■ **Eastern Orthodox** — This faith has a long tradition of encouraging medical healing but believes it should be done according to God's will, not our own, according to Demetrios Demopulos, pastor at Holy Trinity Greek Orthodox Church in Fitchburg, Mass. Therefore, embryos shouldn't be sacrificed in experiments, no matter how worthy the goal is. Demopulos says the prohibition on research using human embryos should be upheld in the public sector and even extended to the private sector.

■ **Protestantism** — Protestant faiths are split on stem cell research. Gilbert C. Meilaender Jr., a Christian ethicist at Valparaiso University in Indiana, says using stem cells from aborted fetuses or spare embryos is an example of the strong using the weak. Society is trying to benefit some members at the expense of others who have already been condemned to die, in this view.

However, Ronald Cole-Turner, a professor of theology at the Pittsburgh Theological Seminary and chair of the United Church of Christ committee on genetics, believes stem cell research should continue because it promises great benefit. His major concern is that the medical benefits will be distributed only by means of the market and won't be available to underprivileged members of society.

[1] See "A Look At . . . Science and Religion," *The Washington Post*, June 13, 1999, p. B3.

---

body's faulty genes with healthy DNA. Biologists currently perform gene therapy by loading the healthy DNA onto viruses that provide a means of transport. However, the body's immune system often rejects these treatments. This has frustrated medical efforts to weed out recessive genes that cause conditions like sickle-cell anemia. However, stem cell-based gene treatments have the potential to be far more efficient because they could carry the patient's own DNA with only the undesired, recessive gene altered. With stem cells' capacity to multiply, some genetic diseases that are now incurable could be defeated. However, such techniques would likely prompt a new debate over medical ethics because they would essentially alter human heredity. [22]

Oversight System

The prospect of stem cell researchers tinkering with human genetics has prompted differing views of how far the government should go in regulating the field. If federal funding for stem cell research is approved, the AAAS believes existing government agencies can oversee potential applications of the technology. The Food and Drug Administration would have the authority to regulate the development and use of human stem cells used as biological products to diagnose, treat or cure a disease. Similarly, the National Bioethics Advisory Commission and the separate Recombinant DNA Advisory Committee could work with physicians, patient disease groups, religious leaders, Congress and funding agencies like NIH to assure that appropriate safeguards are in place, the AAAS says.

The bioethics commission believes there should be a system of national oversight supplemented by local independent review boards to ensure that research can proceed under specific conditions. The ethics panel believes supervision of scientists who derive stem cell lines should begin at the local level so the university or other sponsoring institution and other interested parties take responsibility for ensuring the researchers' ethical conduct. The local boards also could review consent documents and oversee the sharing of research materials with foreign institutions.

On a national level, the ethics panel is urging HHS to establish a national oversight panel of scientists and representatives from other fields to ensure that research is conducted in an ethically acceptable manner. "In an ethically sensitive area of emerging biomedical research, it is important that all members of the research community, whether in the public or private sectors, conduct the research in a manner that is open to appropriate public scrutiny," the ethics panel says in its report endorsing federal funding of stem cell research.

Echoing some of the panel's conclusions, Dartmouth ethics expert Green says, "We need to have federal funding of this research, but the best researchers have to remain under open scrutiny as they continue to develop the field. Scientists have to be aware of the need to draw ethical lines, and that people [opposed to their work] aren't just a bunch of medieval anti-Copernicans." ∎

CURRENT SITUATION

Startling Discovery

Until recently, most scientists dismissed the notion that transplanting brain cells could cure serious head injuries or neurological disorders such as Alzheimer's and Parkinson's diseases. Now they are reconsidering the possibilities in light of some startling new evidence.

Researchers in Sweden and the United States over the past year have uncovered pathways in which the brain produces a small but consistent number of new nerve cells, contradicting the long-held belief that the adult brains of humans and other primates can only lose cells, not gain them. [23] At the center of the activity are neural stem cells that can grow into a wide variety of brain cells.

The news was startling because scientists previously thought that the complexity of the human brain prevented the constant production of new cells; essentially, the addition of extra cells would only disrupt the organ's orderly flow of electrical signals. But researchers working with adult macaque monkeys found that stem cells appear to stimulate creation of new nerve cells in the fluid-filled ventricles deep in the brain. The new cells then migrate over a week or more to the cortexes, where they subsequently send out connec-

tions to other nerve cells. The researchers now are trying to interrupt production of the new cells to see if the animals' behavior changes.

"Doctors might ... be able to stimulate stem cells to migrate into areas where they usually do not go and to mature into the specific kinds of nerve cells required by a given patient," neuroscientists Gerd Kempermann and Fred H. Gage of the Salk Institute for Biological Studies in La Jolla, Calif., wrote recently in *Scientific American*. "Although the new cells would not regrow whole brain parts or restore lost memory, they could, for example, manufacture valuable amounts of dopamine [the neurotransmitter whose depletion is responsible for the symptoms of Parkinson's disease] or other substances."

The findings have inspired a new burst of research into the brain's functions, long one of the biggest mysteries in biology. But while the discoveries ignited popular interest and inspired news headlines such as "Can I Grow a New Brain?" researchers caution that the brains of Alzheimer's victims and stroke patients don't appear to try to repair themselves, indicating the regenerative efforts may not be enough to overcome the most serious brain injuries. And they dismiss the futuristic scenario of whole-brain transplants as virtually impossible due to the sheer number of cells and the complex ways they are arrayed. [24]

If the latest research continues to appear promising, scientists expect to give animals various tests and learning tasks to see whether they can influence the stem cells to channel brain cells to various parts of the organ. One study performed on rats showed that if the rodents were trained in tasks involving a brain part called the hippocampus, which influences learning, memory and emotion, more new cells migrated to the part.

Key Questions About Stem Cells and Embryos

Following are some of the questions being raised by ethicists and other concerned Americans about current embryo research:

Why is so much attention being focused on stem cells? Scientists for decades knew that the cells existed, but only recently have been able to isolate them in laboratories. Watching how the cells differentiate into body parts gives researchers the best glimpse yet into the mysteries of early human development. Furthermore, learning how to "train" the cells to evolve into desired tissue could bring a host of promising new medical treatments. But some religious leaders and anti-abortion groups oppose the practice of extracting the cells from embryos and aborted fetuses, which they believe have the same moral status as a human being. Moreover, they worry that scientific advances may prompt researchers to clone embryos strictly so they can be tapped for their stem cells.

Can't scientists obtain stem cells from another source? Yes. Stem cells can also be extracted from adult tissue or from biological materials like umbilical cord blood. However, biologists say these stem cells are different from the ones that are extracted in the embryonic stage and display less of a tendency to differentiate. Thus, their usefulness in research is limited. Opponents of embryonic research say federal money should be directed toward finding new uses for this variety of stem cells.

Isn't there already a ban on using embryos in federally funded research? Yes. President Clinton and Congress have both forbidden taxpayer funding for research with human embryos, regardless of their source. However, lawmakers have also enthusiastically supported research on fetal tissue, as long as investigators don't have a connection with the abortion that provides the tissue source. This has created a curious dichotomy and made it more difficult for lawmakers to sort out whether stem cells actually fall under a funding ban, and whether Congress even has the legal authority to weigh in on the research.

Will stem cell research eventually allow people to clone themselves? It's not inconceivable. However, most experts believe stem cell technology will be primarily used to generate an endless supply of spare parts, such as heart muscle tissue, bone or cartilage. It also could be used in tandem with gene therapy to eliminate undesirable genetic traits in a person that give rise to diseases. That poses a new set of ethical questions, such as are we creating a new bioengineered subspecies of man.

Why are Geron Corp. and other biotechnology companies so interested in the field? Some of the companies want to turn people's ordinary cells into stem cells, then treat them so they can replicate indefinitely. This could provide a source of replacement tissue for deteriorating and diseased tissue and help reverse the aging phenomenon. Other companies want to study how stem cells differentiate to prevent miscarriages and birth defects or help infertile people conceive children.

While stem cells are showing new promise for brain research, they simultaneously are being shown to have less-than-anticipated utility in other areas of medicine. New research is showing that a cancer treatment consisting of high doses of chemotherapy accompanied by stem cell transplants may be no better than ordinary chemotherapy for women with advanced stages of breast cancer. [25]

The regimen was thought to be effective for patients whose breast cancer had spread to other parts of the body. Aggressive chemotherapy would kill the tumor, along with the undesired side effect of killing healthy bone marrow. Afterward, rapidly dividing stem cells previously filtered from the patient's blood would be transplanted back into the body to take up the bone marrow's function and grow new blood cells. Breast cancer is the primary reason such "autotransplants" are now performed. However, a recent study of 1,188 women with metastatic breast cancer treated in North America, Brazil and Russia found the treatment could not reverse the disease in the most serious cases.

"Everyone expected this to be the miracle," says Mary Horowitz, scientific director of the Autologous Blood and Marrow Transplant Registry of North America at the Medical College of Wisconsin and one of the study's authors. [26] She said the results would help breast cancer patients make more informed decisions, perhaps discouraging those with slim odds of survival from trying it as a last resort. ■

OUTLOOK

Future of Cloning

As science continues to challenge people's definitions about what it means to be human, it is likely that more controversial public policy decisions will be made surrounding issues of birth and death. Embryo research provides an important crucible, in the opinion of many experts, because it challenges society to find ethically acceptable applications of its rapidly expanding knowledge about the human condition.

The scientific discoveries surrounding stem cells actually are less of a concern to many people than the potential applications of the work — and what limits should be placed on the technology. Such worries were raised last fall when a Worcester, Mass., company, Advanced Cell Technology, created stem cells by cloning the nucleus of a human cell into a cow egg. The cow eggs are much easier to obtain than human eggs and could provide a more practical way of transplanting a person's own stem cells to replace damaged tissue.

However, critics worried that the company had created a strange cow-human hybrid and called for new controls on cloning technology. Company officials responded that the cells in question could not possibly grow into a viable creature and that they were strictly interested in biomedical applications. [27]

Cloning is the likely "next step" in the stem cell saga.

Science journalist Gregg Easterbrook, a senior editor at *The New Republic*, writes that, while stem cell research is in itself scientifically promising, it really serves as a means of accumulating the technical know-how to eventually clone human beings. This may not be something to necessarily fear, in Easterbrook's view, because cloned individuals could not be created as anything but

babies and would still be subject to the character-shaping effects of their generation's particular upbringing. Dictators would not be able to make carbon copies of themselves, as has been suggested in popular fiction and Hollywood movies. Instead, there would be beneficial effects, such as providing the means for infertile people to conceive and raise children.

"We should not be squeamish about cloning just because it mixes reproduction, technology and the new," Easterbrook writes. "Owing to the stem cell breakthrough, there now stands the prospect that our children

Harold Varmus, director of the National Institutes of Health, discusses the possible uses of stem cells during hearings before the Senate Appropriations Subcommittee on Labor, Health and Human Services and Education on Dec. 2, 1999.

will not only live healthier lives but that their children will be the final generation of Homo sapiens, supplanted by Homo geneticus or whatever comes next. . . . If all goes well, the advent of control over our own cells might offer our grandchildren many things we would wish for them." [28]

Bioethicist Dorothy C. Wertz of the Shriver Center in Waltham, Mass., predicts human cloning will become a treatment primarily used in fertility clinics, similar to egg donation or in-vitro fertilization. She notes both of those techniques were initially criti-

cized as ethically unacceptable but gradually became commonplace.

"The most likely use of cloning would be by people who cannot have children in the usual way and who want to have a child who is like themselves, rather than inviting an unknown stranger's genes into the family," Wertz wrote in the *Gene Letter*, a scientific journal. "Eventually, cloning on a limited basis will become an accepted reproductive technology." [29]

But such acceptance won't begin without more clear-cut rules governing reproductive medical research. President Clinton in 1994 prohibited federal funding from being used to clone human beings, saying, "each human life is unique, born of a miracle that reaches beyond laboratory science." [30] Federally funded scientists could extract DNA from fetal tissue until late last year, when NIH temporarily banned work that used fetuses to create stem cells. Meanwhile, it isn't clear whether Congress or any federal agency can regulate embryo research done in private — or the donation of embryos from thousands of fertility clinics.

Dartmouth ethics expert Green says a widespread ban on cloning and similar technologies won't work because no one will get all countries to agree on what is ethical science. People who want to seek out cloning procedures will travel to countries where the technology is tolerated, while research in countries with cloning bans will be stifled. He believes it's better to permit such research but subject it to strict ethical guidelines.

"There's a deep ethical need to draw lines, defend human life but not just be ignorant and resistant to

AFP Photo/Luke Frazza

At Issue:

Should the federal government fund research involving stem cells derived from embryos remaining after infertility treatments?

NATIONAL BIOETHICS ADVISORY COMMISSION

FROM "ETHICAL ISSUES IN HUMAN STEM CELL RESEARCH," EXECUTIVE SUMMARY, SEPTEMBER 1999.

*r*esearch involving the derivation and use of human ES [embryonic stem] cells . . . remaining after infertility treatments should be eligible for federal funding. An exception should be made to the present statutory ban on federal funding of embryo research to permit federal agencies to fund research involving the derivation of human ES cells from this source under appropriate regulations that include public oversight and review. . . .

The current ban on embryo research is in form of a rider to the appropriations bill for the Department of Health and Human Services (DHHS), of which the National Institutes of Health (NIH) is a part. The rider prohibits use of the appropriated funds to support any research "in which a human embryo [is] destroyed, discarded or knowingly subjected to risk of injury greater than that allowed for research on fetuses in utero." . . .

The ban, which concerns only federally sponsored research, reflects a moral point of view either that embryos deserve the full protection of society because of their moral status as persons or that there is sufficient public controversy to preclude the use of federal funds for this type of research. . . . In our view, the ban conflicts with several of the ethical goals of medicine and related health disciplines, especially healing, prevention and research. These goals are rightly characterized by the principles of beneficence and non-maleficence, which jointly encourage pursuing social benefits and avoiding or ameliorating potential harm.

Although some may view the derivation and use of ES cells as ethically distinct activities, we do not believe that these differences are significant from the point of view of eligibility for federal funding. That is, we believe that it is ethically acceptable for the federal government to finance research that both derives cell lines from embryos remaining after infertility treatments and that uses those cell lines.

Although one might argue that some important research could proceed in the absence of federal funding for research that derives stem cells from embryos remaining after infertility treatments (i.e., federally funded scientists merely using cells derived with private funds), we believe that it is important that federal funding be made available for protocols that also derive such cells.

Relying on cell lines that might be derived exclusively by a subset of privately funded researchers who are interested in this area could severely limit scientific and clinical progress.

RICHARD M. DOERFLINGER

Associate director for policy development, Secretariat for Pro-Life Activities, National Conference of Catholic Bishops

FROM TESTIMONY BEFORE THE SENATE APPROPRIATIONS SUBCOMMITTEE ON LABOR, HEALTH AND HUMAN SERVICES AND EDUCATION, DEC. 2, 1998.

*i*n discussions of human experimentation, the researcher's temptation is to think that if something technically can be done it ethically should be done — particularly if it may lead to medical benefits or advances in scientific knowledge. A civilized society will appreciate the possibilities opened up by research but will insist that scientific progress must not come at the expense of human dignity. When this important balance is not maintained, abuses such as the Tuskegee syphilis study or the Cold War radiation experiments become a reality.

In deciding whether to subsidize various forms of human experimentation, legislators are not merely making an economic decision to allocate limited funds. On behalf of all citizens who pay taxes, they are making a moral decision. They are declaring that certain kinds of research are sufficiently valuable and ethically upright to be conducted in the name of all Americans — and that other kinds are not.

By such funding decisions, government can make an important moral statement, set an example for private research and help direct research toward avenues which fully respect human life and dignity as they seek to help humanity. . . .

A remaining question involves the other avenues for advancing stem cell research, or for advancing the medical goals to which this research is directed, without exploiting developing human beings. Last year, for example, we proposed to Congress that there may be nine promising alternatives to the use of cloning to provide stem cells — and eight of these seem to involve no use of embryonic stem cells at all.

In the same few weeks that these embryo experiments garnered such national attention, significant advances were reported in two of these areas: the use of growth factors to help hearts grow new replacement blood vessels and the use of stem cells from placental blood to treat leukemia and other illnesses.

It would be sad, indeed, if Congress' attention were to focus chiefly on those avenues of research which garner front-page news precisely because they are ethically problematic. Instead, Congress has an opportunity to use its funding power to channel medical research in ways which fully respect human life while advancing human progress.

change," Green says. "If we can't develop a basic understanding of things like stem cells, it will be an impediment to our progress as a society." ∎

Notes

[1] See David Masci, "The Cloning Controversy," *The CQ Researcher*, May 9, 1997, pp. 409-432.

[2] See Adriel Bettelheim, "Biology and Behavior," *The CQ Researcher*, April 3, 1998, pp. 289-312.

[3] For background, see Roger A. Pedersen, "Embryonic Stem Cells for Medicine," *Scientific American*, April 1999, pp. 68-73.

[4] See *CQ Almanac 1995*, pp. 11-55-11-60.

[5] See Charles Marwick, "Funding Stem Cell Research," *Journal of the American Medical Association*, Vol. 281, No. 8, p. 224 (Feb. 24, 1998).

[6] Testimony before the Senate Appropriations Subcommittee on Labor, Health and Human Services and Education, Dec. 2, 1998.

[7] For background, see Sarah Glazer, "*Roe v. Wade* at 25," *The CQ Researcher*, Nov. 28, 1997, pp. 1033-1056.

[8] See National Bioethics Advisory Commission, "Ethical Issues in Human Stem Cell Research," September 1999.

[9] From the Andre Hellegers Lecture, Kennedy Institute of Ethics, Georgetown University, December 1998.

[10] Quoted in Paul Smaglik, "Stem Cell Scientists Caution Clinical Applications Remain Years Away," *The Scientist*, Vol. 12, No. 23, Nov. 23, 1998, p. 1.

[11] See *CQ Almanac 1998*, p. 19-3.

[12] See Paulette Walker Campbell, "Fight Over Stem Cell Research Is Unlikely to Tie Up Spending Bill," *The Chronicle of Higher Education*, Oct. 15, 1999, p. A36.

[13] See Gina Kolata, "When a Cell Does an Embryo's Work, a Debate Is Born," *The New York Times*, Feb. 9, 1999.

[14] Pedersen, *op. cit.*

[15] See "Two Republicans Endorse Stem Cell Research Funding," Reuters, July 30, 1999.

[16] See Nicholas Wade, "Scientists Cultivate Cells at Root of Human Life," *The New York Times*, Nov. 6, 1998, p. A1.

[17] Pedersen, *op. cit.*

[18] See Adriel Bettelheim, "Cancer Treatments," *The CQ Researcher*, Sept. 11, 1998, pp. 785-808

[19] See Rick Weiss, "Stem Cell Discovery Grows Into A Debate," *The Washington Post*, Oct. 9, 1999, p. A1.

[20] See testimony before the Senate Appropriations Subcommittee on Labor, Health and Human Services and Education, Dec. 2, 1998.

[21] See Gregg Easterbrook, "Medical Evolution," *The New Republic*, March 1, 1999, pp. 20-25.

[22] Easterbrook, *op. cit.*

[23] See Gerd Kempermann and Fred H. Gage, "New Nerve Cells for the Adult Brain," *Scientific American*, May 1999, pp. 48-53.

[24] See David Brown, "Brain Regenerates Cells, Study Says," *The Washington Post*, Oct. 15, 1999, p. A2.

[25] See Philip A. Rowlings et al., "Factors Correlated With Progression-Free Survival After High-Dose Chemotherapy and Hematopoietic Stem Cell Transplantation for Metastatic Breast Cancer," *Journal of the American Medical Association*, Vol. 282, No. 14, (Oct. 13, 1999), pp. 1335-1343.

[26] Quoted in Marilynn Marchione, "Study Shows When Treatments for Breast Cancer Are Most Effective," *Milwaukee Journal Sentinel*, Oct. 13, 1999, p. 1.

[27] See Faye Flam, "Despite Objections, Hopes Rise for Material That Could Repair Human Ailments," *The Philadelphia Inquirer*, June 27, 1999.

[28] Esterbrook, *op. cit.*

[29] See "Conclusion: The Future of Cloning," *Gene Letter*, Vol. 3, Issue 1, August 1998

[30] See "Human Cloning Discouraged," The Associated Press, March 4, 1997.

FOR MORE INFORMATION

Center for Bioethics and Human Dignity, 2065 Half Day Road, Bannockburn, Ill. 60015; (847); 317-8180, www.bioethix.org. This nonprofit group is spearheading opposition to federally funded stem cell research on material derived from embryos, arguing the work entails destroying human beings.

Geron Corp., 230 Constitution Dr., Menlo Park, Calif. 94025; (650) 473-7700; www.geron.com. This biotechnology company funded the recent research into stem cells and licensed patents from the academic institutions where the work took place. It hopes to combine stem cell technology with cloning to create new anti-aging products.

National Institutes of Health, 1 Center Dr., Building 1, Suite 126, Bethesda, Md. 20892; (301) 496-2433; www.nih.gov. This branch of the Department of Health and Human Services supports and conducts biomedical research into causes and prevention of disease and would oversee federally supported research on stem cells and embryos. It now is devising guidelines on stem cell research.

Patients' Coalition for Urgent Research, 2021 K St., N.W., Suite 305, Washington, D.C. 20006; (202) 293-2856. This coalition of more than 30 patient advocacy and disease groups actively lobbies for federal funding for embryo and stem cell research, citing myriad potential health benefits.

Bibliography

Selected Sources Used

Books

Cook-Deegan, Robert, *The Gene Wars: Science, Politics and the Human Genome*, W.W. Norton, 1996.
The former director of the Biomedical Ethics Advisory Committee gives a firsthand account of efforts to launch the Human Genome Project and the politics surrounding the biomedical research community.

Lyon, Jeff, and Peter Gorner, *Altered Fates: Gene Therapy and the Retooling of Human Life*, W.W. Norton, 1996.
Two reporters explore the possibility of curing thousands of genetic conditions by transplanting properly coded genes for defective ones. They also explore the genetic roots of aging, psychology and intellect and discuss the biomedical possibilities from cloning human embryos.

McGee, Glenn, (ed.)., *The Human Cloning Debate*, Berkeley Hills Books, 1998.
Numerous perspectives on the promise and challenges from cloning in the wake of the 1997 creation of Dolly, the sheep. Special emphasis on the philosophical implications of human cloning.

Quesenberry, Peter J. (ed.), *Stem Cell Biology and Gene Therapy*, Wiley-Liss, 1998.
A somewhat technical look at stem cell research and gene therapy. Topics covered include preparations of stem cells, possible therapies and new clinical applications.

Articles

"Comment: Stem Cell Research," Mary Woodard Lasker Charitable Trust, 1998.
A comprehensive review of key scientific, policy and ethical issues surrounding stem cell research and how it may relate to the 1995 congressional ban on embryo research. Included are perspectives from politicians, religious leaders, government officials and prominent scientists.

Hoffman, Paul, "Can I Grow A New Brain?" *Time*, Nov. 8, 1999, p. 94.
This portion of *Time*'s Visions 21 series focuses on the use of neural stem cells to repair damage and even re-create parts of the brain.

Marwick, Charles, "Funding Stem Cell Research," *Journal of the American Medical Association*, Vol. 281, No. 8, p. 224 (Feb. 24, 1999).

Account of how the National Institutes of Health decided it can fund research on stem cells from human embryonic tissue, despite the statutory ban on research involving human embryos.

Pedersen, Roger A., "Embryonic Stem Cells for Medicine," *Scientific American*, April 1999, pp. 68-73.
A stem cells researcher at the University of California at San Francisco details the far-reaching potential of stem cell-derived therapies if scientists are able to coax the cells into making perfectly matched tissues for transplantation.

Smaglik, Paul, "Stem Cell Scientists Caution Clinical Applications Remain Years Away," *The Scientist*, Nov. 23, 1998, p. 1.
Biologists still have years of work before patients will receive either stem cell-derived tissue transplants or stem cell-based gene therapy, scientists agree.

Wade, Nicholas, "Scientists Cultivate Cells at Root of Human Life," *The New York Times*, Nov. 6, 1998, p. A1.
The first report of the isolation of human embryonic stem cells and an early analysis of the thicket of ethical and legal questions that the discovery prompted.

Weiss, Rick, "Stem Cell Discovery Grows Into A Debate," *The Washington Post*, Oct. 9, 1999, p. A1.
The new field of stem cell research faces major tests in the laboratory and in Congress as the fiscal 2000 federal budget cycle draws to a close.

Reports

American Association for the Advancement of Science, "Stem Cell Research & Applications," Aug. 18, 1999.
After hearing from scientists, religious leaders and government officials, the association endorses federally funded stem cell research, saying it holds enormous potential for contributing to mankind's understanding of basic human biology.

National Bioethics Advisory Commission, "Ethical Issues in Human Stem Cell Research," September 1999.
A White House ethics panel examines pressing issues surrounding stem cell research and concludes the federal government should have a funding and oversight role.

10 Human Genome Research

MARY H. COOPER

I magine an instruction manual, the kind that comes with, say, a new computer. Now imagine the same manual expanded to several hundred volumes the size of the Manhattan phone book. Then try to imagine the same set of instructions shrunk so small it could easily fit on the head of a pin.

That's roughly the amount of information contained in the human genome — the "book" of genetic instructions that directs development. The genome comprises all the body's genetic material, long strands of deoxyribonucleic acid (DNA) that are distributed among the 23 sets of chromosomes contained in almost every one of the 100 trillion cells that make up a human being. Each of the genome's approximately 100,000 genes, which are carried on the chromosomes, orders the manufacture of one or more proteins. It is these proteins that carry out all the body's vital functions. (*See diagram, p. 178.*)

Decoding the body's complex genetic instructions has been the focus of an intensive effort by both public and private laboratories. In the very near future — perhaps as early as this spring — scientists are expected to complete the monumental task of mapping most of the human genome, passing a new milestone in the history of science.

"The scientific community has pursued this as their Holy Grail for years," says Richard A. Gibbs, director of the Human Genome Sequencing Center at Baylor College of Medicine in Houston. "They've worked hard, doggedly pursuing this, and it's driven the whole field to the point it's at now. And no wonder — we like to say it's the most exciting project ever."

From *The CQ Researcher*, May 12, 2000.

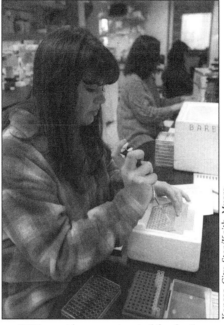

DNA samples are extracted for further testing at Washington University in St. Louis, Mo., one of four U.S. labs working on decoding the human genome.

Kansas City Star/Keith Myers

Genome research has greatly expanded a relatively new field of study called genomics, the study of genes and their function in health and disease. The quest to sequence, or decode, the human genome was launched in 1990 by the Human Genome Project — a joint endeavor of the U.S. Department of Energy and the National Institutes of Health (NIH). Originally, the deadline for completing the project was 2005, but advances in computer technology pushed the completion date up to 2003.

The pace of human genome research received a major boost in 1998, when J. Craig Venter, a gene researcher at NIH, left the public project to start up a private company, Celera Genomics Inc., committed to completing the genome by 2001.

Venter's challenge kicked off a race between public and private labs that produced a rapid succession of key discoveries. Last December, the Human Genome Project for the first time published the genetic code of an entire human chromosome, Chromosome 22. * In March, a joint project between Celera and researchers at the University of California at Berkeley completed the genome of the most complex organism to date — *Drosophila melanogaster*, a tiny fruit fly that contains a large number of genes similar to those in humans. On April 6, Celera announced that it had finished decoding 99 percent of the human genome, placing it well ahead of the public effort.

Whatever the outcome of the public-private competition, scientists agree that sequencing the genome is just the first step in an entirely new phase of scientific research that is destined to revolutionize biological sciences and the practice of medicine.

"We have to understand that the sequence of the genome represents just the building blocks," says Eric S. Lander, director of the Whitehead/MIT Center for Genomic Research at the Massachusetts Institute of Technology, the largest of the five major sequencing centers in the Human Genome Project. "We don't yet understand how those building blocks work together."

To visualize the enormity of the work that lies ahead, Lander likens the human genome to a list of parts for a Boeing 777, which contains about 100,000 components, the same as the estimated number of human genes.

"The parts list would not tell you how the thing flies, and it certainly wouldn't tell you how to make it turn

---

* The Human Genome Project reported May 8 that it has decoded Chromosome 21, which is responsible for Down syndrome. Some 350,000 people in the United States have Down syndrome, the most common genetic cause of mental retardation.

'Deposits' in Gene 'Bank' Skyrocketed

Rapid advances in computer technology have greatly accelerated researchers' efforts to decode the human genome. Nearly 5 million gene sequences are now filed in GenBank, a publicly accessible database on the Internet, compared with fewer than 40,000 sequences a decade ago.

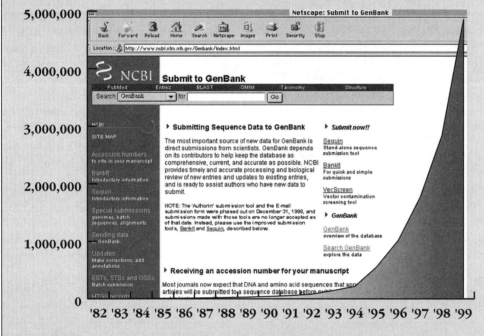

Number of sequences

5,000,000

4,000,000

3,000,000

2,000,000

1,000,000

0

'82 '83 '84 '85 '86 '87 '88 '89 '90 '91 '92 '93 '94 '95 '96 '97 '98 '99

Source: National Institutes of Health

way to understand what genomics is about is getting us to the starting line, where for the first time we can find out what's really wrong in a disease, rather than merely treat the symptoms," Lander says. "The Human Genome Project is just an infrastructure-building project. Now get set — the infrastructure is finally here, and biology is ready to explode in many, many directions."

The explosion in scientific research and discovery is not without collateral damage, however. Even before the genome's completion, controversies are building over a number of legal, social and ethical problems that are emerging in its wake.

A major issue involves ownership of the genome and its components. Academic labs and private companies such as Incyte Genomics Inc. and Human Genome Sciences (HGS) are applying for thousands of patents on human genes and gene fragments that may bring windfall profits if future research links them to common diseases and, hopefully, to new drugs. Celera is also applying for thousands of patents, but its main focus is making its genome-sequencing data and analysis available to paying clients with deep pockets, mainly drug companies and research organizations.

Private labs, drug companies and others involved in the emerging biotechnology industry say commercial applications of basic scientific re-

left," he says. "Well, that's where we are with the human genome. We have a wonderfully exciting century ahead of us figuring out precisely how this works, and by its end, we will."

Along the way, researchers expect to unravel the mysteries of many diseases that can be traced to genetic defects. "Any two human beings, regardless of ethnic or racial self-identity, are 99.9 percent the same at the genetic level," explained Francis S. Collins, director of the National Human Genome Research Institute and head of the public project. "But certain changes in the sequence, some as subtle as a single 'letter' change, contribute to disease or dis-

ease risk. Today, to find the misspelling or misspellings that contribute to common diseases, such as cancer, Parkinson's disease, asthma, depression or heart disease, researchers must study pedigrees and search through large chromosome 'neighborhoods' using the genetic map.

"But having the reference sequence, and new technologies for finding those places in the genome that vary among us, means that assembling a catalog of common genetic variants is now possible and will greatly speed the process of disease-gene discovery." [1]

Researchers eagerly anticipate a new era in biology and medicine. "The best

search benefit the public because they speed the development of new treatments.

"We have two races going on today," says Charles Ludlum, vice president for government affairs at the Biotechnology Industry Organization (BIO), the industry's main lobby. "We have a race to identify the genetic information and to secure patents, and we have a race by the patent-holder to develop the invention into a commercial product. Those two races are exactly what you want if you're a patient with a genetic disease."

Critics of the privatization of genetic information argue that the genome belongs in the public domain. They point to the Human Genome Project, which releases its sequencing data daily via GenBank, a database that is freely available to anyone with access to the Internet. [2] Many academic researchers also argue that patenting genetic material will slow the pace of medical research while enriching a few patent-holding companies and their stockholders.

The patenting issue came to a head on March 14, when President Clinton and British Prime Minister Tony Blair jointly called for the release of "raw" genetic data into the public domain. Although the statement merely summarized existing policy on gene patenting, it prompted a massive sell-off of stock in genomic companies as investors wrongly assumed that existing gene patents might be voided as a result of some new policy.

Some experts say the controversy over gene patenting is a symptom of something more worrisome, an overemphasis on the importance of genes in human health and disease.

"There's an assumption in this debate that we are our genes," says Martin Teitel, executive director of the Council for Responsible Genetics, which studies the ethical and legal implications of new genetic technologies. Teitel and others fear that employers and insurers may use genetic profiles to refuse employment or coverage.

"Genetic determinism is loose in the land, but there is still an awful lot that science doesn't understand," Teitel says. "When you start reducing people to their genes, you start going down roads that are terribly misleading, and things like discrimination and loss of privacy may come as a result."

Although many states have laws against genetic discrimination, Congress is only beginning to consider the broader legal and social implications of genomics research.

As researchers close in on their quest to fully decode the human genome, these are some of the issues that policy-makers are considering:

Should the government issue patents on human genetic material?

As the discovery of new genes has accelerated in recent years, so too has the pace of gene-patent applications by research organizations hoping to cash in on their discoveries. The U.S. Patent and Trademark Office (PTO) has been inundated with thousands of applications for patents, not only for whole genes but also gene fragments known as ESTs (expression sequence tags) and SNPs (single nucleotide polymorphisms, pronounced "snips").

And it's not just private companies that have applied for gene patents: Of the top five organizations that have received gene patents, two are public labs. (*See table, p. 185.*)

Although patent law clearly permits the patenting of genetic material, a lively debate has emerged over the wisdom of allowing individuals or companies to "own" the essence of human life.

"The human genome is, by definition, something that is common to every person," Teitel says. "If we hold anything in common, it's got to be that; it's what makes us who we are. As soon as you patent it, you privatize it, and philosophically, I have a problem with that."

The Genetic Bill of Rights issued by Teitel's organization declares, "All people have the right to a world in which living organisms cannot be patented, including human beings, animals, plants, microorganisms and all their parts." [3]

While most gene patents are being issued to U.S. companies and public labs, the most vocal criticism of genetic commercialization comes from Europe. Demonstrators have filled the streets in a number of countries to protest imports of U.S. genetically engineered foods, and protesters recently destroyed genetically altered crops in Britain. [4]

Though the main focus of concern in Europe is the potential health threat of so-called "Frankenfoods," skepticism of privatizing genetic material is on the rise.

"There is a considerable groundswell in the U.K. of opinion that doesn't like the concept of patenting genes," says Don Powell, a spokesman for the Sanger Center, near Cambridge, one of the five major genome-sequencing centers that comprise the Human Genome Project. "There are 100,000 genes in the genome, so there's more than enough to go around. Simply in terms of human benefit, the more people who are working in this area, the better."

Gene patents were not an issue in 1952, when lawmakers passed the Patent Act, which broadly defined patentable material. In 1980, the Supreme Court agreed with that approach in its landmark decision in *Diamond v. Chakrabarty.*

"The Supreme Court said that anything under the sun that is made by man is eligible to be patented, and that's where we stand today," says John Doll, the director of biotechnol-

Understanding the Human Genome

The genome is the complete genetic code of one person. The genetic code that determines whether a person has brown or blue eyes — and all the person's other inherited characteristics — lies in a long molecule, DNA, that can duplicate itself during cell division with almost perfect accuracy.

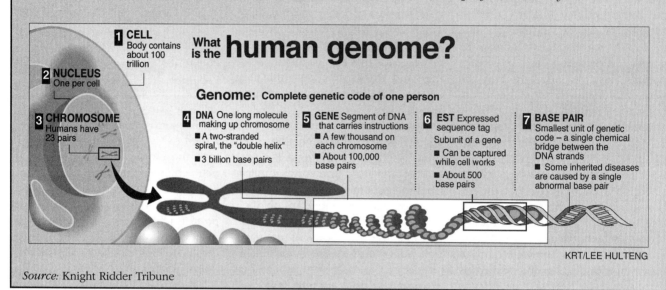

KRT/LEE HULTENG

Source: Knight Ridder Tribune

ogy patent examination. "I see a lot of comments that genetic material should not be patented, but the people who drafted the Patent Act clearly had a very liberal and broad interpretation as to what patentable subject matter was. And that was simply that if it occurs naturally in nature, it should not be patented, but if it has been influenced by the hand of man, it is clearly eligible to be patented."

Doll emphasizes that the government does not issue patents on living human matter. "When you patent a human gene, you're not patenting what's in your arm," he says. "What you're patenting is an isolated and purified chemical compound that is not naturally occurring in nature. If all you have to do is draw material from your arm in a blood sample, it probably is not patentable. But once you isolate it, purify it, give it some utility and functionally characterize it, then it's a patentable invention."

The biotechnology industry views patenting as an essential incentive for research. "The people who view patents from a moral point of view do not understand what patents are," the BIO's Ludlum says. "The only thing you can patent is a man-made invention in a lab, where the gene or gene sequence is extracted from the chromosome, purified, isolated and characterized in terms of its function. This is an industrial invention that can require substantial brilliance and funding."

Even then, Ludlum says, holding a patent on a gene does not confer "ownership" of that gene. "Once you secure a patent," he says, "you simply have a right to protect your investment vis-à-vis commercial competitors." That right ends when the patent expires, 20 years after the application is filed.

Biotech entrepreneurs also say they would never embark on the research and development of new drugs, which can cost up to $350 million over 12 years, without patent protection. [5]

"What all of us want is to speed the treatment and cure of disease," writes William A. Haseltine, chairman and CEO of Human Genome Sciences Inc., a Rockville, Md., biopharmaceutical company. "That is precisely what gene patents do, by ensuring somebody who is willing to invest in the development of a gene-based drug or treatment that he can have a return on that investment. Absent patents, these new drugs will not be developed." [6]

Many researchers agree that the ability to patent genetic material has helped spur research that has already begun to yield important results. But they also express concern about access to patented material that may be crucial to their work.

"It all really depends on whether or not it's going to actually impede the progress of those of us in basic research," says Chris T. Amemiya, associate professor and director of

Using Gene Testing to Uncover Disease

Medical research has already traced the causes of some diseases — cystic fibrosis, Duchenne muscular dystrophy and Huntington's disease, to name but a few — to flawed genes. Genetic mutations also are known to increase the risk of developing heart disease, diabetes, cancer and other common illnesses.

Human genome research is speeding the recognition of the genetic links to disease. In 1997 alone, scientists used the portions of the genome that had already been sequenced to isolate 16 disease genes. Future research is expected to uncover a hereditary link for as many as 5,000 diseases — and gene tests for each one of them.

The virtues of gene testing are clear. Women whose close relatives have had breast or ovarian cancer, for example, may derive considerable relief if they test negative for mutations on the BRCA1 and BRCA2 genes, which have been linked to certain forms of the diseases. Even those who test positive may benefit by taking immediate steps to reduce their risk by eating a better diet, exercising and making other lifestyle changes and ensuring that any future tumor is detected early by getting frequent mammograms.

Gene testing offers no guarantees, however. A negative result does not mean you won't get the disease. Also, test results are only as reliable as the people who run them. A false positive result may prompt a person to opt for preventive surgery before the disease takes hold, only to learn that the result was negative after all. [1]

And what about genetic diseases for which there is no known cure or treatment? Perhaps the most devastating example is Huntington's chorea, a degenerative neurological disease named for George Huntington, a physician who first described it in 1872. Huntington's typically begins at age 30 to 40 with mild psychotic and behavioral symptoms that lead to muscular spasms, dementia and death within an average of 17 years. About 30,000 Americans have Huntington's, and about 150,000 more are at risk of inheriting it from a parent. [2]

In the late 1970s, Nancy Wexler, a Columbia University neurologist whose mother and three uncles had Huntington's, began searching for its genetic roots. She focused her search on three rural villages in Venezuela where there was an unusually high incidence of the disease. In 1983, thousands of blood samples later, the genetic defect responsible for Huntington's was traced to Chromosome 4.

It took 10 more years to identify the actual gene, and by 1986 a test was available to determine whether an individual with a family history of Huntington's is destined to get the disease. Scientists hope further research will lead to a cure.

But for now, the link between the genetic mutation and Huntington's is so strong that a positive test result for the disease amounts to a virtual sentence to a premature and agonizing death. Parents with Huntington's are also burdened with the knowledge that their children may well be doomed to the same fate. That's because Huntington's, unlike the vast majority of conditions, is caused by a dominant gene.

"The cause is in the genes and nowhere else," states science writer Matt Ridley. "Either you have the Huntington's mutation and will get the disease or not. This is determinism, predestination and fate on a scale of which Calvin never dreamed." [3]

Huntington's illustrates the dilemma posed by human genetic research — scientists are learning about the origin of diseases faster than they are learning how to prevent or cure them. In such cases, the wisdom of gene testing is questionable. Wexler calls the dilemma "the Tiresias complex," recalling the words of the blind seer Tiresias in Sophocles' "Oedipus the King": "It is but sorrow to be wise when wisdom profits not."

As Wexler explains, "Do you want to know how and when you are going to die, especially if you have no power to change the outcome? How does a person choose to learn this momentous information? How does one cope with the answer?" In fact, very few people have availed themselves of the gene test for Huntington's. [4]

In most other cases, a positive result from a gene test does not necessarily mean the individual will succumb to the disease. "Fortunately, Huntington's is a very rare example," says J. Craig Venter, president of Celera Genomics Inc., the leading private company involved in sequencing the human genome. "It was thought that cystic fibrosis was an absolutely genetically determined disease, and that if you had changes in the spelling of the so-called cystic fibrosis gene you would get cystic fibrosis. Further studies have proven that that's not true. There are different diseases associated with the same gene, such as chronic pancreatitis, and there's even no disease associated with those same genetic changes."

"Genetics tools have concentrated on the few very, very rare events that do seem to go awry when there's a problem with one gene," Venter says. "Huntington's disease is one of the rare diseases that's in that category, but that's not how most biology works. That's because of the complex interactions that all our proteins have with other proteins. We don't work one protein at a time."

---

[1] For one such example, see Anne Underwood, "When 'Knowledge' Does Damage," *Newsweek*, April 10, 2000, p. 62.

[2] From the National Institutes of Health Web site, www.ncbi.nlm.nih.gov.

[3] Matt Ridley, *Genome* (1999), p. 56.

[4] N.S. Wexler, "The Tiresias Complex: Huntington's Disease as a Paradigm of Testing for Late-Onset Disorders," *FASEB Journal* (Federation of American Societies for Experimental Biology), July 1992, pp. 2820-2825.

Most States Prohibit Genetic Discrimination

Many states passed laws in the late 1990s to prevent discrimination based on a person's genetic makeup. Forty-four states now prohibit health insurance companies from refusing coverage to those at high risk for certain medical conditions, such as cancer, because of their genetic history. Sixteen states prohibit genetic discrimination in employment.

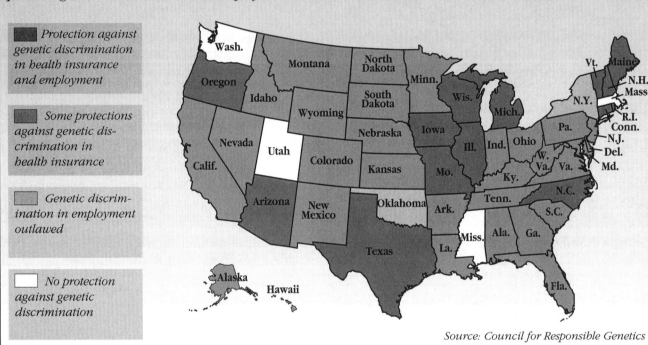

Protection against genetic discrimination in health insurance and employment

Some protections against genetic discrimination in health insurance

Genetic discrimination in employment outlawed

No protection against genetic discrimination

Source: Council for Responsible Genetics

developmental genetics at the Center for Human Genetics at Boston University School of Medicine. "Are we going to not be allowed to study these genes at all, or with certain restrictions? That's the big question that everyone is asking."

The question is likely to become even more pressing in the future, as researchers move beyond the study of single genes to trying to determine how they interact.

"Basically, what people are interested in is understanding not just the function of a single gene but how that function interacts with the functions of other genes," Amemiya says. "Delineating these biochemical pathways is extremely important. But if there are restrictions put on the use of the genes that are part of these biochemical pathways,

that could severely hamper that progress and impact all of us in basic research."

While computer technology has been essential to genome research, some scientists say it also makes it too easy to obtain patents on genetic material. "In the old days, one thought about patents as protecting novel, creative ideas, and society granted a monopoly to an inventor as a way of incenting that person to make an invention," Lander says. "Today we have the ability to make automatic discoveries by running machines and in a completely automatic fashion generate data and then file patents on it. This kind of work is so straightforward that anyone can do it, and society is getting very little for its bargain."

By contrast, the work required to

determine the function of a gene, and then to use it in medical therapies, is extremely difficult, Lander says. "But if we've already given away the basic monopoly right to the person who has merely reported the sequence, then we have, in fact, diminished the economic reward for the difficult and expensive step of finding function and fashioning of therapy.

"That's just economically foolish," Lander continues. "It's not a question of trying to deny the people who did the trivial work a patent; it's a question of making sure that we have something there to dangle in front of the people who are going to have to do the multimillion-dollar work on each gene."

Critics renewed their call for tougher standards in issuing gene patents on Feb. 15, when Human Genome Sciences announced that it had been granted a patent for a gene that it said encodes a protein that may enable HIV, the AIDS virus, to penetrate and infect cells. The same day, an AIDS researcher reported that the company's description of the CCR5 gene that was filed with the Patent Office contained four sequencing errors.

"By looking at the sequence and those four mistakes that are in the sequence, I knew that the mistakes that are in the patent had arisen solely by [human] sequencing error," says Christopher C. Broder, a professor of microbiology at the Uniformed Services University of the Health Sciences, a medical school for military officers in Bethesda, Md. Broder and his team had separately identified the CCR5 gene from their own research and discovered its link to AIDS.

"I agree that patents on genes are viable," Broder says. "However, the invention should include not only the gene's identification but a functional analysis, so you know what role it plays. Edison invented the light bulb; he didn't find it on the forest floor."

The CCR5 gene patent is only one of 7,500 patent applications filed by HGS as of mid-April, not to mention other genomic firms such as Incyte and Celera. "There's no way that they know the functional data for all of these things," Broder says. "It's just a way to get their foot in the door. If we hadn't come across the fact that these genes were involved in HIV entry, then HGS would be sitting on a patent that would just be gathering dust."

Will the sequencing of the human genome open the door to genetic discrimination?

Like so many scientific advances of the past, the genomic revolution poses a serious problem: Human acquisition of information may be proceeding at a faster pace than society is able to use it wisely. The discovery and harnessing of atomic energy unleashed a nearly 50-year Cold War and lingering fears of nuclear annihilation. Likewise, for all its potential for treating and preventing disease, genome research is yield-

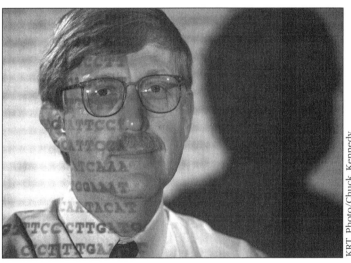

Francis S. Collins, director of the National Human Genome Research Institute at the National Institutes of Health, isolated the first human gene. The projected letters represent part of the description of the cystic fibrosis gene he discovered in 1989.

ing information that could result in widespread discrimination against individuals based on their genetic makeup. Ethicists paint a bleak future in which employers, insurers and governments could use personal genetic information as a weapon of discrimination, creating an underclass of genetically "flawed" individuals. (*See story, p. 186.*)

"My biggest concern about this new information is the potential abuse of it," Celera's Venter says. "I wish we could say we don't have to worry about that, but recent events

in human history suggest that we don't have a very good track record as a species. People who want to discriminate and hate won't get much justification for that from the genetic code because they'll find that they're far more like their enemies than different. But at the same time, insurance companies, employers and governments can and already do use this information to discriminate."

The privacy issue has already emerged in Britain, where the government is considering a proposal for the country's nationalized health system to set up a unified database containing all citizens' genetic information in an effort to make health care more efficient.

"The National Health Service would be able to look at the best ways of dispensing medicine on the basis of the database of human DNA sequences," says the Sanger Center's Powell. "But there's a great deal of concern about this, and the government has called for open and public talks about how we're going to set that up and how we're going to safeguard privacy."

Freedom from genetic discrimination is a central goal of the Council for Responsible Genetics, whose Genetic Bill of Rights also proclaims the right to prevent the inclusion of an individual's genetic information in the kind of database Powell describes without voluntary informed consent.

Teitel, the council's executive director, says the threat of genetic discrimination arises from the mistaken assumption that our genetic makeup contains everything anyone needs to know about us.

"The root of the problem is determinism, this idea that we are our genes," he says. "It's the silly idea that if my gay gene is switched on, then I'm gay, or my fat gene makes me fat or I indulge in risky behavior because my risk-taking gene is switched on."

Gene research has identified a number of genes in which polymorphisms, or coding abnormalities, are known to cause certain diseases, such as Huntington's disease, a devastating neurological disease with no known cure. "But for all the rest of known diseases, the genes operate in a kind of collective," Teitel says. "The genes code for proteins, and those proteins influence each other, so therefore everything is contextual."

To prevent misuse of genetic information, some advocates are calling for two types of regulation. "We need protection on the confidentiality of genetic information to make sure that outsiders can't get the information in the first place," Ludlum of the BIO says. "Then we need protections against discrimination, so that if they have the information they cannot use it to discriminate."

Congress partly addressed the concern about discrimination with the 1996 Health Insurance Portability and Accountability Act, which helps workers keep their health insurance when they change jobs. The law bars group insurers such as health maintenance organizations (HMOs) from denying coverage on the basis of pre-existing conditions. It also bars them from using genetic information as evidence of disease in the absence of a medical diagnosis indicating the disease is in progress.

"This is the first law to ban discrimination based upon genetic information," says Ludlum, whose organization supported the provision. "We still have problems in the individual health-insurance market, but today it is illegal to discriminate on the basis of genetic information in

the group health-insurance market. The next step is to deal with discrimination in other contexts, such as employment and education."

Some researchers caution that exaggerated concerns about privacy and discrimination may needlessly impede their work. "Getting the initial human DNA for the sequencing project was fraught with ethical land mines and what-ifs," says Gibbs of the Human Genome Project's Baylor Center. He also says ethical concerns may make it hard for individuals to gain access to their own genetic information when they want to find out what they can do to avoid certain gene-related maladies.

Someone who discovers through testing that he has a genetic predisposition to heart disease, for example, can reduce the likelihood of getting sick through diet and exercise. Conversely, a woman who tests negative for the faulty BRCA1 or BRCA2 gene linked to breast cancer can find considerable relief from fear of coming down with a potentially fatal disease.

"I'm a big advocate of due process in order to protect individuals," Gibbs says, "but it seems that many of the ethicists underpin their arguments for ensuring due process with the notion that nobody can ever be smart enough to make their own decisions."

In Gibbs' view, it is by no means certain that genome research will tip the scales in favor of insurance companies at the expense of individual rights. For one thing, he says, individuals could gain the upper hand by taking out insurance to cover diseases they know from gene testing that they may suffer from in the future, but about which the insurer is unaware. For another, the additional information provided by genomic data may actually make the insurance system fairer by more accurately defining risks.

"There may be real potential here for insurance to be better managed

through this kind of knowledge," he says. "You'd still need to have legislation in place to prevent the exclusion of different groups who are at risk, but in a large sense, there's a positive thing going on here, and that is that management of risk will become better articulated."

In the long run, gene research also may actually end up being the solution to discrimination, at least by insurers. "Insurance companies indirectly use genetic information all the time when they take your blood pressure or your family history in trying to limit their risk," Venter says. "That's understandable, because they'll go out of business otherwise."

But once personalized genomes become available for individuals, and tests are created to scrutinize them, Venter predicts, the rationale for private insurance companies will disappear.

"Once we've sequenced all of our genomes, we will all be uninsurable because we all have genes in our genetic code that would indicate a propensity for some disease in the future," he says. "This is probably the single, best justification for nationalized health insurance." ■

BACKGROUND

Peas and Fruit Flies

The genome revolution traces its roots to Gregor Mendel, a Moravian monk whose experiments in breeding garden pea plants during the 1860s laid the groundwork for modern genetics. Mendel discovered basic principles of heredity by crossing different varieties of plants with distinctive characteristics such as seed

Chronology

1860s-1900s
Gregor Mendel and Charles Darwin define the basis of modern biology and genetics.

1859
Charles Darwin presents his theory of evolution in *The Origin of Species.*

1863
Gregor Mendel, a Moravian monk, states that inherited traits are controlled by invisible elements, later called genes.

—— • ——

1900s-1940s
Successive discoveries show that genes contain the instructions for making proteins and that mutations are the result of altered genes.

1927
American geneticist Hermann Joe Muller discovers genes can undergo mutations.

1940
American scientists George Beadle and Edward Tatum discover that each gene specifies the production of a specific enzyme.

1943
American chemist Linus Pauling discovers that sickle-cell anemia is caused by a fault in the gene that orders the production of the protein hemoglobin.

—— • ——

1950s-1980s
The discovery of DNA's struc- ture marks the beginning of modern genetics.

1952
The Patent Act defines patentable material, excluding naturally occurring matter.

Feb. 28, 1953
English scientist Francis Crick, co-discoverer with American James Watson of the structure of deoxyribonucleic acid (DNA), proclaims, "We've discovered the secret of life."

1980
The U.S. Supreme Court, in *Diamond v. Chakrabarty,* approves the principle of patenting genetically engineered life forms.

—— • ——

1990s The quest to sequence the human genome begins.

Oct. 1, 1990
Led by Watson, the Human Genome Project sets out to identify and publish the complete sequence of DNA in the human genome by 2005.

1995
Congress bans federal funding of research on human embryonic stem cells.

1996
The Health Insurance Portability and Accountability Act bans discrimination by group health insurers based upon genetic information.

1997
Scottish scientists report cloning a sheep, named Dolly. The U.S. scientific establishment adopts a voluntary moratorium on human-cloning research.

May 9, 1998
U.S. gene researcher J. Craig Venter starts Celera Genomics Inc. with the goal of sequencing the human genome in three years.

Aug. 17, 1998
Incyte Pharmaceuticals announces that it will sequence "all commercially relevant" information on the human genome within two years.

April 1999
The SNPs Consortium, a public-private joint venture, is formed to identify more than 300,000 gene fragments called single nucleotide polymorphisms.

March 15, 1999
The Human Genome Project shortens its deadline for completing the genome and promises a "working draft" of the sequence by spring 2000.

December 1999
The Human Genome Project completes the first human chromosome ever sequenced, Chromosome 22.

March 7, 2000
Following the earlier death of a teenager undergoing experimental gene therapy, the Food and Drug Administration and the NIH tighten oversight of gene-therapy experiments in humans.

March 24, 2000
Celera and publicly funded labs in Europe and at the University of California at Berkeley publish the genome of the fruit fly — the most complex organism sequenced to date.

shape and color. Although the resulting hybrids always resembled just one parent plant, when the hybrids self-fertilized the missing traits reappeared consistently in about a quarter of the next generation.

Mendel's results proved that inherited traits are not diluted at reproduction but pass to the next generation intact in predictable proportions according to whether they are dominant or recessive. His law of segregation describing that principle held that inherited traits were controlled by invisible elements, later called genes.

The significance of Mendel's discoveries went unrecognized in his lifetime. In 1859, Charles Darwin published *The Origin of Species*, in which he presented the theory of evolution that was to define modern biology. Darwinism seemed initially to contradict Mendel's law of segregation by suggesting that environmental forces are responsible for the myriad changes in inherited traits that constitute evolution. How could mere environmental changes, critics asked, affect such immutable elements as genes?

The answer came in 1927. By bombarding fruit flies with X-rays, Hermann Joe Muller, an American geneticist, discovered that genes could be changed, undergoing mutations that were visible in new physical characteristics. That also suggested that genes contained structures that were capable of mutation.

In 1940, two other Americans, George Beadle and Edward Tatum, found that certain organisms exposed to X-rays failed to produce a certain enzyme and that one gene specifies the production of one enzyme. Three

years later, American chemist Linus Pauling built on their theory and discovered that sickle-cell anemia, a debilitating condition found in people of African descent, was caused by a fault in the gene that orders the production of the protein hemoglobin. By the mid-1940s, it had become clear that genes contain the instruc-

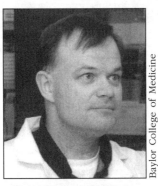
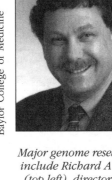
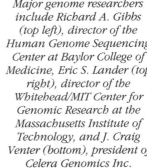

Major genome researchers include Richard A. Gibbs (top left), director of the Human Genome Sequencing Center at Baylor College of Medicine, Eric S. Lander (top right), director of the Whitehead/MIT Center for Genomic Research at the Massachusetts Institute of Technology, and J. Craig Venter (bottom), president of Celera Genomics Inc.

tions for making proteins and that mutations were the result of altered genes making altered proteins. [7]

But the way genes made proteins remained an enigma until the 1950s, when two scientists traced the mechanism to deoxyribonucleic acid, or DNA. James Watson, an American, and the English scientist Francis Crick poured over earlier findings on DNA until they discovered the molecule's structure — an immensely long double helix connected by base pairs resembling a circular ladder that is found in the chromosomes within the cell's nucleus.

Watson and Crick also found that the base pairs forming the steps on

the DNA ladder are made up of just four bases — adenine, cytosine, guanine and thymine — represented by the letters A, C, G and T. They then found that the four-letter code yields combinations of the four letters that constitute a 20-letter alphabet, which is the same number of amino acids that make up proteins. Their accomplishment, often called the most important scientific discovery in history, prompted Crick to declare on Feb. 28, 1953, "We've discovered the secret of life."

By 1965, the whole genetic code had been cracked, vindicating the theories put forth by Mendel, Darwin and their successors and forming the basis of modern genetics. Within two decades, scientists were able to set a realistic goal of actually stringing together the 3 billion letters representing the sequence of base pairs that spells out the human species.

Mapping the Genome

Although it is expected to have its greatest impact on medicine, the Human Genome Project was actually the brainchild of scientists at the Department of Energy. Researchers at the department's Los Alamos and Lawrence Livermore national laboratories came up with the idea to map the entire genome in the early 1980s. Their goal was determining whether the children of survivors of the atomic bombing of Hiroshima and Nagasaki had mutations in their DNA as a result of their parents' exposure to radiation.

The Energy Department launched

several pilot projects on the human genome in 1987 and initially requested $15 million for the work. Congress appropriated $10.7 million in fiscal 1988 and separately added $17.2 million for the National Institutes of Health (NIH) to launch its own genome studies. In 1989, the two agencies decided to merge their efforts.

Under Watson's leadership, the Human Genome Project began its work on Oct. 1, 1990, as a coordinated effort between the Energy Department and the NIH to identify and publish the complete sequence of DNA in humans. The two agencies initially estimated the project would take 15 years and $3 billion.

In addition to sequencing the 3 billion chemical bases comprising human DNA and identifying all of the estimated 100,000 genes in the human genome, the project promised to make its findings freely available to the public via the Internet. When it began pilot sequencing studies in 1996, the project began depositing all its gene information in GenBank. A portion of the project's funds is used to study the complex ethical, legal and social issues that emerge as a result of its findings.

Concerns about the project's impact stirred controversy from the beginning. Even some scientists denounced the effort as one based more on "hype and glitter, rather than on scientific merits," and warned that it would "drain talent, money and life from smaller, worthier biomedical endeavors." [8]

Despite the outcry, the project proceeded. The Energy Department began its portion of the research in three genome centers at the Lawrence Livermore, Los Alamos and Lawrence Berkeley labs, all of which were merged into the Joint Genome Institute in Walnut Creek, Calif., in January 1997.

The NIH, which has received nearly three-quarters of the funding

Top Five Gene Patent Holders

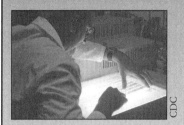

The five biggest holders of U.S. patents on human genetic material include three drug companies, a federal agency and the University of California. Overall, the number of gene patents jumped from just 12 in 1980 to 5,200 in 1999.

Patent Holder	Patents Issued 1977-1999
Incyte Pharmaceuticals Inc.	315
University of California	219
U.S. Department of Health and Human Services	183
SmithKline Beecham Corp.	137
Genentech Inc.	136

Source: U.S. Patent and Trademark Office

for the project, contracted out its part of the work to university research centers, under the leadership of its National Human Genome Research Institute. International efforts, funded largely by the Wellcome Trust, a British charity, are also under way in England, France, Germany, Japan and China. Most of the Human Genome Project's work is being carried out at sequencing centers at the Massachusetts Institute of Technology's Whitehead Institute, Washington University's School of Medicine in St. Louis, Baylor College of Medicine in Houston, the Joint Genome Institute and the Sanger Center.

Private-Sector Challenge

Rapid advances in sequencing technology enabled the Human Ge-

nome Project to speed up the genome's completion by two years. Added pressure for haste came from two companies founded in 1998 that are bent on finishing the work even faster. While working at the Institute for Genomic Research, a nonprofit institution in Rockville, Md., Venter developed an innovative computer sequencing system that promised to reveal the genome's basic structure much faster than the public project's technique.

Venter's "whole genome shotgun" method involves breaking up the entire genome into tiny segments and randomly sequencing them with no idea of their place on a chromosome. Using powerful computers and complex mathematical formulas, the segments are then assembled in their proper order. [9]

In contrast, the Human Genome Project's principal method has involved the use of gene "markers,"

Eugenics' Dark Past — And Bright Future

To some skeptics, human genome research evokes a nightmarish flashback to Nazi Germany, where official policy was premised on the supposed genetic superiority of the Aryan race. Hitler's death camps, where millions of Jews, gypsies and other people who did not match the Nazi model of genetic "purity" were exterminated, were history's most ghastly examples of genetic policy run amok.

Rarely emphasized in American history books is the fact that Hitler seems to have taken his cue from the United States. The German "Law for the Prevention of Offspring with Hereditary Diseases," adopted in 1933, was based on similar legislation then on the books throughout much of the country.

Eugenics, or the "science" of improving the human race through selective breeding, was the brainchild of Sir Francis Galton of Britain. He conceived the idea in 1883 based on his first cousin Charles Darwin's theories of evolution and natural selection. The idea quickly took root in the United States, where in 1907 the Indiana legislature passed the first law authorizing the sterilization of individuals considered unfit to reproduce. Supporters founded the American Eugenics Society, which in 1926 declared that "some Americans are born to be a burden on the rest" in the absence of similar legislation in other states. [1]

The American eugenics movement gained strength from the U.S. Supreme Court's 1927 ruling in *Bell v. Buck* upholding Virginia's eugenics law. Enacted in 1924, it required the sterilization of the "insane, idiotic, imbecile, feebleminded or epileptic." In his opinion in the case, Chief Justice Oliver Wendell Holmes reflected the belief common at the time that mental disabilities were likely to be inherited. "It is better for all the world if, instead of waiting to execute degenerate offspring for crime, or to let them starve for the imbecility, society can prevent those who are manifestly unfit from continuing their kind," he wrote.

By the 1930s, nearly two-thirds of the states had adopted similar laws, calling for the sterilization of the insane, the mentally retarded and other residents of mental institutions, as well as prison inmates who were repeat offenders, in the belief that their disabilities or antisocial behavior were inheritable traits.

Although the Holocaust discredited the U.S. eugenics movement, the pace of forced sterilizations did not begin to slow until the 1960s. It was not until 1979 that Virginia overturned its eugenics law and closed the last remaining institution enforcing the practice, the Colony for the Epileptic and Feebleminded, in Lynchburg. By then, more than 60,000 Americans had been sterilized.

Supporters of eugenics are a distinct minority in American public opinion today. The cover page of a Web site advocating "humanitarian eugenics," for example, warns users that the ideas expressed therein are "politically incorrect." Among these are arguments that human intelligence is largely hereditary and that mankind is evolving into a less intelligent species because "the least intelligent people are having the most children." [2]

But some observers of the meteoric advance in scientists' ability to identify and manipulate human genes say public vigilance still is needed to protect individual rights to privacy and protection from genetic discrimination. Article 6 of the "Genetic Bill of Rights," issued this year by the Council for Responsible Genetics, a nonprofit organization in Cambridge, Mass., reads: "All people have the right to protection against eugenic measures such as forced sterilization or mandatory screening aimed at aborting or manipulating selected embryos or fetuses."

President Clinton has called on Congress to address the potential threats to civil liberties posed by genetic information. "Clearly, there is no more exciting frontier in modern scientific research than genome research," Clinton said after barring federal agencies from discriminating against employees on the basis of genetic information.

"But," he added, "it will also impose upon us new responsibilities and, I would argue, only some of which we now know — only some of which we now know — to ensure that the new discoveries do not pry open the protective doors of privacy." [3]

Yet some scientists warn against allowing fears about the potential abuses of genetic research to impede its progress. "[Y]ou should never put off doing something useful for fear of evil that may never arrive," wrote James Watson, who with Francis Crick won a Nobel Prize in medicine and physiology for discovering the structure of DNA.

"If appropriate go-ahead signals come [from genetic engineering]," Watson continued, "the first resulting gene-bettered children will in no sense threaten human civilization. They will be seen as special only by those in their immediate circles, and are likely to pass as unnoticed in later life as the now grown-up 'test-tube baby,' Louise Brown, does today.

"If they grow up healthily gene-bettered, more such children will follow, and those whose lives are enriched by their existence will rejoice that science has again improved human life." [4]

---

[1] Bill Baskervill, "Forced Sterilization Leaves Bitter Legacy," *The Seattle Times*, March 26, 2000. For a thorough history of the eugenics movement, see Philip R. Reilly, *The Surgical Solution: A History of Involuntary Sterilization in the United States* (1991).

[2] From Future Generations, at www.eugenics.net.

[3] From remarks before a meeting of the American Association for the Advancement of Science, Feb. 8, 2000.

[4] James D. Watson, "All for the Good: Why Genetic Engineering Must Soldier On," *Time*, Jan. 11, 1999.

which are identifiable physical locations on chromosomes, to draw a map of the genome. DNA from a randomized set of donors is divided into small pieces from known locations in the genome and then sequenced. These sequenced pieces are then arranged at their known spots in the genome.

The work is divided among the project's five centers; the Sanger Center, for example, is working on eight specific chromosomes. After selected portions of the genome are sequenced, the markers are used to locate the pieces within the genome itself.

"The difference between the two approaches is that we subdivided the problem into small, manageable pieces at the outset to greatly simplify putting together the result," explains Gibbs of the Human Genome Project's Baylor center, "whereas Celera's tactic has been to start with the whole thing, randomly attack it and then sort the whole mess out in a computer at the end. But we're all on the same road to Rome, and there are more similarities than differences, and these technical differences are things that only a sequencer could love."

On the basis of his discovery, Venter obtained backing from the Perkin-Elmer Corp. (now PE Corp.) of Norwalk, Conn., to start up a new company. On May 9, 1998, they announced the formation of Celera Genomics, whose goal was to "substantially complete the sequencing of the human genome in three years" using "breakthrough DNA analysis technology." The cost of the private venture was estimated to run between $150 million and $300 million, a fraction of the genome project's total cost.

Venter's enterprise launched a wave of protest in the academic community, where researchers feared the new venture would cannibalize the genome project's findings.

In the tradition of academic research, the genome sequencing centers published their findings daily on the Internet, for the benefit of researchers around the world.

Celera promised to make its raw genome data available once completed, but said it would provide its findings and interpretations based on the genome only to subscribers for unspecified fees.

Within days of Celera's announcement, the Wellcome Trust promised to double its funding of the Sanger Center's research in an effort to allow researchers there to sequence a third of the genome, up from one-sixth as previously planned. The charity also offered to increase funding even more as scientists involved in the public effort accused Venter of "cherry-picking" and trying to "run off with the prize." [10]

As if confirming the academics' suspicions, a second company, Incyte Pharmaceuticals (now Incyte Genomics) of Palo Alto, Calif., announced on Aug. 17, 1998, that it would sequence "all commercially relevant" information on the human genome within two years.

The Human Genome Project responded to the two new, private challenges by accelerating its own deadline for completing work on the genome from 2005 to 2003 and promising to produce a "working draft" of the sequence by the end of 2001.

On March 15, 1999, it shortened its timetable even further, announcing it would produce at least 90 percent of the genome by the spring of 2000. Not to be outshown, Celera responded on Oct. 20 — less that two months after it had begun its work — that it had already sequenced and provided to its subscribers some 1.2 billion base pairs of human DNA. ■

CURRENT SITUATION

New Legislation

The fast pace of genetic research has left policy-makers scrambling to devise policies to deal with the social, legal and ethical fallout left in its wake. The Senate is currently considering legislation that would lift a 1995 ban on federal funding of research on human embryonic stem cells — cells that can evolve into different types of tissue and may lead to cures for a number of maladies, such as spinal-cord injuries and Parkinson's disease. [11]

The development of cloning technology, essential for genome sequencing and a host of gene-based therapies, raised the specter of future attempts to clone humans and prompted the U.S. scientific establishment in 1997 to adopt a voluntary moratorium on human-cloning research. On March 7, following the September death of a teenager undergoing experimental gene therapy at the University of Pennsylvania, the Food and Drug Administration and the NIH tightened federal oversight of gene-therapy experiments in humans. [12]

Concerns related more directly to genome research also have prompted new laws and regulations. To address the claims of critics who say it is too easy for private genomics companies to apply for and obtain patents, the Patent Office has issued new guidelines for issuing gene patents.

"Under the law, every invention must be new and useful before it will be granted a patent; that is, it has to have a utility," says Doll of the Patent Office. "Our new guidelines state that to be acceptable, the utility must be specific, substantial and credible."

Doll cites as an example a design for a protein with a particular amino-acid profile to be used to feed a type of animal that needs very high lysine content. "That would still be patentable under the new guidelines," he says. "But don't come in with an isolated protein and say it may be a regulatory agent in uncontrolled cell growth associated with a particular form of cancer, and then say that by the way, since you really don't know what it does, you're going to use it as an animal supplement."

Critics' Concerns

But critics say the guidelines don't go far enough. "If you discovered some new proteins and told me that they could be used as packing peanuts in cardboard boxes, that would not be a substantial utility, and the Patent Office shouldn't allow that any more than it should allow a patent on the use of a protein as landfill," says Lander of the MIT center. "But that is what's happening right now."

The new Patent Office guidelines do raise the bar by requiring that raw sequences must be accompanied by computer analysis to qualify for patents, but Lander says that further experimentation should also be required.

"The Patent Office has the authority to interpret this bar so that it serves the basic purpose of the law," he says. "I think we do a great disservice to society by giving away monopolies for simply pressing the return button on a computer."

Lander calls on Congress to hold hearings to bring further attention to the issue. "I don't think it needs to change the patent law," he says, "but I do think Congress has ways to make clear that the patent system was not intended to be an inflexible, doltish

system that gives away the store."

Investors in booming biotechnology stocks thought that President Clinton and Prime Minister Blair had come to a similar conclusion when they issued a joint statement on gene patents on March 14. The two leaders said that "raw fundamental data on the human genome, including the human DNA sequence and its varia-

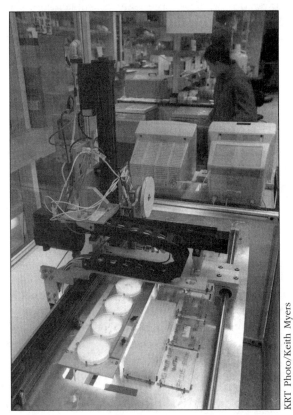

A "plaque-picker" robot at Washington University in St. Louis, Mo., saves hundreds of hours of human labor in genetic research by extracting DNA samples grown in colonies of bacteria. Previously, researchers did extractions by hand using toothpicks.

tions, should be made freely available to scientists everywhere."

Although the statement did no more than confirm existing policy, investors panicked, selling off their holdings in genomics companies and sending biotechnology stocks into a $30 billion tailspin for several days. On April 6, the House Science

Energy and Environment Subcommittee held hearings to consider another aspect of the patent debate — concerns that gene patents may impede basic research.

"I am concerned that researchers at universities, hospitals or companies may find themselves having to negotiate complicated and expensive license agreements in order to do research on patented genes," said Rep. Jerry F. Costello, D. Ill., ranking minority member of the subcommittee. "Some of them may abandon research that could result in life-saving discoveries because they fear legal ramifications, an outcome that could be very detrimental to health-care research and innovation."

Concerns about privacy and the threat of discrimination based on individual genetic information have prompted relatively little action by federal lawmakers, however, apart from the 1995 provision barring group-health insurers from denying coverage to individuals based solely on their genetic risk for disease. Most of the regulation in this area has fallen to state governments, many of which have passed a variety of laws aimed at thwarting genetic discrimination. (*See map, p. 180.*)

"Between 1997 and 1999 a lot of states passed laws on this issue that had not previously had laws on the books," says Sophia M. Kolehmainen, director of the human genetics program at the Council for Responsible Genetics. "So this is definitely a new trend." According to her program's

At Issue:

Does patenting human genes impede medical research?

JONATHAN KING

Professor of molecular biology, Massachusetts Institute of Technology, and board member, Council for Responsible Genetics

WRITTEN FOR *THE CQ RESEARCHER*

*t*he genetic engineering revolution has led to extraordinary progress in understanding life on a molecular basis — advances that stem from 50 years of publicly funded biomedical research into protecting human health and alleviating the ravages of disease. Knowledge has flowed from shared resources and open communication.

The Human Genome Project, an attempt to read all the gene sequences in human DNA, represents one of the most dramatic of these research efforts. These sequences are the blueprints for biological structure and function. Recently, some institutions and private companies began competing with the international, publicly funded endeavor in hopes of keeping the results in private hands — a move made possible by a U.S. Patent and Trademark Office (PTO) decision to include gene sequences under utility patent laws.

Our genes are passed down to us through our parents, who received them from their parents. They represent millions of years of evolution. They are in the deepest possible sense "products of nature" — historically excluded from patenting. Genes were not invented by individuals, corporations or institutions. Granting patents on them represents an egregious misuse of the system and a theft of the common biological heritage of all human beings.

Contrary to the claims of venture capitalists and patent lawyers, gene patenting sharply retards progress in the biomedical arena. Patenting introduces chilling secrecy where openness is essential, slowing and misdirecting biomedical progress.

Scientific findings that have been reported publicly are deemed "prior art" and cannot be patented. As a result, individuals and corporations planning to file for gene patents do not report their results, even informally, until they have successfully passed through the expensive patent process.

That has created researchers who refuse to answer questions from their colleagues because they have patent claims pending. Biomedical researchers and health-care institutions are being denied access to human gene sequences unless they pay steep license fees.

PTO's decision to extend patents to human gene sequences took place outside of public debate and congressional oversight. Congress has the power to pass, modify or repeal patent laws, and it should explicitly exclude gene sequences from the patent process as a matter of sound social and scientific policy.

J. CRAIG VENTER

President and chief scientific officer, Celera Genomics Inc., Rockville, Md.

FROM HOUSE TESTIMONY, APRIL 6, 2000.

*p*harmaceutical and biotech companies use [human] genes as the direct means of producing drugs such as insulin and as "targets" to develop drugs. The cost of taking a single drug through the U.S. Food and Drug Administration approval process can range from $300 million to $800 million. Having patents on the drugs allows [companies] a period of time when they can exclusively use these patented discoveries for commercial purposes. This provides them a period in which to try and recover their drug-development costs. This rationale for patenting is one that is fully accepted and supported by the [National Institutes of Health]. . . .

However, [Celera Genomics Inc.] and many of our pharmaceutical partners are very concerned that the patenting of random genome and [gene] fragments by many companies and research institutions will restrict their access to key targets required for drug development. An important aspect of Celera's policies is the non-exclusive licensing of drug targets.

How does Celera respond to the concerns of scientists who worry that patenting gene sequences and putting such basic information in private hands will discourage research. . . ?

Under the U.S. and European patent systems, researchers are free to conduct basic research for non-commercial purposes on others' patented discoveries. While some hypothesize that patents on genes will generally inhibit research, the facts indicate otherwise. For example, a patent was granted on the BRCA1 gene associated with breast cancer in 1993. Since that time, over 721 basic research papers have been published on the BRCA1 gene, and [many] further patent applications on important inventions, including genetic tests related to the BRAC1 gene, have been filed. . . . Also, Celera's policy of licensing genes on a non-exclusive basis will assure that gene discoveries are available to many — not just one. . . .

When PR Corp. and I announced the creation of Celera in May 1998, it was based on a shared vision of sequencing the human genome as the basis of accelerating a revolution in biology and health care. Financed exclusively by private investment, we brought together unique technologies and capabilities within a start-up enterprise to pursue this seemingly impossible goal. With hundreds of others joining in this effort, Celera already has exceeded its own expectations and continues to evolve as a participant in this exciting revolution.

statistics, 44 states have enacted laws that provide some level of protection against genetic discrimination in health insurance, including individual health-insurance policies ignored by the federal ban. Some states have minimal protections. Alabama, for example, bars insurers from discriminating on the basis of genetic information related to cancer alone. Others, such as Maine, cover all types of genetic data.

"In those states you can tell that there was a big debate," Kolehmainen says. "It's obvious that they really thought about the issues, and they covered everything." A smaller number of states have passed laws barring genetic discrimination by disability insurers and life insurers as well.

On Feb. 8, President Clinton addressed another potential source of genetic discrimination by prohibiting federal government agencies from discriminating against employees or job applicants on the basis of individual genetic information. But Clinton's directive is limited to federal agencies, and Congress has yet to extend this protection to the general work force. Meanwhile, 16 states have passed laws barring genetic discrimination in employment.

Nearing Completion

The Human Genome Project expects to complete its "working draft" of the genome within weeks. Indeed, says Lander, "The genome race is over. The genome sequence is out there. With some 80 percent of the genome already freely available on the Web, no researcher is standing there waiting for the genome to be sequenced. This is one of the great triumphs of public funding. It created biotechnology, genomics and the genome project and delivered all of these things ahead of schedule."

As the Human Genome Project nears its goal of publishing a "working draft" of the genome, Celera is holding to its commitment to publish its completed version before the end of the year, though Venter says the

> "The private sector has said it is going to make the data available, but the terms under which they are going to be available will certainly slow down research progress."
>
> — *Eric S. Lander, director, Whitehead/MIT Center for Genomic Research*

project's plans may force his company to come out with a less complete version earlier than planned.

"If people are led to believe that their very incomplete version of the genome is really the complete thing, we'll probably have to publish sooner than we would like to," Venter says. "The public doesn't seem to distinguish what a rough draft is compared with an accurately completed genome, and that confusion is dangerous to our business."

Friction between public and private research efforts reached a peak in March, when talks aimed at reaching an agreement to pool their data and collaborate on human genome sequencing broke down over Celera's insistence that any collaboration include agreements to protect the company's commercial interests. [1] But Venter says he plans to make its version of the genome freely available as long as users agree not to redistribute the data. "We're not patenting the genome," he says. "We're sequencing it and giving it to the public for free."

Lander remains skeptical. "The private sector has said it is going to make the data available, but the terms under which they are going to be available will certainly slow down research progress," he says. "Everybody can have access to the data, but no other researcher will be able to take Celera's data and put it on the Web site with further analysis. I stand very firmly by the notion that the American people will be better served by a sequence of the human genome that is freely available for redistribution, and that's what we in the public project are doing."

Despite the friction between the public and private labs over the quality of work each is pursuing, some of the most promising findings are coming from collaborative projects. In April 1999, for example, 10 large drug companies, IBM, Motorola and the Wellcome Trust announced the formation of a new consortium whose goal is to identify more than 300,000 SNPs that may be associated with disease and provide targets for further study of biological processes and development of new gene therapies. All the data generated by the consortium are deposited in a publicly available database. The consortium has already identified nearly 150,000 SNPs, more than half of which have been mapped and deposited in its Internet database. [14]

Another joint project, between Celera and publicly funded labs in Europe and at the University of California at Berkeley, recently completed the fruit fly genome, the most complex organism that has been sequenced to date. [15] Because *Drosophila* is one of the most commonly used organisms in biomedical research, the publication and free availability of its genome is expected to enrich human genome research as well.

For Venter, the project proved the effectiveness of his shotgun sequencing technique, which he plans to use for sequencing genomes of other organisms after the human genome is completed, including the mouse, another key lab animal, and rice, the world's most important food source. ■

OUTLOOK

Enormous Potential

A s the mapping of the human genome nears completion, scientists agree that the real work in human genetics lies ahead. "This whole idea of the race to the finish line is silly," says Lander of the Whitehead/ MIT Center. "We're actually racing to the starting line. We do not know today what is the actual cause of diabetes, asthma, heart disease or many other common diseases. I expect that within as few as 20 years we will in fact know what is the mechanism that has gone awry in each of those diseases."

Once those genetic causes have been identified, using the human genome as a guide, the next step will be to fashion therapies to treat them

Geneticist Beverly S. Emanuel, working in her lab at the Children's Hospital of Philadelphia, led a five-year effort to develop a physical map of Chromosome 22.

more effectively — or even prevent them from occurring altogether. That will be done by replacing faulty genes with good ones — instead of merely treating the symptoms of disease as we do today. That effort will require an enormous investment in research and development.

"We will need many, many billions of dollars invested in genome research over this century," says biotech spokesman Ludlum. "Right now it's thought at least 5,000 diseases are genetic in nature, and there are probably more than that. Once we have the genomes of individual patients, more research will be required to determine why some people respond to and tolerate certain drugs and others do not."

Hints of what the future holds are heard almost daily with reports of breathtaking gene-related discoveries. The recent report from France that three infants with severe immune disorders apparently have been restored to health using gene therapy provides new hope for this branch of medicine at a time when safety concerns have slowed gene-therapy applications in the United States. [16]

New animal-cloning studies in Massachusetts suggest that cloning using certain techniques may actually produce younger cells, a finding of potentially sweeping implications for the future of organ transplantation. [17] The birth of the world's first litter of cloned pigs offers hope that thousands of patients awaiting organ donations may one day receive a "xenotransplant" organ from another species. [18]

Researchers recently discovered that people with Down syndrome have a low incidence of most types of cancer, suggesting that the same genetic flaw that causes this form of mental retardation may hold the key to finding a genetic cure for cancer. [19]

In the context of such enormous potential, one thing that public and private genomics researchers agree on is that their current disputes eventually will be forgotten.

"This controversy will all go away," says Celera's Venter. "What people will remember are the scientific achievements and the impact they will have on hopefully moving forward on cancer treatments and other things that we are all striving for." ■

Notes

[1] Collins testified March 30 before the Senate Appropriations Subcommittee on Labor, Health and Human Services and Education.

[2] http://www.ncbi.nlm.nih.gov/Genbank/GenbankOverview.html.

[3] Council for Responsible Genetics, 2000.

[4] For background, see Kathy Koch, "Food Safety Battle: Organic vs. Biotech," *The CQ Researcher*, Sept. 4, 1998, pp. 761-784.

[5] Biotechnology Industry Organization, *Editors' & Reporters' Guide to Biotechnology*, www.bio.org. For background on pharmaceutical research costs, see Adriel Bettelheim, "Drugmakers Under Siege," *The CQ Researcher*, Sept. 3, 1999, pp. 753-776.

[6] William A. Haseltine, "21st Century Genes," *The Washington Post*, March 28, 2000.

[7] Information in this section is based on Matt Ridley, *Genome* (1999), pp. 38-53.

[8] Natalie Angier, "Great 15-Year Project To Decipher Genes Stirs Opposition," *The New York Times*, June 5, 1990.

[9] For a detailed description of different sequencing techniques, see U.S. Department of Energy and Human Genome Project, "To Know Ourselves," 1996.

[10] Aisling Irwin, "The Gene Genie Racing To Grab A Fast Billion," *The Daily Telegraph* (London), May 14, 1998.

[11] For background, see Adriel Bettelheim, "Embryo Research," *The CQ Researcher*, Dec. 17, 1999, pp. 1065-1088.

[12] For background, see Craig Donegan, "Gene Therapy's Future," *The CQ Researcher*, Dec. 8, 1995, pp. 1089-1112.

[13] Justin Gillis, "Celera Leaves Door Open to Genetic Research Deal," *The Washington Post*, March 8, 2000.

[14] "The SNP Consortium Exceeds First-Year Goals to Identify and Map Set of Gene Markers," *PR Newswire*, May 1, 2000.

[15] Mark D. Adams et al., "The Genome Sequence of *Drosophila melanogaster*," *Science*, March 24, 2000, pp. 2185-2195.

[16] See Gina Kolata, "Scientists Report the First Success of Gene Therapy," *The New York Times*, April 28, 2000.

[17] See Rick Weiss, "Dolly's Premature Aging Not Evident in Cloned Cows," *The Washington Post*, April 28, 2000.

[18] See Rick Weiss, "In Organ Quest, Cloning Pigs May Be the Easy Part," *The Washington Post*, March 20, 2000.

[19] H. Hasle, I.H. Clemmensen and M Mikkelsen, "Risks of Leukaemia and Solid Tumours in Individuals with Down's Syndrome," *Lancet*, Jan. 15, 2000, pp. 165-169

FOR MORE INFORMATION

Biotechnology Industry Organization (BIO), 1625 K St., N.W., Suite 1100, Washington, D.C. 20006; (202) 857-0244; www.bio.org. This organization for biotechnology companies monitors government policies affecting the industry and is involved in the ethical debates surrounding gene research.

Celera Genomics Inc., 45 West Gude Dr., Rockville, Md. 20850; (240) 453-3000; www.celera.com. Founded in 1998, this company is the main private concern involved in sequencing the human genome.

Council for Responsible Genetics, 5 Upland Rd., Suite 3, Cambridge, Mass. 02140; (617) 868-0870; www.gene-watch.org. This nonprofit organization promotes a comprehensive public interest agenda for biotechnology.

National Human Genome Research Institute, National Institutes of Health, 31 Center Dr., MSC-2152, #4B09, Bethesda, Md. 20892-2152; (301) 402-0911; www.nhgri.nih.gov. The institute, together with the Energy Department, is responsible for U.S. involvement in the international Human Genome Project, which seeks to map all genes in humans.

U.S. Patent and Trademark Office, Department of Commerce, 2121 Crystal Park II, Suite 906, Arlington, Va. 22202; (703) 308-4357; www.uspto.gov. The office administers the 1952 Patent Law by reviewing applications and issuing patents on inventions, including gene patents.

Bibliography

Selected Sources Used

Books

Hubbard, Ruth, and Elijah Wald, *Exploding the Gene Myth: How Genetic Information Is Produced and Manipulated by Scientists, Physicians, Employers, Insurance Companies, Educators, and Law Enforcers*, Beacon Press, 1999.

The authors suggest that the revolution in human gene research not only has been overhyped by self-serving researchers and the media, but also poses new threats to civil liberties from a number of sources.

Jones, Steve, *Darwin's Ghost: The Origin of Species Updated*, Random House, 2000.

A geneticist re-examines Darwin's 1859 classic in view of subsequent discoveries in his field. Although genetic research has revealed the existence of a far more complex system than Darwin could have imagined, it has upheld and expanded upon his theory of evolution.

Kitcher, Philip, *The Lives to Come: The Genetic Revolution and Human Possibilities*, Simon & Schuster, 1996.

A science historian examines a number of practical and philosophical questions raised by the explosion of new discoveries in gene research.

Lewontin, Richard, *The Triple Helix: Gene, Organism and Environment*, Harvard University Press, 2000.

A noted population geneticist cautions against excessive confidence that genomics will uncover all mysteries surrounding human physiology because of the unpredictable impact of environmental events on the interaction between DNA, proteins and protein receptors.

Ridley, Matt, *Genome: The Autobiography of a Species in 23 Chapters*, HarperCollins, 1999.

Science writer Ridley uses one gene from each of the 23 human chromosomes to tell the story of genetics, its many applications in science and the potential impact of gene research on our knowledge of human physiology.

Articles

"In-gene-uous: In Genomics, the British and American Governments Are Meddling in Things That Do Not Concern Them and Neglecting Those That Do," *The Economist*, March 18, 2000.

In contrast to the recent joint declaration by President Clinton and Prime Minister Tony Blair affirming that raw genomic data should be placed in the public domain, this editorial defends the right of private companies to withhold the results of their research.

Adams, Mark D., et al., "The Genome Sequence of Drosophila melanogaster," *Science*, March 24, 2000, pp. 2185-2195.

A public-private venture completed most of the genome of the fruit fly, the most complex organism to be so described to date. The collaborative effort between Celera Genomics and nonprofit labs including one at the University of California at Berkeley is described in accompanying articles as promising for future joint ventures in genomic research.

Begley, Sharon, "The Race to Decode the Human Body," *Newsweek*, April 10, 2000, pp. 50-58.

This cover story, together with several companion articles, describes public and private efforts to complete the human genome this year.

Little, Peter, "The Book of Genes," *Nature*, Dec. 2, 1999, p. 467-468.

The sequence of human Chromosome 22, published in the same issue of *Nature*, marks the first phase of a biological revolution that eventually may enable scientists to identify all the proteins in the human body and their function in health and disease.

Reports and Studies

National Bioethics Advisory Commission, "Cloning Human Beings," June 1997.

The commission, set up to advise the president on ethical issues posed by gene research and therapeutics, examines the implications of cloning technology for potential efforts to clone whole humans.

National Bioethics Advisory Commission, "Ethical Issues in Human Stem Cell Research," September 1999.

Following the successful isolation and culture in 1998 of stem cells, which offer hope of new cures for debilitating diseases, the commission reviews the ethical implications of using human embryos to produce these cells for research and treatment.

U.S. Department of Energy and Human Genome Project, "To Know Ourselves," 1996.

The Energy Department, one of the partners in the federally funded Human Genome Project, presents a comprehensive overview of the principles of genetics, as well as descriptions of various techniques used to map the genome.

11 Global AIDS Crisis

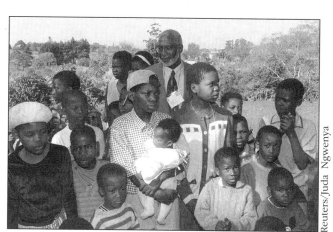

U.S. Surgeon General David Satcher visits with children orphaned by AIDS during the 13th International AIDS Conference in Durban, South Africa, in July.

Reuters/Juda Ngwenya

Selina Abongo, a Kenyan farmer in her 70s, has reached that point in life when most people want to retire. Instead, she finds herself raising children again. [1]

Once, Abongo had eight kids of her own. But four died, as well as a daughter-in-law, all felled by AIDS. So now she cares for her orphaned grandchildren.

"This is the picture you get in every village you go to: a grandmother made almost prisoner by orphans," says Ambrose Misore, a Kenyan government health worker. [2]

Thousands of Kenyans die each month from AIDS, leaving spouses, children and jobs behind. But with 14 percent of the country's adult population infected by HIV or AIDS, millions more will die in the coming decade.

As grim as the situation is in Kenya, the infection rate is even higher in other African nations. The worst hit is Botswana, where an estimated 36 percent of all adults between the ages of 15 and 49 are infected. South Africa, Zambia and Zimbabwe aren't far behind.

The global AIDS epidemic has already killed nearly 20 million people — roughly twice the casualties in World War I. Another 34.3 million are infected with the HIV virus and are likely to die within the next decade. Moreover, an additional 5 million people are being newly infected with the virus each year. Most of the victims live in sub-Saharan Africa, where 25 million people currently have HIV or AIDS.

In the United States, Europe and other developed countries, the disease is becoming much more manageable. Infection rates are low and

stable, and new treatments are dramatically prolonging the life spans of sufferers. Even more encouraging, pharmaceutical companies are developing a host of new drugs designed to make AIDS a chronic, or treatable, disease.

But in the developing world, the situation is very different. AIDS therapy generally costs more than $10,000 per year, far too expensive to be used by most nations in Africa, Asia and elsewhere.

Some AIDS experts have criticized drugmakers for pricing their life-prolonging therapies beyond the reach of almost everyone in the developing world. [3]

"They've developed all of this medicine for 5 percent of the people with AIDS — the 5 percent who can afford their outrageous prices," says Eric Sawyer, a founding member of ACT UP, an AIDS advocacy group in New York City. Sawyer and other health activists charge that the pharmaceutical firms that make AIDS drugs care mainly about profits and are ultimately willing to let millions die in order to preserve the bottom line.

But the pharmaceutical companies say that they have discounted some AIDS drugs and even offered others for free. The problem, they say, is not

drug prices but a lack of health infrastructure in most developing countries.

"You can't just drop drugs into a country," says Mark E. Grayson, senior communications director for the Pharmaceutical Research and Manufacturers of America. "You have to have storage facilities, distribution and a plan for treatment — something most of these countries just don't have."

Still, many health experts say that preventing the disease from spreading is more important than drugs and treatment. "In every epidemic — including this one — prevention is the key, and the earlier the better," says Don Thea, a development associate at the Overseas Program Office of Harvard University's Kennedy School of Government.

Many non-governmental organizations (NGOs) are working to prevent the disease in sub-Saharan Africa and Asia by promoting safe sexual practices and distributing condoms. But some experts contend that condoms and sex education are not the answer. Indeed, they say, making condoms readily available ultimately might do more harm than good because it encourages people, especially young people, to have sexual encounters with many different partners. Such sexual activity is still very dangerous, they say, even with condoms.

Instead of safe sex, says Steven Mosher, president of the Population Research Institute in Front Royal, Va., governments and organizations should encourage abstinence. "Look, we've been at this for more than a decade now — pushing condoms, etc. — and the disease is out of control," he says. "The message we need to be sending is that if you

From *The CQ Researcher*, October 13, 2000.

Global AIDS Crisis   195

On An Average Day, 1999

- **15,000 new HIV infections worldwide**
- **More than 95% in developing countries**
- **1,700 in children under age 15**
- **About 13,000 in people ages 15 to 49, of whom:**
  - **— almost 50% are women**
  - **— about 50% are ages 15 to 24**

Source: UNAIDS, June 2000

don't have sex, you won't get AIDS. Period."

Actually, many health experts point out, most developing countries, especially in Africa, haven't "been at it" for a decade or even, in some cases, for a year. However, countries that have promoted sex education and condoms aggressively, like Uganda and Thailand, have brought HIV infection rates down dramatically in recent years.

"People need to know how to protect themselves," says Jeff Jacobs, director of government affairs at AIDS Action, a group that advocates more spending for AIDS research and education. "That's the most important thing."

Jacobs and others also dispute the notion that abstinence should be the centerpiece of HIV prevention efforts. "Abstinence can be a very small part of an HIV-prevention campaign, but it's not going to change enough behavior to be very effective," he says.

In some parts of Africa, the debate over prevention is not very relevant, since little or nothing is being done to stop the spread of the disease. "This epidemic has been raging for 20 years and, still, nothing or not enough is being done," says Alan Whiteside, director of the Health, Economics and HIV/AIDS Research Division at the University of Natal in Durban, South Africa. As a result, he says, "hundreds of millions of Africans are going to die," leaving tens of millions of orphans and a continent wracked by disease, social breakdown and poverty.

What does this grim scenario mean for the United States? Beyond humanitarian concerns, many officials, including Vice President Al Gore, say the AIDS epidemic has significant national-security implications. For one thing, they argue, the United States receives one out of every six barrels of imported oil from Africa, as well as many key minerals, such as titanium. In addition, AIDS may eventually ravage Asia as brutally as it has Africa, leaving one of the world's most important economic regions in turmoil.

But others argue that the AIDS epidemic in Africa doesn't really threaten the security of the United States. "If AIDS were to destabilize Africa, that would be a tragedy, but the stability of Africa is not vital to the U.S.," says Jack Spenser, a policy analyst for defense and national security at the Heritage Foundation, a conservative think tank. "Although we get certain things from the continent, our economy isn't fundamentally linked to it."

Whatever its implications for the United States, the AIDs epidemic portends hard years ahead for the developing world. As the world community responds to the tragedy, here are some of the questions being asked:

Are pharmaceutical companies doing enough to make AIDS drugs available in the developing world?

On May 11, five major drugmakers met in Geneva, Switzerland, with officials from the United Nations, the World Health Organization (WHO) and the World Bank to announce an initiative to reduce the cost of treating HIV and AIDS in developing countries. The companies — including Merck, Bristol-Myers Squibb and Glaxo Wellcome — offered few specifics, promising only to "work with committed governments . . . to broaden access while ensuring rational, affordable, safe and effective use of our drugs."

Despite the lack of details, some public health officials were jubilant. "It's a breakthrough in the sense that for the first time, a group of pharmaceutical companies are open to significantly decreasing the price of their products in poor markets," said Peter Piot, head of UNAIDS.* [4]

Currently, that price is very high — roughly $10,000 to $15,000 a year for the three-to four-drug combination therapy used in the developed countries. These drugs, known as protease inhibitors, or anti-retrovirals, can significantly delay the onset of AIDS, giving thousands of infected people new hope (*see p. 205*).

But for the vast majority of HIV/AIDS sufferers in Africa, Asia and Latin America, the combination therapy is out of reach. In most sub-Saharan African countries, per capita gross domestic product (GDP) is less than $1,000 per year. [5] Even in Uganda and Ivory Coast, where the cost of the therapy has been discounted to $5,000 annually, only the rich can afford treatment.

---

* The U.N., World Trade Organization and World Bank created UNAIDS in 1996 to coordinate the global fight against the disease.

The Toll in Africa

More than 10 percent of the people ages 15 to 49 in 14 African nations are infected with HIV. Nearly all of the severely afflicted nations are in Southern and Eastern Africa. Of the world's 34.3 million adults and children with HIV/AIDS in 1999, an estimated 24.5 million were in sub-Saharan Africa.

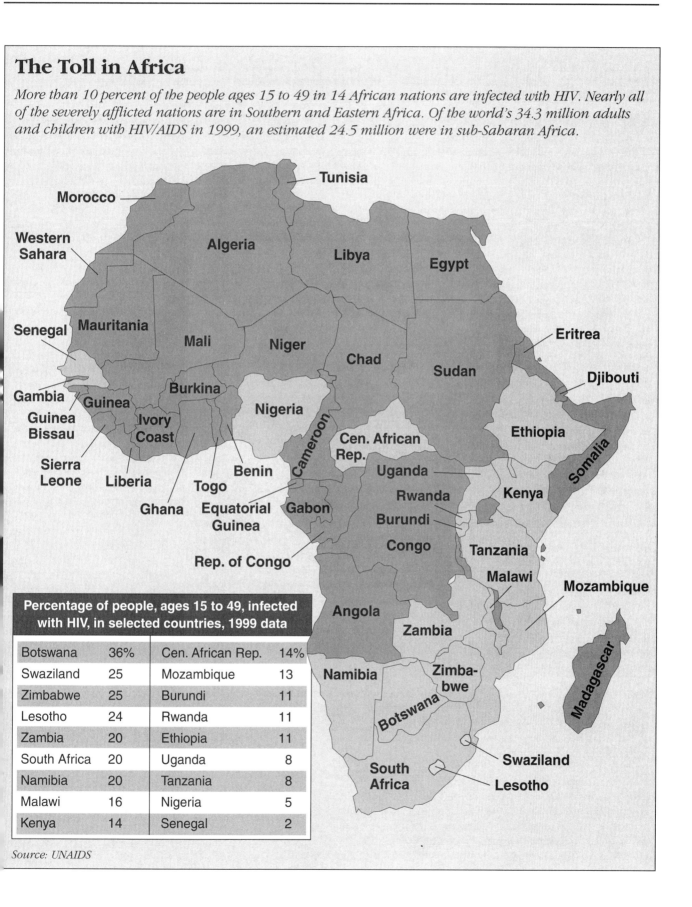

Percentage of people, ages 15 to 49, infected with HIV, in selected countries, 1999 data

Country	%	Country	%
Botswana	36%	Cen. African Rep.	14%
Swaziland	25	Mozambique	13
Zimbabwe	25	Burundi	11
Lesotho	24	Rwanda	11
Zambia	20	Ethiopia	11
South Africa	20	Uganda	8
Namibia	20	Tanzania	8
Malawi	16	Nigeria	5
Kenya	14	Senegal	2

Source: UNAIDS

Does AIDS Threaten "Natural Disaster" in Asia?

With more than two-thirds of the world's AIDS cases, it's understandable why much of the world's attention is on Africa.

But more and more, experts are beginning to worry about Asia, where more than 6 million people are HIV-infected or have AIDS. Moreover, the number of infections is increasing rapidly, nearly doubling in the last five years, according to the Joint United Nations Program on HIV/AIDS (UNAIDS).

"There's a chance that this disease could get out of control in a country like India or China, with their huge populations," says Jeff Jacobs, director of government affairs at AIDS Action, an AIDS advocacy group. "If something like that happened, imagine the cost."

Until now, the AIDS spotlight in Asia has focused on Thailand, which seemed particularly at risk because of its huge sex industry. Indeed, the country has the highest number of reported HIV/AIDS cases in East Asia, more than 1 million.

Yet, Thailand has become something of an AIDS success story. When it became apparent in the early 1990s that the virus was spreading rapidly, the government initiated a massive AIDS education campaign and distributed millions of condoms, paying special attention to sex-industry workers. The efforts paid off, lowering new infection rates from 60 cases per 100,000 population in 1994 to 48 per 100,000 in 1998.

Other Asian countries, among them the Philippines and Vietnam, also have launched major efforts to halt HIV's spread. A government-run café in Ho Chi Minh City even offers condoms and clean needles to patrons along with coffee.

But Jacobs is among many experts especially worried about larger Asian countries. In India, for instance, AIDS prevention efforts are scattered or non-existent. Slightly more than 2 percent of India's population — 4 million people — have HIV or AIDS, and the epidemic is spreading quickly. Moreover, the disease is not confined to high-risk groups, such as prostitutes, intravenous drug users and gay men, but has hit several sectors of Indian society, including young urban workers and professionals.

"India has a real problem on its hands because it already has a high rate of sexually transmitted diseases (STDs)," says Richard Laing, an associate professor of international health at Boston University's School of Public Health. Because STDs facilitate HIV transmission, "This really could lead to trouble for India."

In China, an estimated 600,000 people have contracted HIV or AIDS, fewer than 1 percent of all adults. But new cases are increasing by 30 percent annually. And, as in India, the disease is no longer the provenance of traditional high-risk groups but is spreading to the general population, affecting everyone from rural workers to urban professionals.

Recently, Zeng Yi, an AIDS researcher in China, warned that his country is facing a "natural disaster" if the government doesn't act more forcefully to stop the epidemic. [1] Currently, China spends less than Thailand on AIDS prevention, even though it has 20 times the population.

"The central government doesn't seem to realize how serious this is," said Qui Renzong, a bioethicist at the Chinese Academy of Social Sciences. "We have not yet had an effective risk-reduction strategy because [government] departments are very conservative. They think chastity is more important than condom use." [2]

Some experts predict that parts of Asia could begin to see a decline in economic activity, much like what has occurred in Africa, if the disease is allowed to spread unchecked.

Speaking of HIV carriers in India, Dr. Rohto Sob, a consultant with the World Health Organization says: "This is your working population. In the long run, industrial production will be hit as it has in Africa."

But others are more hopeful. "I'm heartened by the fact that the virus has been in Asia for more than 20 years and, so far, hasn't gotten out of control like it has in Africa," Laing says.

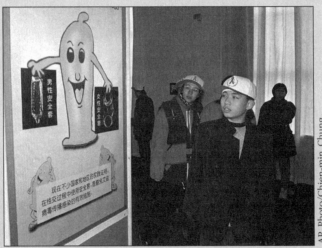

A poster promoting condom use at a World AIDS Day exhibition in Beijing in 1998 catches the eye of students. Beijing's first public exhibition on the disease featured photographs of drug users and AIDS patients.

AP Photo/Chien-min Chung

---

[1] Quoted in Julie Chao, "Prostitution Boom in China Poses Growing Threat to Public Health," *The Atlanta Journal-Constitution*, Sept. 26, 2000.

[2] Quoted in Elizabeth Rosenthal, "Scientists Warn of Inaction As AIDS Spreads in China," *The New York Times*, Aug. 2, 2000.

The situation has prompted angry criticism of the drug industry by many AIDS experts. "That announcement in Geneva was all smoke and mirrors, a big public relations exercise to get the media off their backs," says ACT UP's Sawyer. "It's been half a year since the announcement, and they've basically done nothing to bring prices down and won't in the future."

Sawyer and others say the big drugmakers are focused only on markets where people can pay the highly inflated prices they charge for AIDS drugs. The fact that roughly 95 percent of HIV/AIDS sufferers live in the developing world is of little concern to them, they add.

"These companies have drugs to fight AIDS, and they're basically preventing almost everyone with the disease from having access to them," says Peter Lurie, deputy director of Public Citizen's Health Research Group. "They've done this for one reason and one reason alone: to keep profits enormously high."

But companies that produce AIDS drugs say the criticism is unfounded and unfair, and that their pledge to make AIDS drugs more affordable is not an empty promise.

"This is not just a PR stunt," says Tom Bombelles, director of international government relations at Merck, one of the world's largest pharmaceutical firms. "We're committed to doing everything we possibly can to give people access to treatment and care."

Bombelles says that just two months after the Geneva announcement, Merck pledged $50 million to provide drugs and health-care support to beleaguered Botswana. And the German drug company Boehringer Ingelheim is providing free Virammune (nevirapine), which reduces chances that a pregnant woman with HIV will pass the virus on to her fetus.

"We're meeting with the president of Botswana to work out how to move forward on this," Bombelles says. "I don't call that smoke and mirrors. Do you?"

Drugmakers and their supporters also point out that they are spending billions of dollars each year to develop new and better AIDS treatments, making it financially difficult simply to give the medicine away without any remuneration. "Merck spent over a billion dollars just to develop Crixovan, one of the protease inhibitors that's working so well right now," Grayson says.

Jacobs of AIDS Action concedes that Merck and other drugmakers have taken "a step in the right direction this year with the announcement in Geneva." But, he adds, "when you think about the kinds of profits they're making, you realize that they could afford to be much more caring and compassionate than they've been."

Drug company profits are high, critics say. For example, in the first six months of the year, Merck earned $3.2 billion on revenue of $18.3 billion and Bristol-Myers Squibb earned $2.3 billion on revenues of $10.5 billion. With those profits, Sawyer says, "$50 million or $100 million spread out over so many years isn't very generous at all."

Critics also contend that drug companies are loath to drastically lower the price of AIDS drugs for fear of sparking a drive to reduce prices in the United States and other developed countries. "There's very strong evidence that drug prices are much too high in this country and that there is significant price gouging going on," Lurie says. "If they lower prices dramatically in places like Africa, they would demolish the whole facade that they need to charge high prices."

But supporters of the pharmaceutical industry say that critics like Sawyer and Lurie are trying to blame them for a problem drug companies cannot solve by themselves. "It's hard to say that companies need to do more when there's so much that needs to be done," Grayson says.

For instance, he and others contend, giving away sophisticated AIDS drugs does little good if there isn't a health-care infrastructure in a country to distribute the medicine and monitor patients. "AIDS treatment isn't just about parachuting drugs into a country," Bombelles says.

Indeed, according to Peter Piot, head of UNAIDS, "90 to 95 percent of Africans who carry the virus don't even know they're infected." [6] Even if everyone with HIV was identified, experts say, most countries in the developing world wouldn't have the doctors, nurses or hospitals to treat them.

"You need to be able to deliver these drugs in the right dosage, at the right time and to the right people, and in most parts of Africa that's out of the question right now," the University of Natal's Whiteside says.

In addition, many of the same countries, especially in Africa, also suffer from endemic government corruption, making it even harder to establish and deliver health-care services.

"Look, a recent World Bank study found that 88 percent of the drugs purchased for South Africa either didn't reach a patient or were inappropriately administered," Grayson says. [7]

Finally, drug-industry supporters argue, some developing nations are uninterested or at times even hostile to offers of help. South African President Thabo Mbeki, for example, recently turned down an offer to distribute Virammune to pregnant women with HIV or AIDS.

Should sexual abstinence be the primary focus of efforts to prevent the spread of AIDS in the developing world?

In the ongoing battle against AIDS, Senegal is one of Africa's rare success stories. On a continent where 25 to 30 percent of the adult population in some areas has HIV or AIDS, Senegal has managed to keep the infection rate at 2 percent.

Touching All Corners of the Globe

Since the global epidemic started in the 1980s, nearly 20 million adults and children have died from AIDS, as of the end of 1999. About three-quarters of the deaths were in sub-Saharan Africa. Meanwhile, some 34 million people are estimated to have HIV/AIDS around the world, including nearly 1 million in North America and more than 5 million in Southeast Asia.

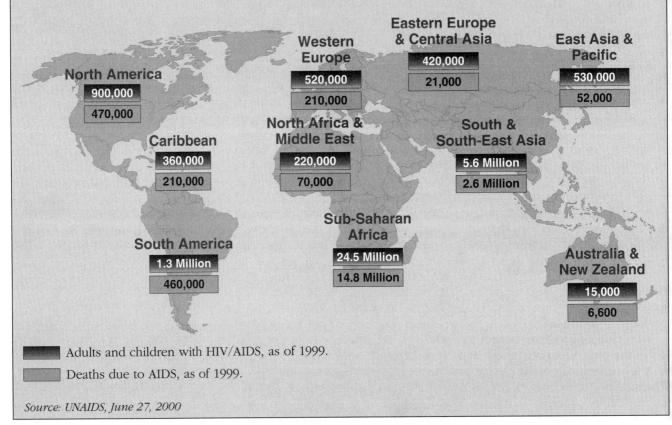

Eastern Europe & Central Asia
420,000
21,000

Western Europe
520,000
210,000

East Asia & Pacific
530,000
52,000

North America
900,000
470,000

Caribbean
360,000
210,000

North Africa & Middle East
220,000
70,000

South & South-East Asia
5.6 Million
2.6 Million

South America
1.3 Million
460,000

Sub-Saharan Africa
24.5 Million
14.8 Million

Australia & New Zealand
15,000
6,600

Adults and children with HIV/AIDS, as of 1999.

Deaths due to AIDS, as of 1999.

Source: UNAIDS, June 27, 2000

Senegal owes its impressive statistics in part to Ibrahima Ndoye; a gynecologist who initiated a nationwide campaign against AIDS in 1987, when the country only had 45 reported cases. Ndoye's program focused on increasing the distribution of condoms among almost all segments of Senegalese society, from classrooms to health clinics to brothels. As a result, condom distribution rose dramatically in Senegal, from 800,000 in 1988 to more than 7 million by 1997. [8] An AIDS education program was part of the approach as well.

Senegal's condom-distribution strategy has been widely praised as a model for other countries seeking to lower HIV infection rates.

"Condoms should be like a loaf of bread or a Coca-Cola, and we want to make sure that people can talk about them that way and find them in the same places," says Ivor Williams, a public health worker in Botswana. [9]

Supporters of condom distribution like Williams say that condoms are the only reliable way for sexually active people to protect themselves from HIV. But others argue that condom use is ultimately not effective in preventing the spread of HIV.

"Pushing the condom message is a value-free message, and that's why it's not going to work," says Robert McGinnis, vice president for national security and foreign affairs at the

Family Research Council. "Instead, we need to be sending people, particularly young people, a strong abstinence message."

McGinnis contends that making condoms readily available does more harm than good in the long run because it encourages people to become promiscuous. "There's an implied message when we encourage condom use," McGinnis says. "People see it as a green light to have more sex with more partners."

And that leads people into dangerous territory. "It's true, of course, that condoms decrease your chance of getting HIV per sexual encounter," says Mosher of the Population Research Institute. "But they also increase the number of sexual encounters, hence increasing your chances of getting the disease over the long haul."

According to Mosher and McGinnis, condom users are still very much at risk for several reasons. First, many will only use condoms "sometimes." In addition, many people in the developing world are poorly educated and don't learn how to properly use prophylactics, or they break during intercourse.

Finally, McGinnis says, a condom, even when used properly, "is not an iron bar between you and your partner." For instance, he says, "it doesn't block some sexually transmitted diseases like syphilis," which is known to facilitate the transmission of HIV between partners.

The only alternative, opponents of the condom strategy say, is to focus on teaching sexual abstinence until marriage.

"The only reliable way to avoid contracting AIDS through sexual contact is by maintaining a lifelong monogamous relationship," the Rev. Franklin Graham told the Senate Committee on Foreign Relations on Feb. 24. "But just as important, we must recognize that the ability to adopt such dramatic lifestyle changes is almost impossible without the moral conviction that sex outside of a marriage between a man and a woman is contrary to God's law," added Graham, who is president of Samaritan's Purse, a Christian aid organization, and the son of evangelist Billy Graham.

Graham and others contend that religious groups must play an active role in convincing people to abstain from sex outside of marriage. They note that many countries that have

had success in stemming the spread of HIV — like Senegal, Uganda and the Philippines — have had strong abstinence campaigns directed from churches and mosques. "Kids don't need condoms, they need good val-

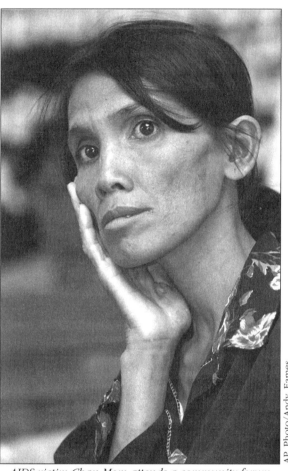

AIDS victim Chan Mom attends a community forum marking World AIDS Day in Phnom Penh, Cambodia, in 1999. The 34-year-old woman contracted the AIDS virus from her husband.

ues, the kind you get from your church," McGinnis says

But Jacobs of AIDS Action says that supplanting safe-sex education with exhortations to abstinence is dangerous and naïve. "It's like moving forward with your eyes shut because it doesn't recognize . . . the reality on the ground," he says.

That "reality," Jacobs and others say, is that poverty forces young people in

Africa to grow up fast, leading them to become sexually active at very young ages. "Adolescence is a Western, middle-class term that doesn't really exist in places like Africa," says Ron MacInniss, director of the Global AIDS Project at the Global Health Council.

MacInniss and others point out that even in the affluent West, which has the resources to shelter children much more than in the developing world, sexual activity often begins soon after puberty. "How can we honestly expect that young Africans are all going to abstain when our own young people don't?" Jacobs asks. "Besides," he adds, focusing primarily on abstinence "simply detracts from the message of safe sexual practice, the message that's going to save their lives."

In addition, condom advocates say, a health policy that stresses abstinence over condoms is completely unrealistic for more mature adults, in part, because many who give and get the virus are married. "A lot of the victims of this disease are married women who think they're already in a monogamous relationship, but, as it turns out, they're not," says Carol Miller, director of public policy at the Global Health Council. "People like this need condoms to protect themselves."

Finally, opponents of abstinence disagree with the contention that offering people sex education and condoms encourages them to have more sex than they normally would. "That's a complete fallacy, and it's been disproved in studies," Miller says. She cites a study by the Institute of Medicine that shows that providing young people with sex education doesn't lead to promiscuity. [10]

But others say that combining elements of both abstinence and sex-education campaigns is the best approach. "Condoms are only one part of the equation because you must also change sexual practices in order to succeed," says Richard Laing, an associate professor of international health at Boston University's School of Public Health.

Laing points to Uganda, which distributed condoms but also initiated a campaign to discourage promiscuity. "They worked to make sure that young girls started having sex at a much later age, and that's produced real results."

Is the spread of AIDS in the developing world a security threat to the United States?

In 1991, the Central Intelligence Agency released a study on the likely impact of HIV/AIDS. It painted a grim picture, estimating that by the turn of the millennium 45 million people, mostly in Africa, would either be dead from the disease, or infected — more than the number of combatants killed in both world wars. In fact, the total number of people killed or infected by the year 2000 was 8 million higher, or 53 million. [11]

The report made little impact in intelligence and military circles. Nor did the public release of an unclassified version of the document by the State Department in 1992.

But now, almost a decade later, AIDS is squarely on the national-security agenda. Clinton administration officials, including National Security Adviser Samuel R. "Sandy"

Berger and U.S. Representative to the United Nations Richard Holbrooke, regularly paint the AIDS epidemic in geopolitical terms. Moreover, on Jan. 10, Democratic presidential nominee Al Gore told the U.N. Security Council that, "today, in sight of all the world, we are putting the AIDS crisis on the top of the world's security agenda." [12]

Those who agree with Gore argue that AIDS needs to be seen as more than just a health crisis, since it has the potential to destabilize all of

Balloons in the shape of the ribbon symbolizing AIDS are hung in Pasay City, the Philippines, to celebrate World AIDS Day and increase awareness of the disease.

AP Photo/BullitMarquez

Southern Africa and beyond.

"Using the national-security label is appropriate because this disease could bring down nations, and not just in Africa," says Jacobs of AIDS Action. "This disease is also starting to spread in Southeast Asia, which is so important for the global economy. If it spread in India and China as fast as it did in Africa, these two vitally important nations could spiral out of control, dramatically affecting our national interests."

Even in Africa, vital interests are at stake, supporters say. "We get a lot of oil, diamonds, gold, titanium and other

vital minerals from Africa," McGinnis says. "These natural resources not only help fuel our economy, but some, like titanium, are a necessary part of the weapons we build, like missiles and fighter planes."

Finally, those who view AIDS as a national-security issue argue that if left alone AIDS could mutate into a virus that posed much greater dangers to the entire world. "People think it doesn't matter because it's just an African problem," MacInniss says, "but when you have a deadly virus that's constantly mutating and running out of control, we don't know what will happen."

But the Heritage Foundation's Spenser says that makes no sense. "Look, AIDS doesn't threaten the security of the United States," he says, "and that's how we should be determining whether something is or isn't an issue of national security."

Spenser argues that labeling AIDS as a national-security concern is merely a tactic to enhance the issue's importance and drain resources from real security needs.

"Liberals always define national security to fit their interests," he says, pointing to the use of the American military for peacekeeping and other humanitarian missions. "Our already-scarce military resources should be used to protect our vital interests and allies, not on other distractions."

Frank J. Gaffney Jr., director of the Center for Security Policy, agrees. "Instead of broadening our definition of national security to include things like AIDS, we should be focused on preparing for the next 'no kidding' national-security problem, like the next war."

Chronology

1980s AIDS first appears and develops into a global crisis.

June 1981
U.S. Centers for Disease Control and Prevention (CDC) documents the first cases of a mysterious immune-system disorder in five homosexual men in Los Angeles.

July 1982
After determining that the disease also occurs in heterosexuals, the CDC names it AIDS — Acquired Immune Deficiency Syndrome.

1983
Scientists from the CDC and National Institutes of Health discover AIDS patients in Zaire. Evidence suggests that the virus is being spread through heterosexual contact.

1984
Scientists at the Institute Pasteur in France and National Cancer Institute in Bethesda, Md., announce that they have separately isolated the virus that causes AIDS, later named the human immunodeficiency virus (HIV).

1985
The Food and Drug Administration (FDA) approves the first blood tests to detect the presence of antibodies to HIV. To reduce the risk of spreading the disease through transfusions of tainted blood, U.S. blood banks introduce blood-screening tests.

1985
Movie star Rock Hudson dies of AIDS, raising awareness of the disease in the United States.

1987
FDA approves the first anti-AIDS drug, AZT. Senegal begins an AIDS-prevention campaign that has succeeded in containing the spread of the virus.

1988
The first World AIDS Day Summit is convened. An estimated 5 million people in sub-Saharan Africa have HIV or AIDS.

———— • ————

1990 to Present AIDS begins to spread rapidly through the developing world, especially sub-Saharan Africa, while scientists in the West begin making progress on treatments.

1990
Central Intelligence Agency conducts a study of the global impact of AIDS and predicts that 45 million will die or be infected by the year 2000.

1991
The total number of people with HIV/AIDS in sub-Saharan Africa reaches 10 million.

1992
Ugandan President Yoweri Museveni begins a major AIDS-prevention campaign that succeeds in bringing the HIV infection rate down by the late 1990s.

1995
The first protease inhibitors, or anti-retroviral drugs, are released.

1996
UNAIDS is established. By year's end, more than 20 million Africans have HIV or AIDS.

1997
The Joint United Nations Program on HIV/AIDS reports that the disease is more widespread than previously thought, estimating 30 million people may be living with HIV/AIDS and that 16,000 new infections are spawned each day.

1999
The number of people with HIV/AIDS in sub-Saharan Africa reaches nearly 25 million.

January 2000
U.N. Security Council convenes a meeting on the global AIDS crisis, chaired by Vice President Al Gore.

May 2000
Five large pharmaceutical firms announce discounted prices on AIDS drugs for the developing world.

July 2000
South African President Thabo Mbeki attends the 13th International AIDS Conference and refuses to acknowledge that the HIV virus causes AIDS.

August 2000
President Clinton signs a law authorizing more than $300 million for AIDS prevention and treatment in the developing world.

September 2000
World Bank creates $500 million fund to help sub-Saharan Africa battle the epidemic.

2001
Preliminary results from Phase 3 AIDS vaccine trials will be released.

Moreover, Spenser and Gaffney don't think AIDS will spread in Asia or the rest of the world in the way it has through sub-Saharan Africa. "This disease is slowing down in Asia and elsewhere as countries acknowledge its existence and begin educating their people about it," Spenser says.

And while they acknowledge that the United States does have some strategic interest in Africa, they doubt the AIDS epidemic will threaten those interests, at least in the near term.

"If Africa were to self-destruct, of course there could be repercussions that might affect our national security and require some sort of military action down the road," Gaffney says. "But it hasn't self-destructed. Instead it's just one of a host of things that could impact our security sometime in the future and shouldn't be assumed to be a national security problem when it isn't right now."

Opponents also dispute the idea that the AIDS epidemic could disrupt the flow of strategic minerals to the United States. "Just because AIDS is sweeping across parts of Africa doesn't mean we won't be able to get the resources we need," Spenser says. "There will always be people who will extract the strategically important minerals we need because they are huge export earners for these countries." ■

BACKGROUND

Out of Africa

It is generally believed that humans first contracted HIV decades ago in Africa. The earliest evidence of the virus in humans was recently found in a blood sample from 1959.

It was taken from a man in the Belgian Congo (now the Democratic Republic of Congo) in Central Africa. [13]

Scientists think the HIV virus spread from chimpanzees to human beings, although they don't know exactly how. In his 1999 book *The River*, journalist Edward Hooper claimed that humans first contracted the virus from a tainted oral polio vaccine that was administered to children in Central Africa in the mid-1950s. [14] But efforts to confirm that hypothesis have turned up no connection between the vaccine and HIV.

The disease first came to the attention of the health community in 1981, when CDC scientists documented a strange, immune-system disorder in five homosexual men from Los Angeles. Initially, the condition seemed confined to members of the gay community and was dubbed Gay-Related Immune Deficiency, or GRID. But the following year, when new cases of the disease appeared in heterosexual women, drug users and Haitian immigrants the condition was renamed Acquired Immune Deficiency Syndrome (AIDS.)

It was not until 1984 that scientists first identified HIV, the virus that causes AIDS. French and American researchers discovered it simultaneously. By this time, scientists understood that the virus was generally transmitted via semen during sexual relations, in blood by drug users using dirty needles or by transfusions of contaminated blood.

By the mid-1980s, public awareness of the disease in the United States and other Western countries had begun to grow, spurred by the death in 1985 of movie star Rock Hudson, the first major public figure to succumb to AIDS. That same year, the Food and Drug Administration approved the first tests capable of detecting the presence of antibodies to HIV in the blood.

In 1987, the first anti-AIDS drug, AZT, came on the market. Although

it was released with great fanfare, it only helped some people with the disease, and only for a few years. In addition, AZT proved highly toxic, forcing some patients to stop treatment prematurely.

The next big advance in AIDS treatment did not come until 1995, when a number of drug companies released a new class of medicines known as protease inhibitors. They stopped the disease by blocking an enzyme in cells used by the virus to replicate itself. They also were somewhat less toxic than AZT, and hence easier to take.

Researchers found that protease inhibitors were most effective when patients were given a "cocktail" of three or even four different types at the same time. Even AIDS patients who were very ill responded. While the new drugs gave hope to many living with AIDS or HIV, they were not a cure.

The Gathering Storm

AIDS in Africa first came to the attention of Western researchers in 1983, two years after it appeared in the United States. A CDC team visited a hospital in Kinshasa, Zaire (now Congo) and found dozens of young men and women dying, their bodies literally wasting away.

Although there was no test for AIDS at the time, the scientists found the same low levels of infection-fighting T-cells in the victims' blood as they had in AIDS sufferers in the United States. The Africans were also fighting pneumonia and the other opportunistic infections that afflicted Americans with AIDS.

But there was one crucial difference between the African and U.S. sufferers: "There were so many women [in Africa]. It said to me it's heterosexual," said Piot of UNAIDS,

Mbeki's Controversial Stand on AIDS

When South African President Thabo Mbeki mounted the podium to open the recent international AIDS conference in Durban — the first ever held in a developing country — many hoped he would use the historic occasion to end a simmering controversy.

For more than a year, Mbeki had been saying that there is no proven link between HIV and AIDS, in spite of the overwhelming scientific evidence to the contrary. Instead, he claimed that HIV is just one of a host of factors that cause AIDS. In particular, he has pointed to poverty as the main culprit.

A week before the conference, 5,000 AIDS researchers and physicians had signed an open letter that stated, unequivocally: "HIV causes AIDS." Dubbed "The Durban Declaration," it went on to say: "It is unfortunate that a few vocal people continue to deny the evidence. This position will cost countless lives." [1]

But Mbeki refused to acknowledge that HIV always causes AIDS. Instead, he restated his position: "It seemed to me that we could not blame everything on a single virus."

The speech was not well-received. Hundreds of delegates walked out when the president addressed the issue. "It is a travesty," said William Blattner, co-founder of the Institute of Human Virology, angrily leaving the stadium where Mbeki was speaking. [2]

In the ensuing months, the president has stuck to his guns, weathering a storm of criticism from a wide range of sources including the media, churches and the medical profession. A recent headline in a South African newspaper begged: "Just Say 'Yes' Mr. President." [3]

Critics of Mbeki contend that his refusal to acknowledge the connection between HIV and AIDS further muddies the water in a country where ignorance about the disease is already rife. "When he questions whether HIV causes AIDS, it fosters an environment where denial can continue to rage unabated," says Eric Sawyer, co-founder of ACT UP, an AIDS advocacy group in New York City. "People can say: 'Well, if the president isn't worried about HIV, why should I be?' "

Others are even less charitable, speculating that the president is willfully denying a connection between HIV and AIDS for political reasons. "In South Africa, more than 4 million people are infected with HIV," says an AIDS researcher. "It's hard to tell them that they're going to die, that there's little you can do to save them, and then expect them to vote for you in the future."

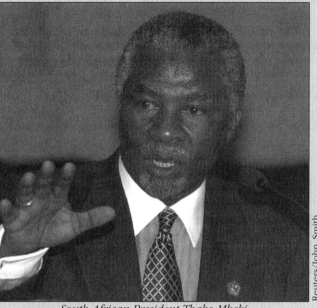

South African President Thabo Mbeki

Reuters/John Smith

[1] Sabin Russell, "Mbeki's HIV Stand Angers Delegates," *San Francisco Chronicle*, July 10, 2000.

[2] Quoted in *Ibid*.

[3] Karen MacGregor. "Mbeki Loses Authority Over Aids Stance," *The Independent*, Sept. 24, 2000.

who led the CDC team in 1983 and is the co-discoverer of the Ebola virus. "That means that everyone is at risk," he said. "Until then, I never thought a whole country, a whole population, could be involved." [15]

When Piot and his team tried to publicize the results of their work, they were virtually ignored by the international public health community. Scientist Jonathan Mann — who showed that the disease in Africa was quickly spreading among all social groups — also received little attention. Throughout the mid-1980s, health officials focused instead on the prevalence of HIV and AIDS among gays and drug users in the United States and Europe.

Only in the last years of the decade did the worldwide implications of the disease begin to become apparent, thanks to Piot, Mann and others. The first World AIDS Day Summit was held in 1988 and, for the first time, the United States, the U.N. and other organizations began to put resources into understanding and combating the epidemic in the developing world.

Even so, political considerations and bureaucratic infighting at WHO, USAID and other organizations slowed the developed world's response to the disease. More important, by the early 1990s it became

How HIV Kills

The HIV virus attacks T-cells, or lymphocytes, which help fight infections. By destroying these vital cells, the virus reduces the body's ability to fend off other diseases. After a number of years with HIV, the body's T-cell count becomes very low. At less than 200 T-cells per cubic millimeter of blood, the patient is considered to have full-blown AIDS. The weakened immune system makes the patient susceptible to opportunistic, often lethal infections, such as tuberculosis and pneumonia. Death may also be caused by dementia and wasting syndrome, which may be caused by the virus itself. The two major AIDS viruses, HIV-1 and HIV-2, operate in much the same way. But HIV-1, the primary virus in Africa, is easier to transmit than HIV-2 and has a shorter gestation period between infection and the onset of AIDS. HIV-2 is more common in North America and Asia.

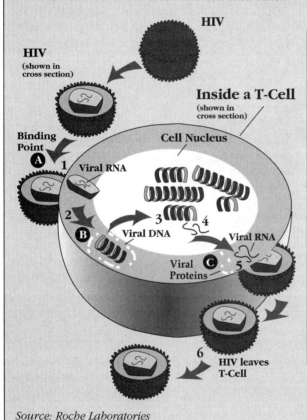

How the AIDS Virus Attacks a T-Cell

1. Virus enters cell, losing its protein coat.

2. Viral RNA is converted to viral DNA.

3. Viral DNA is replicated.

4. DNA is converted back to RNA.

5. Viral proteins are produced.

6. New viruses, produced when proteins and RNA combine, leave demolished T-cell and enter bloodstream.

Drugs That Fight AIDS

Ⓐ gp120 vaccine seeks to prevent binding of HIV to cell wall.

Ⓑ AZT and other drugs known as nucleotide analogs attack virus by blocking conversion of viral RNA into DNA.

Ⓒ Antiviral drugs called protease inhibitors block production of HIV enzyme essential to virus replication.

Source: Roche Laboratories

apparent that in the developed world, AIDS was unlikely to significantly spread to the broader heterosexual community. The news lessened the sense of urgency that had begun to characterize response to AIDS in the late 1980s.

In Africa and elsewhere in the developing world, the disease also was largely ignored, even as it spread like wildfire throughout the 1980s and '90s. With the exception of a few countries, notably Senegal, Uganda and Thailand, governments formulated few, if any, HIV-prevention policies. Ironically, some of the most affluent African states, like South Africa and Kenya, did the least.

In the late 1990s, the problem of AIDS in the developing world slowly began to be noticed by policy-makers, both in Africa and the West. In 1996, UNAIDS was created to coordinate the global fight against the disease. Meanwhile, Kenya, Botswana and other African nations began to take tentative steps toward formulating prevention programs.

The issue has received an unusual amount of attention this year. In January, the U.N. Security Council held a special meeting, chaired by Vice President Gore, to discuss the epidemic. The meeting attracted a lot of attention and underscored the international interest in the disease.

Six months later, former South African President Nelson Mandela helped focus world attention on the disease once again, at the 13th International AIDS Conference in Durban.

"We have to rise above our differences and combine our efforts to save our people," Mandela said. "History will judge us harshly if we fail to do so — and right now."

Mandela's impassioned plea and the attendant media attention were seen as a sign that AIDS is now atop the international community's health agenda.   ■

CURRENT SITUATION

Recent Initiatives

On Aug. 19, President Clinton signed legislation into law that authorized more than $300 million to fight AIDS, primarily in Africa. Among the prevention and education programs to be funded are those that provide testing for the HIV virus, counseling for HIV/AIDS suffers and drugs to prevent mother-to-child transmission of HIV. [16]

Clinton's pledge came on the heels of an announcement in July by the U.S. Export-Import Bank. It promised $1 billion in loans to sub-Saharan African countries to finance needed health-care infrastructure and to purchase AIDS drugs. [17] (See "At Issue," p. 209.)

In September, the World Bank weighed in, announcing the creation of a $500 million loan fund for sub-Saharan African countries battling the AIDS epidemic. The money will support HIV-education programs, condom distribution and training of health-care workers. [18]

Two countries with high HIV infection rates, Kenya and Ethiopia, will receive the first loans — for $50 million and $60 million, respectively. Nigeria, Zimbabwe and Zambia are among the nations likely to receive loans next.

"What I'm trying to do is get money out there as quickly as I can," said World Bank President James D. Wolfensohn. "I honestly don't think in a crisis as grave as this that money is going to be a problem." [19]

In addition to these initiatives, there has been a slew of other recent efforts by public and private groups. The Bill and Melinda Gates Foundation has pledged $50 million for health-care and education programs in Botswana in conjunction with another $50 million for Botswana pledged by Merck. And Bristol-Myers Squibb plans to spend $100 million over five years on anti-AIDS drugs and other assistance for Southern Africa.

According to international AIDS experts, the recent offers of assistance reflect a new attitude and awareness that the epidemic, especially in Africa, is going to require a massive and costly response. "There does seem to be a tide of change on this issue of late," says MacInniss of the Global AIDS Project.

According to the World Bank, however, sub-Saharan Africa alone will need up to $3 billion per year to bring the epidemic under control and provide at least some treatment for Africans already afflicted. And HIV is spreading rapidly in Asia, a continent with roughly half the world's population.

"We're finally starting to go in the right direction and take this thing seriously, but it's all much too little, much too late," says Harvard University's Thea. "I read recently that the U.S. is giving $1.4 billion to Colombia to fight the drug war," he says. "That's the kind of money we should be spending on fighting this epidemic, not a few hundred million."

Focus on STDs

On the plus side, Thea says, much of the new money for Africa will fund prevention and education programs. "Like every epidemic, early prevention efforts are the best way to stop HIV/AIDS from spreading," he says. "Look at what they were able to do in Senegal."

Still, many AIDS experts want more attention paid to treating other sexually transmitted diseases (STDs), like syphilis, which act as conduits for HIV, making it much easier for the virus to be passed on during sexual relations.

"One reason HIV has swept through Africa is that the continent has very high levels of STDs," Boston University's Laing says. "We know that we can reduce the HIV infection rate by as much as half if we aggressively work to treat STDS."

Others argue that a major effort should be made to provide the latest lifesaving drugs to even the poorest in Africa, Asia and elsewhere, and not just for humanitarian reasons.

"Most of the people with HIV or AIDS in places like Southern Africa have families," ACT UP's Sawyer says. "With anti-retroviral drugs, we can keep many of these people alive for another 10, 15 or even 20 years, which will give them time to see their kids to adulthood, see that they are cared for and educated."

But many AIDS experts say that even with a flood of new funds from the West, the epidemic ultimately won't be beaten unless African governments make HIV/AIDS a top priority.

In many countries, taboos against talking about sex or an unwillingness to confront the catastrophic impact of the disease have kept many governments silent. In South Africa, which has seen its HIV-infection rate increase by 2,000 percent in the last decade, President Mbeki won't acknowledge that HIV leads to AIDS. "I think [leaders in

Africa] are having a hard time confronting the horror that faces them," the University of Natal's Whiteside says.

"The leadership in most of these countries needs to face this issue head on and say, 'This problem is real and we need to come to grips with it,'" Thea says. "They need to be like President Museveni of Uganda, who brings up AIDS every chance he gets."

"In most countries," Sawyer adds, "there's still no battle plan to combat this disease."

Economic Impact

This year, for the first time, the International Monetary Fund's "World Economic Outlook" makes special note of the impact of HIV and AIDS on the economies of sub-Saharan Africa. [20]

The news is not good. According to the IMF, AIDS may well wreck many already fragile economies on the continent. Instead of growing, the per capita gross domestic product (GDP) in sub-Saharan Africa is expected to be 5 percent lower by 2010, the report says.

According to UNAIDS, GDP loss will probably be much greater in those countries hardest hit by the disease. For example, in South Africa, GDP is expected to be 17 percent lower by 2010 than it is today.

Part of the problem is blamed on the sheer size of the epidemic. In some countries, a large percentage of the adult population is afflicted. In South Africa and Zambia, for instance, 20 percent of all people between the ages of 15 and 49 are infected. In Zimbabwe and Botswana, the numbers are even higher. In nations with such high infection rates, life expectancy is likely to fall from about 60 years today to 30 by 2010. [21]

Just as important, though, is the fact that 80 percent of those felled by AIDS are between the ages of 20 to 50 — adults in the midst of or just beginning the most productive years of their lives. [22] "You're talking about people with jobs and families," says the Population Research Institute's Mosher.

As a result, AIDS is already having a profound economic impact. Many teachers, doctors and policemen are dying almost as fast as they can be replaced. In Zambia, for instance, 1,300 teachers died in the first 10 months of 1998 — more than two-thirds of the Zambians trained as teachers in a typical year.

"The education profession has been particularly susceptible to this

Prostitutes in Mexico City march during annual Day of the Dead festivities in 1998 in memory of colleagues who have died from the AIDS virus.

disease because a lot of times young teachers are sent to different rural villages, where they're alone and unmarried," Thea says. Since teachers in Africa are part of the educated elite, they tend to be popular with single women in the village. "They

end up having a lot of partners, with predictable results," he says.

The disease also has devastated the health-care field, especially nurses, Laing says. The high attrition rate is exacerbated by another factor, he says. "Many health-care professionals leave because it's so depressing to treat hundreds of people each year who are going to die," he says, referring to the large number of AIDS victims who are clogging the continent's hospitals.

Employers Desperate

The private sector is also suffering. "You've got places in Africa where employers are hiring three or four people for the same job because they know the first two or three are going to die in the next few months," says former Rep. Ronald V. Dellums, D-Calif., president of the President's Advisory Council on HIV/AIDS.

In addition, many large firms are spending a much greater share of their income on benefits for their increasingly sick work force. In Botswana, health-care costs have risen by up to 500 percent. A recent study by Metropolitan Life estimated the cost of paying death-related benefits for companies in South Africa would more than double — from 5.5 percent of payroll in 1997 to 12 percent in 2007. [23]

The continent's farm sector — where most Africans still work — also has been hurt by the epidemic. "At this point, all we have is anecdotal evidence, but from what we do know, things are not looking good," Thea says. "In Zimbabwe, for instance, farm produc-

At Issue:

Should African countries reject loans from the U.S. Export-Import Bank to help treat people with AIDS?

KALUMBI SHANGULA
Secretary of Health and Social Services, Republic of Namibia

FROM *THE WASHINGTON POST*, SEPT. 17, 2000

*t*here is no question that HIV/AIDS is a serious public health problem. AIDS causes slow and agonizing death, leaves family members, relatives and friends of victims traumatized and creates an army of orphans. It has a negative impact on the economy and the demographic structure of a nation. No one knows this better than the governments of southern Africa. . . .

Yet the charge that we are not moving aggressively to deal with AIDS has once again been raised. This time it is because of the decision by Namibia and at least three other African nations not to accept an offer from the U.S. Export-Import Bank to provide loans to buy anti-retroviral drugs to treat HIV infection.

The bank's $1 billion lending program is offered in conjunction with the decision in May by five major pharmaceutical companies to reduce the prices of anti-retroviral drugs for developing countries. We recognize that the bank's proposal, like the pharmaceuticals' offer, was made from a noble impulse to help out in a case of need, and from the realizations that a significant proportion of the world population faces a huge catastrophe if the developing countries take no action.

But our decision not to accept the offer was based on the conviction that the risks our country faced in taking on the burden of a loan outweighed the benefits we would receive from the drugs.

The tragic truth of AIDS is that it is a long, drawn-out disease, lasting 10 years or more from first infection. Anti-retroviral drugs prevent early onset of opportunistic infections and improve the quality of life, but they are not a cure. . . .

If HIV drugs were a cure, many African countries would consider accepting the Ex-Im Bank offer. But given the duration of treatment required and the increasing number of AIDS patients, assuming a loan to purchase anti-retroviral drugs does not make sense for developing countries, many of which are already burdened by foreign indebtedness. It does not make sense for Namibia. It would mean plunging ourselves into perpetual debt from which we would not be able to extricate ourselves. If we do not have the money to buy anti-retroviral drugs directly, where will we get the money to pay back this loan, plus interest? This is a trap into which we cannot afford to fall. . . .

It is wiser to invest in drugs that treat the conditions that are caused by AIDS, to alleviate suffering to the extent that we can.

Reprinted with permission

JAMES A. HARMON
Chairman, U.S. Export-Import Bank

FROM *THE WASHINGTON POST*, SEPT. 17, 2000

*w*ho would not be horrified by the statistics coming out of sub-Saharan Africa? The HIV/AIDS pandemic threatens to bring decades of slow, hard-won progress to an abrupt end. It is a catastrophe that can only be reversed by a massive influx of resources — a staggering need that far outruns available humanitarian aid.

. . . . The historic Durban conference, which . . . drew the international spotlight to Africa's HIV/AIDS struggle, identified longer credit terms and sustainable resources as an essential part of a broader solution. Accordingly, we decided to offer $1 billion a year in financing to the region to build a sustainable, effective infrastructure of health care across sub-Saharan Africa.

This program has been incompletely described as a loan program for African governments to purchase anti-retroviral drugs to treat HIV-infected patients. In reality, it offers countries the opportunity to purchase whatever is needed — from medical equipment to adviser services to hospitals, as well as pharmaceuticals.

. . . . I am frequently asked: Why add to the region's debt? Without a doubt, the international donor community should do more. But in reality, there remains a significant gap between existing need and available aid. The Joint United Nations Program on HIV/AIDS (UNAIDS) estimates that more than $2 billion in annual global investment is necessary. Yet only $300 million has been invested in the effort this year. Bluntly put, today's resource levels are inadequate.

. . . . Without question, however, the success of our program hinges on American companies significantly reducing their prices to put vital medicines and supplies within economic reach. . . . Clearly, the humanitarian need challenges all of us to set aside business as usual. . . . We also hope that our move triggers other export credit agencies in Europe and Japan to make even more resources available.

. . . . Clearly, the Ex-Im Bank is only one piece of a broader solution. Debt forgiveness can give countries more freedom to acquire what they need. . . . The international community should give more direct aid. But the need of others to do more does not negate the moral obligation of all parties to find a way to help.

Too many in the Western world have learned to steel themselves to the hardships in sub-Saharan Africa. It's a habit we should abandon in the 21st century. For Africa to win this war, it will take all of us tackling this vast humanitarian crisis, and doing what is in our power to make a difference.

Reprinted with permission

tion has fallen off for the last few years, because the disease has created a labor shortage."

Experts predict that the grim statistics and anecdotal reports will get much worse before getting better. People who are dying of AIDS today are the ones who had HIV in the early-to-mid-1990s. Now, the number of HIV-positive people in sub-Saharan Africa is much greater than it was even in 1995.

"For Africa, this is Armageddon, and I'm not exaggerating," Thea says. Other experts use similar language. CDC AIDS expert Kevin DeCock called the epidemic "Africa's worst social catastrophe since slavery." [24]

According to the U.S. Census Bureau, AIDS will cause population declines in South Africa, Zimbabwe, Botswana and other countries in the next few years, while Malawi, Namibia and Zambia are among those expected to experience no population growth.

Hardest hit will be the children. Demographers predict that by 2010 there will be more than 40 million AIDS orphans in Africa. Today there are more than 12 million boys and girls (almost all in Africa) without parents because of AIDS. Many are placed with distant relatives or left to fend for themselves.

"We don't know what's going to happen to all of these orphans, but many could become criminals or become part of rogue armies," Miller says, referring to the rebel armies in Africa that conscript children. [25]

OUTLOOK

Vaccine Prospects

An estimated 15,000 people around the world become infected with the HIV virus every day. And the number is expected to double and double again before the rate of infection slows. [26]

"We are at the beginning of a pandemic, not the middle, not the end," says Sandra L. Thurman, director of the White House Office of National AIDS Policy. "We certainly know that before

Song Pengfei, right, walks with his father during a visit to Beijing for HIV treatment. After he contracted the AIDS virus from a blood transfusion, he was banned from school and ostracized by his village.

we're able to stop this pandemic, we'll have hundreds of millions of people infected and dead — and that's the best-case scenario."

Leaders in Africa and the West are hoping that an AIDS vaccine can put a

dent in Thurman's grim prediction. But none of vaccines under development is ready for general or even limited use.

Scientists have been working on a vaccine for more than a decade. Early attempts at bolstering infection-fighting antibodies failed. Today, researchers are focusing on strengthening another part of the immune system — the so-called T cells that go into action against a virus when it evades the antibodies.

Another potential vaccine — developed by the co-discoverer of the AIDS virus, Robert Gallo — would strengthen the mucosal immune system, which works in moist parts of the body, like the mouth and vagina, to fight infection. [27]

Currently, 21 clinical vaccine trials are under way around the world, but only two are in late stage, or Phase III, trials, which test whether the drug actually works. Preliminary results are expected early next year. [28]

One of the Phase III trials is taking place in the United States and Thailand, where 5,400 and 2,500 people, respectively, are testing a vaccine made by Vaxgen, an American drug company. If the vaccine proves at least 30 percent effective at stopping the transmission of HIV, the company will halt the trials and apply for regulatory approval. Even limited protection, scientists say, would be better than nothing.

Another closely watched trial is being conducted in England, using a vaccine developed at the universities of Oxford and Nairobi. The vaccine tries to mimic the T-cell activity of a number of Kenyan prostitutes, whose immune systems have proven resistant to HIV. The trial in England is testing the vaccine for safety. A test of its effectiveness is set to begin in Kenya before the end of the year.

The test in Kenya could be vitally important in slowing the epidemic. Unlike the Vaxgen vaccine, which was developed to fight the strain of AIDS common in North America, Europe and Asia, the drug being tested in England aims to halt type A AIDS, which is prevalent in Africa.

Public health experts are heartened by the work on an AIDS vaccine, but they don't expect a "magic bullet" any time soon. "I think we're still eight to 15 years away from a vaccine that will make a difference," Jacobs of AIDS Action says.

Even if one of the vaccines being tested proves effective, however, it might not remain so for long. AIDS tends to mutate easily, making it resistant to vaccines being used against it and thus very hard to stop over the long term.

The shortage of health-care personnel and lab facilities to vaccinate everyone adds to the challenge. And even if facilities were available, some people would still be very hard to reach, because many Africans live in remote areas, with bad or non-existent roads.

As *Washington Post* reporter Barton Gellman has noted, smallpox was eliminated just 20 years ago, even though an effective vaccine was developed in 1817. [29] And even diseases for which there are vaccines, like measles, still kill millions each year in the developing world.

"In a place like Africa, there are so many obstacles," says Boston University's Laing. "It's not like the U.S., where all the children are in school and easily reachable. So we can't underestimate the challenge of getting this vaccine out there and inoculating people." ∎

FOR MORE INFORMATION

AIDS Action, 1875 Connecticut Ave., N.W., Suite 700, Washington, D.C. 20009; (202) 986-1300; www.aidsaction.org. Monitors and promotes legislation dealing with AIDS research, education and related public-policy issues.

Global Health Council, 1701 K St., N.W., Suite 600, Washington D.C. 20006; (202) 833-5900; www.globalhealthcouncil.org. Seeks to strengthen U.S. participation in international health activities, especially in developing countries.

Joint United Nations Program on HIV/AIDS (UNAIDS), 20 Avenue Appia, CH-1211 Geneva 27 Switzerland; (4122) 791 3666; www.unaids.org. Coordinates responses to the global AIDS epidemic.

U.S. Centers for Disease Control and Prevention (CDC), 1600 Clifton Rd., N.E., Atlanta, Ga. 30333; (404) 639-3534; www.cdc.gov. Surveys national and international HIV/AIDS trends, administers block grants to states for preventive health services and promotes AIDS education programs.

Notes

[1] Ann M Simmons, "Bell Tolling for Kenya Families as AIDS Ravages Nation's Adults," *Los Angeles Times*, March 5, 2000.
[2] Quoted in *Ibid*.
[3] Adriel Bettelheim, "Drugmakers Under Siege," *The CQ Researcher*, Sept. 3, 1999, pp. 753-776.
[4] Quoted in David Brown, "AIDS Drug Discounts Offered to 3rd World," *The Washington Post*, May 12, 2000.
[5] Cited in Michael Waldholz, "African Nations Studying Generic AIDS Drugs," *The Wall Street Journal*, July 13, 2000.
[6] Quoted in Jeffrey Goldberg, "Epidemic Proportions," *The New York Times Magazine*, June 4, 2000.
[7] For background, see Kenneth Jost, "South Africa's Future," *The CQ Researcher*, Jan. 14, 1994, pp. 25-48.
[8] UNAIDS: www.unaids.org.
[9] Drusilla Menaker, "Africa Breaks Silence About AIDS and Sex: Agencies' New Mission Is to Change Thinking," *Dallas Morning News*, Oct. 17, 1999.
[10] D. Kirby, "School-Based Interventions to Prevent Unprotected Sex and HIV Among Adolescents," in Peterson and DiClemente, eds., *Handbook of HIV Prevention*, 2000.
[11] Barton Gellman, "The World Shunned Signs of the Coming Plague," *The Washington Post*, July 5, 2000.
[12] Quoted in Ibid.
[13] Adriel Bettelheim, "AIDS Update," *The CQ Researcher*, Dec. 4, 1998,pp. 1049-1072.

[14] "AIDS Wars," *The Economist*, Sept. 16, 2000.
15 Gellman, *op. cit.*
[16] Ricardo Alonso-Zaldivar, "Clinton Approves $400 Million Bill to Fight AIDS, Other Diseases Around the Globe," *Los Angeles Times*, Aug. 20, 2000.
[17] Michael M. Phillips, "Ex-Im Bank to Help American Businesses Sell AIDS Treatments to African Nations," *The Wall Street Journal*, July 19, 2000.
[18] Michael M. Phillips, "World Bank is Targeting AIDS in Africa," *The Wall Street Journal*, Sept. 12, 2000.
[19] Quoted in *Ibid*.
[20] International Monetary Fund, "World Economic Outlook," 2000.
[21] U.S. Census Bureau.
[22] Figure cited in John Christensen, "Millions of Children in Africa are Struggling to Survive with No Parents As Modern Plague Ravages the Continent," *South China Morning Post*, April 2, 2000.
[23] Figures cited in International Monetary Fund, *op. cit.*, p. 67.
[24] "AIDS to cut African's Life Expectancy to 30 Years," *Star Tribune* [Minneapolis-St. Paul], July 11, 2000.
[25] For background on the refugee problem, see Mary H. Cooper, "Global Refugee Crisis," *The CQ Researcher*, July 9, 1999, pp. 569-592.
[26] Gellman, *op. cit.*
[27] Joannie Schrof Fischer, "Searching for that Ounce of Prevention," *U.S. News & World Report*, July 17, 2000.
[28] "A Turning-Point for Aids?" *The Economist*, July 15, 2000.
[29] Gellman, *op. cit.*

Bibliography

Selected Sources Used

Books

Garrett, Laurie, *The Coming Plague*, Farrar, Straus and Giroux, 1994.

Garrett, a science writer for *Newsday*, gives a good account of researchers' efforts to understand AIDS, from laboratories in the U.S. and Europe to the jungles of Africa.

Hooper, Edward, *The River: A Journey Back to the Source of HIV and AIDS*, Little, Brown, 1999.

Hooper, a former BBC correspondent and United Nations official, searches for the origins of the epidemic and purports to find it in bad batches of an oral polio vaccine administered in Africa in the 1950s.

Articles

"AIDS Wars," *The Economist*, Sept. 16, 2000.

The piece examines recent research into the origins of AIDS. So far, the cause of the disease remains elusive.

Altman, Lawrence K., "Africa's AIDS Crisis: Finding Common Ground," *The New York Times*, July 16, 2000.

Altman argues that poverty is a major factor in the spread of HIV/AIDS throughout Africa.

Bettelheim, Adriel, "AIDS Update," *The CQ Researcher*, Dec. 4, 1998.

Bettelheim gives an excellent overview of the AIDS epidemic in the United States, with illuminating sections on treatment, prevention efforts and the politics surrounding the disease.

Christiansen, John, "Millions of Children in Africa Are Struggling to Survive with No Parents as Modern Plague Ravages the Continent," *South China Post*, April 2, 2000.

Christiansen describes the effect of the AIDS epidemic on African families and examines the disease's general demographic impact on the continent.

Gellman, Barton, "World Shunned Signs of the Coming Plague," *The Washington Post*, July 5, 2000.

Gellman chronicles the ignorance and inaction that surrounded the discovery that AIDS was more than just a disease that afflicted homosexual men and intravenous drug users. In particular, he details the bureaucratic infighting that stalled the World Trade Organization's response to the pandemic.

Jon Jeter, "Free of Apartheid, Divided by Disease," *The Washington Post*, July 6, 2000.

Jeter describes how AIDS threatens to reverse the progress made in post-apartheid South Africa. With nearly one in five South African adults infected with the disease, Jeter writes that "AIDS threatens to slow social change and undo economic development with the staggering costs of caring for the sick, the dying and those they leave behind."

Russell, Sabin, "Mbeki's HIV Stand Angers Delegates," *The San Francisco Chronicle*, July 10, 2000.

Sabin details the controversy surrounding South African President Thabo Mbeki's refusal to publicly acknowledge the direct connection between HIV and AIDS.

Schools, Mark, "In Senegal, Common Sense Spells Success," *The Washington Post*, Jan. 31, 1999.

The article describes how Senegal initiated an aggressive AIDS-prevention campaign soon after uncovering cases of the disease. According to Schools, Senegal's experience proves "that foresight, pragmatism and energy can, even in the midst of deep poverty, hold one of the world's leading infectious killers at bay."

Sternberg, Steve, "AIDS in Africa is Reshaping Whole Populations, Study Says," *USA Today*, July 11, 2000.

The article gives a good sense of how AIDS is altering Africa's demographic future. Citing a recent study by the U.S. Census Bureau, Sternberg concludes that AIDS will "warp whole populations, empty communities and set the stage for vast migrations of men seeking available women."

"A Turning-Point for AIDS," *The Economist*, July 15, 2000.

The piece chronicles recent efforts to prevent the spread of HIV in Africa, including the search for a vaccine.

Waldholz, Michael, "Into Africa: Makers of AIDS Drugs Agree to Slash Prices for Developing World," *The Wall Street Journal*, May 11, 2000.

Waldholz gives a good overview of the controversy surrounding high prices for AIDS drugs, pointing out that even with deep discounts, most will still be out of reach for most Africans.

Reports

"The Status and Trends of the HIV/AIDS Epidemics in the World," U.S. Census Bureau, July 2000.

The report offers a good overview of the global impact of AIDS, now and in the future.

12 Computers and Medicine

ADRIEL BETTELHEIM

Chances are most individuals who browse the Internet's myriad medical Web sites have never heard of Pharmatrak Inc. But it's quite likely Pharmatrak knows quite a bit about some of them.

The Boston company secretly monitors the surfing habits of visitors to Web pages maintained by 11 large drug companies by attaching bits of computer code known as "cookies" to their computers. Using the data, a drug company can break down how often individuals in a particular country download information about one of its products, or gauge precisely how many visitors request details about a certain disease or condition. While the company says it has no intention of trying to identify individual visitors, privacy groups are worried. [1]

"It's one thing to get a banner ad on a commercial Web site targeted to your Web browsing habits, but it's quite another to have a central collection point that allows companies to access and collect information about patients and compare what they are doing," says Sarah Andrews, policy analyst for the Washington, D.C.-based Electronic Privacy Information Center. "It's really an egregious invasion or privacy."

Pharmatrak is but one example of the extent to which computers are driving modern medicine. Over the past five years, health-care providers, insurers, drug companies and research institutions have initiated a massive transformation from a paper-based health-care system to one that increasingly relies on electronic records to manage patient information.

From *The CQ Researcher,* October 27, 2000.

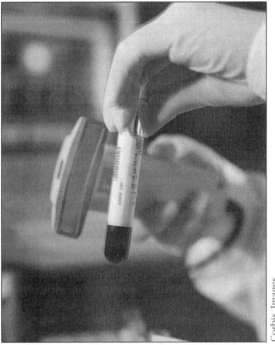

Health-care providers now use barcodes like those in grocery stores to avoid medical errors, such as misidentifying lab samples or prescribing the wrong medication or dosage.

Corbis Images

The changes are being seen in many areas. At a Veterans' Affairs hospital in Washington, D.C., officials use computers to scan bar codes on patient bracelets and medicines to avoid potentially life-threatening mistakes, such as administering the wrong medication or the wrong dosage. The health maintenance organization (HMO) Kaiser-Permanente has outfitted its 16 Denver-area clinics with computers so doctors can write prescriptions on-line, access lab test results by e-mail and quickly compare treatment histories for patients with the same condition.

Patients now can click on medical Web sites such as medscape.com to access articles on subjects such as the efficacy of inhaled steroids in children with asthma or current trends in contraception. They also can fill prescriptions through more than 400 on-line pharmacies — a market analysts predict will ring up $1.4 billion in sales in 2001. Consumers additionally may peruse the Web sites maintained by drug giants such as Pfizer Inc., Glaxo Wellcome PLC and SmithKline Beecham PLC and download information about medications. The companies view the Web sites as increasingly important marketing tools, hoping they will spur more patient inquiries and prompt doctors to prescribe their drugs.

But medicine's move to cyberspace is arousing significant concerns. Experts say that the large-scale collection of patient information raises questions about who has access to individuals' medical histories and whether that information could be used to deny employment or health insurance. Recent cases of identity theft, hacker attacks on commercial Web sites and more innocent technological snafus have reinforced the perception that personal information is not secure. In one widely publicized incident last year, the University of Michigan Medical Center accidentally transferred patient records on to Internet sites while it was updating a computerized scheduling system. The records — containing names, addresses, Social Security numbers and treatments for medical conditions — sat undetected for about a month until a student searching for information on a doctor accidentally stumbled across them.

The privacy issue is expected to become more complicated in light of the recent decoding of the human genome by teams of private and government scientists. [2] The development could lead to the storage of individuals' DNA sequences in cyberspace, where access to their genetic profile could yield information not only about current medical conditions but also whether they or

Web Users Worry About Their Health Information

A majority of today's Web users say they are willing to provide Internet sites with their e-mail address and other basic personal information but are much less comfortable about disclosing their health information and consumer habits. And few Web users want Web sites to share personal information with other sites and advertisers.

	User willing to provide this information to site they are using	User willing to let Web site share this information with other sites
e-mail address	90%	18%
Gender	87	27
Name	82	15
Favorite color	72	22
Ethnicity	61	18
Address	55	8
Promotions you respond to	50	31
Ads you click on	28	48
Products you buy on the site	26	55
Employer	21	2
Health information	18	3
Credit card information	11	0

Source: California HealthCare Foundation and Internet Healthcare Coalition, "Ethics Survey of Consumer Attitudes About Health Web Sites," September 2000

their children are predisposed to specific gene-based diseases.

"Today, at least there is a signed paper trail," says Gregory E. Hedges, technology risk consultant for accounting giant Arthur Andersen. "On the Internet, there is no inherent accountability. Implementing electronic evidence of secure communications is hugely complex and necessary."

The privacy concerns are at the center of a broader public-policy debate over regulating the Internet. Many politicians, consumer groups and regulators are calling for new federal security standards and guidelines for proper conduct in cyberspace, convinced that the

Internet is becoming an increasingly intrusive element in people's daily lives. A 2000 Gallup survey commissioned by the Washington, D.C.-based Institute for Health Freedom found 92 percent of 1,000 adults polled object to allowing government agencies or other parties to review their medical records without their permission. The concerns were felt in the 106th Congress, where lawmakers took up nine medical privacy bills, though they failed to enact any sweeping legislation. [3]

The Department of Health and Human Services (HHS) this fall is expected to release guidelines that will allow government agencies, law enforcement officials and government

researchers expanded access to medical databases. The guidelines came as the result of the Health Insurance Portability and Accountability Act of 1996, which, among other things, mandated Congress to develop national medical-privacy standards by August 1999. When Congress missed the deadline, the task fell to HHS, which says its standards will address consumer rights to see medical records, outline penalties for violating patients' privacy and require repositories to take adequate security measures.

However, privacy groups, such as the Andover, Mass.-based National Coalition for Patient Rights, say the draft rules will not give patients any meaningful control over their medical histories. Moreover, they could allow doctors, insurers and other parties to share patient information without prior consent if it is for treatment, payment or other functions deemed "health-care operations."

Internet firms and medical-information providers argue the best remedy is self-regulation, saying excessive federal meddling will create a legal morass and confusing disclosure standards. Instead, they point to models such as a July 2000 agreement between DoubleClick Inc. and other on-line advertisers to give computer users more notification when they are being monitored and expanded options to disable cookies. Companies such as Pharmatrak do not have to abide by the agreement because they are not advertisers.

"We think the private sector has done a good job of responding to privacy concerns during the seminal growth of electronic commerce," Scott Cooper, manager of technology policy for computer maker Hewlett-Packard Co., told a recent Senate Commerce Committee hearing on Internet privacy. "Self-regulation and credible third-party enforcement, such as the Better Business Bureau privacy seal program, is the single most important step businesses can take to ensure that consumers' privacy will be respected and protected on-line."

The sheer scope of the issue tends to discourage tough government regulation of on-line medical information. It would be difficult for a federal agency such as the Federal Trade Commission (FTC) to monitor the vast number of Web sites already in existence for violations of fair business standards. Moreover, politicians and regulators fear impeding the explosive growth of electronic commerce, which is being increasingly driven by health-care services.

The New York City market re-search firm Jupiter Communications predicts annual health-care spending on the Internet will reach $10 billion in 2004, compared with $200 million in 1999, as more people get comfortable shopping on-line and Internet vendors adopt more sophisticated marketing strategies.

As policy-makers and health-care professionals ponder the increasing influence of computers on health care, here are some questions they are asking:

Is computerized health information compromising patient privacy?

In Orlando, Fla., a woman went to her doctor for a series of routine tests and three weeks later received a mailing from a drug company promoting a treatment for her high cholesterol. In Boston, a temporary employee of the Dana-Farber Cancer Institute stole patients' personal information and allegedly used one person's name and data to obtain $2,500 in phone services. In Jacksonville, Fla., the 13-year-old daughter of a hospital employee accessed the home phone numbers of former emergency room patients. She then called the patients and, as a prank, told them that they were diagnosed with HIV/AIDS. [4]

These medical-privacy stories, all culled from news reports over the past five years, are frequently cited by interest groups and individuals concerned about the collecting of large amounts of patient data on computers. While anecdotal, they raise concerns about whether sufficient protections are in place to accommodate medicine's rapid push into cyberspace and whether patient privacy is being compromised.

"Without trust that the personal, sensitive information they share with their doctors will be handled with some degree of confidentiality, people will not fully participate in their own health care," Janlori Goldman, director of the Health Privacy Project at Georgetown University's Institute for Health Care Research and Policy, testified before the Senate Health, Education, Labor and Pensions Committee in April. Goldman cited cases in which patients lie to their doctors, provide inaccurate information or engage in "doctor-hopping" to avoid building a consolidated medical record in one place.

To be sure, experts like Goldman say the computerization of medical information has brought many benefits. Storing large numbers of records in electronic form allows physicians and researchers to analyze and transmit data more efficiently, sort public-health information for demographic or population trends and engage in "outcomes research" — the study of different treatments of particular diseases or conditions to determine what works best. Such innovations are helping cash-strapped health-care providers, such as rural medical centers, which have been hurt by cuts in Medicare payments and, in many cases, cannot afford to keep specialists on staff.

Computer records also can be protected from eavesdropping easier than paper records by using passwords to limit access and stripping personal identifiers before sharing them with third parties. A 1997 National Research Council study for the National Library of Medicine found that adequate technology to protect patients' data is readily available and not particularly expensive. Indeed, evidence suggests the use of anti-hacker firewalls, multiple ID entry systems and other safeguards is widespread, even through there are few incentives to install them. [5]

But experts say variations in state privacy laws and the lack of a national set of rules for medical privacy still create the potential for compromising a patient's privacy. In particular, they worry about the use of medical records for marketing purposes and unauthorized access by third parties.

Part of the problem is that privacy laws are mostly directed at the individuals who keep the information, but do not necessarily deter the release of such information. Hence, a doctor may not be able to identify a person with a bladder-control problem on the basis of doctor-patient confidentiality, but if the information falls into the hands of an unregulated third party, there is no prohibition against sharing the information.

Lists of filled prescription drugs are a special area of concern, particularly because they often are not even considered part of one's medical record. The chain drug stores CVS and Giant Food in 1998 admitted to making patient prescription records available for use by a direct-mail firm and a drug company. The two companies said they wanted to track customers who do not refill prescriptions and to send them letters encouraging them to do so. Both backed off after a public outcry.

In another instance, Utah-based RxAmerica, a so-called pharmacy-benefits manager (a company that runs prescription-drug benefit programs for health insurers), used patient data to solicit business for its parent company, American Drug Stores. Only a few states, such as Wisconsin and Rhode Island, have tougher prohibitions dealing not just

with the information "keeper" but with the act of disclosure.[6]

Health-care providers and public-policy experts all agree new safeguards need to be drafted but predictably disagree over the details. Health insurers, hospitals and medical-research groups such as the Biotechnology Industry Organization generally prefer Congress to develop privacy legislation that would both protect patients and consumers and enable the groups to obtain on-line health information when necessary. Insurers, for example, say they need ready access to records so they can

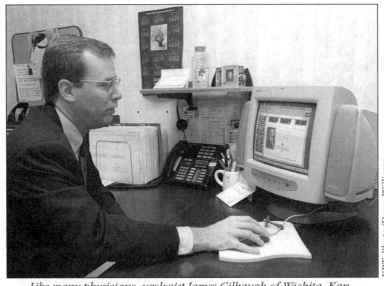

Like many physicians, urologist James Gilbaugh of Wichita, Kan., downloads medical information from the Internet. To ensure patients' privacy, however, he does not communicate with them about their health over the Internet or with e-mail.

KRT Photo/Dave Williams

determine eligibility for benefits, adjust premiums for risk and detect and prevent fraud.

"It is vital that information-sharing continue among health plans and insurers, health-care providers and health-care clearinghouses [which process and transmit claims] for purposes of treatment, payment and health-care operations," says Charles N. Kahn III, president of the Health Insurance Association of America

(HIAA). "Overly restrictive barriers to such exchanges are potentially harmful to patients."

However, Congress was unable to meet the 1999 deadline for developing national, medical-privacy standards and continues to be split over issues such as the right to sue companies that violate privacy rights and privacy for teens getting abortions. The HHS regulations due this fall attempt to strike a middle ground — and help harmonize the varying state regulations by establishing basic minimum standards. But they have both health-care providers and privacy groups anxious.

HIAA's Kahn says draft rules the department released last year on "protected health information" are overly restrictive and would require expensive record keeping and inspections. The American Hospital Association has warned the rules could drive up overall health care costs.[7]

On the other side, some privacy groups worry the HHS rules will be too permissive because the draft regulations only covered health-care providers, health plans and clearinghouses. The Health Privacy Project's Goldman is concerned the rules will not allow patients to control how health information is used for treatment, payment and other health-care operations. She and other like-minded advocates also believe Congress should get involved, largely to fill the gaps the proposed rules will leave.

"We hope that Congress will view the proposed regulations as minimal protections and pass legislation that

Should Physicians' Disciplinary Reports Be Public?

While most of the controversy over medical records and computers centers on patient privacy, a separate debate is raging over whether the public should be able to access information about doctors who have been disciplined for misconduct by states or hospitals.

At issue is the National Practitioner Data Bank, a 10-year-old computer database maintained by the federal government (www.npdb-hipdb.org) that was created by a federal law requiring regulators, insurers and hospitals to report malpractice, fraud, sexual misconduct and other abuses. The complete database can only be accessed by the reporting entities. The public can view a stripped-down version with the names removed.

Consumer groups, some lawmakers and the Clinton administration have tried to open the database to the public, arguing that consumers should be able to identify a physicians who may have been disciplined in one state or lost their hospital privileges, then moved elsewhere to continue practicing. However, groups such as the American Medical Association (AMA) — the influential trade and lobbying group for doctors — have fought such efforts, contending information in the database is misleading, incomplete and will only scare off consumers.

The issue has received increased attention since a 1999 Institute of Medicine (IOM) report that stated medical errors cause the deaths of up to 98,000 patients every year. The House Commerce Committee in September devoted a hearing to the database access issue, during which a California man testified that viewing such information would have saved his wife, who died during cosmetic surgery in 1997. The doctor, William Earle Matory Jr., had been sued for malpractice four times.

"Doctors routinely require consumers to give patient histories before treatment," said House Commerce Committee Chairman Thomas Bliley, R-Va. "I think that patients should have the right to obtain physical histories before placing their very lives in the hands of a doctor." [1]

Bliley vowed to pass legislation opening the data bank before the end of the 106th Congress. But his efforts did not generate much enthusiasm. Democrats charged Bliley was using the issue to retaliate against the AMA for supporting a so-called patients' bill of rights that would allow consumers to sue managed-care companies over treatment decisions.

AMA officials say the database was never supposed to be open to the public and that its contents can be misleading. For instance, many hospitals choose to settle malpractice cases simply to avoid lengthy and costly litigation — not necessarily because there is overwhelming evidence that a doctor did anything wrong.

"The full-time faculty at Harvard Medical School and Johns Hopkins have more cases than anyone else you could find," AMA President-Elect Richard Corlin, a California gastroenterologist, told *The Philadelphia Inquirer* in October. "They're all very good doctors."

Corlin related a case of his own that he said was on the database, in which an instrument broke inside a patient and the patient had to undergo surgery. He noted the incident had nothing to do with his competence, but with the poor quality of the Japanese-made instrument. However, the incident is listed in the data bank next to his name. [2]

However, media analyses of the publicly available portion of the database have turned up numerous cases of repeat offenders, raising questions about whether the consumers would be better served by full disclosure. One review by The Associated Press found that nearly 500 doctors and dentists each have been the subject of at least 10 disciplinary actions or malpractice suits over the past 10 years.

A number of Internet sites provide more limited information about doctors and disciplinary actions. State agencies such as the Florida Department of Insurance (www.doi.state.fl.us) and the New York State Health Department (www.health.state.ny.us) keep information about doctors and other health-care providers, sometimes including malpractice settlement records. The Association of State Medical Board Executive Directors (www.docboard.org) maintains a site with links to those states that keep publicly available information about doctors. Meanwhile, Health Care Choices (www.healthcarechoices.org), a consumer group, tracks the number and types of surgeries performed by doctors in several states.

---

[1] See David Pace, "Congress Urged to Open MD Database," *The (Newark) Star-Ledger*, Sept. 21, 2000, p. 49.

[2] See Shankar Vedantam, "Pennsylvanians Demand Easier Access to Doctor Reprimand Records," *The Philadelphia Inquirer*, Oct. 15, 2000.

---

establishes the patient's right to privacy, restores and protects informed consent and does not pre-empt states from passing stronger privacy protection in the future," says Peter Kane, executive director of the National Coalition for Patient Rights.

Is it safe to purchase drugs on-line?

To unsuspecting consumers, the Web sites Worldwidemedicine.com and Focusmedical.com looked like bona fide on-line clinics for the treatment of sexual dysfunction. The sites boasted they had a full-service clinic, full-time staff and worked with a worldwide network of physicians. In the event that drugs were needed for treatment, the sites claimed prescriptions were filled on premises.

In reality, the sites were examples

The Most-Trusted Sites for Privacy

Among health-related Web sites, research institutes and medical associations were trusted the most by consumers — and drugstores the least — to keep their personal health information private, according to a recent survey. But no site was trusted by a majority of the respondents.

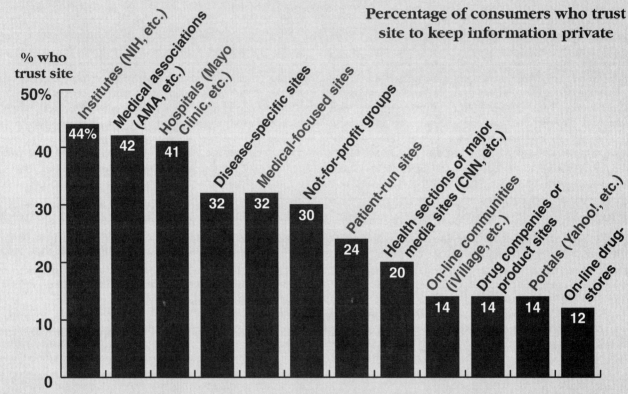

Percentage of consumers who trust site to keep information private

% who trust site

Institutes (NIH, etc.) — 44%
Medical associations (AMA, etc.) — 42
Hospitals (Mayo Clinic, etc.) — 41
Disease-specific sites — 32
Medical-focused sites — 32
Not-for-profit groups — 30
Patient-run sites — 24
Health sections of major media sites (CNN, etc.) — 20
On-line communities (iVillage, etc.) — 14
Drug companies or product sites — 14
Portals (Yahoo!, etc.) — 14
On-line drug-stores — 12

Source: California HealthCare Foundation and Internet Healthcare Coalition, "Ethics Survey of Consumer Attitudes About Health Web Sites," September 2000

of Internet pharmacies that made false claims about their facilities and charged consumers unfairly, according to an FTC settlement with the operators of the Web sites filed in July. Actually, the FTC charged, there was no clinic, and the network of physicians consisted of one doctor in a distant state who reviewed requests for Viagra and was paid $10 for each request that he approved.

Meanwhile, customers of the Web sites were charged $75 for a "medical consultation" that required them to answer questions about their medical histories. Approximately 11,000 customers who used the sites later re-ceived an unsolicited e-mail saying their credit cards would be charged $50 for "Y2K remediation" — an illegal charge without prior authorization. The settlements, which do not constitute an admission of guilt, bar the companies and individuals from continuing their current practices.

Similar incidents have raised questions about the safety of buying prescription drugs on the Internet. With at least 400 businesses now dispensing drugs on-line, Internet pharmacies are one of the most robust sectors of electronic commerce, with sales expected to reach $1.4 billion by 2001 and more than $15 billion by 2004. Large drug-store chains including CVS and Walgreen's have recently established a presence on the World Wide Web, joining established e-pharmacies such as Planetrx.com and drugstore.com. Many people, especially the elderly and busy professionals, use these legitimate vendors because they can be more convenient, less expensive and offer more privacy. Industry executives say the computerized format, when used properly, can deliver dividends that are unavailable in traditional "bricks-and-mortar" drugstores. [8]

"Filling prescriptions over the Internet will save time, help reduce errors caused by illegible handwriting and confusion about drugs that sound alike and automatically screen for potential drug interactions," says Planetrx Chairman and Chief Executive Officer William J. Razzouk.

But experts note there is tremendous variation in the way the drugstores operate. Customers cannot be certain about the quality or purity of the drugs they buy — or even whether they are legal. They also do not know how the site collects and uses personal information about its customers. And some of the more questionable sites don't advise patients about potential health risks from adverse drug reactions, including the potential dangers Viagra presents to heart patients taking other medications. Many in this latter category allow consumers to purchase drugs without any pretense of a prescription. [9]

The risks of on-line purchases have been seen in several high-profile cases in the past year. The drug 1,4, butanediol — an industrial solvent alternately marketed on the Internet as a sleep aid, aphrodisiac and muscle-builder — was implicated in the death of a 21-year-old Tampa, Fla., man in May. The substance affects the central nervous system and can slow the heart rate and breathing. A chemical cousin, gamma hydroxy buteric acid, that was banned by the FDA in 1990 and also is sold on-line has been linked to more than a dozen other deaths in the 1990s.

Questions also have been raised about dietary supplements marketed on the Internet containing the stimulant ephedra, which causes chest pains and palpitations and may have caused the death of a 26-year-old Clearwater, Fla. woman this year. The FDA proposed regulating ephedra-containing supplements in 1997 but backed off after the U.S. General Accounting Office questioned the agency's scientific rationale. [10]

On-line drug sales also are increasingly seen as a conduit to import illegal substances into the United States. The U.S. Customs Service seized 9,725 packages with prescription drugs last year, compared with 2,145 packages in 1998. The number of pills, tablets and other medications impounded rose to 1.9 million from 760,728 in 1998. Most of the drugs seized had not been approved for use in the United States, did not comply with labeling requirements or were substandard — meaning they fell below Food and Drug Administration (FDA) standards for quality and purity. [11]

Texas Attorney General John Cornyn announces in August he has charged two on-line pharmacies with threatening consumers' health by selling dangerous drugs on the basis of an on-line consultation.

AP Photo/Jack Plunkett

Federal and state governments as well as private industry are taking steps to establish some standards. The Park Ridge, Ill.-based National Association of Boards of Pharmacy in 1999 established a self-policing program that confers a seal of approval on those Internet pharmacies that comply with licensing and inspection rules of their state and the states to which they dispense drugs. The participating pharmacies also have to meet industry privacy standards, have quality-assurance policies and be able to demonstrate security

On the federal level, the FDA has been increasingly active in the area of on-line drug sales. Since mid-1999, the agency has included consumer tips on the safe purchase of drugs on its Web site, www.fda.gov. The agency's role increased in December 1999, when President Clinton announced a new $10 million effort to protect patients who buy drugs on-line. The move would give the FDA enforcement power to prosecute Web sites selling unapproved or counterfeit drugs and create new civil penalties for wrongdoing. The FTC continues to police unscrupulous business practices but tends to refrain from challenging those things that fall within the traditional doctor-patient relationship, such as communications about treatment decisions.

State governments also are flexing their muscles. Kansas, Missouri, Illinois and Michigan, among others, have filed permanent injunctions to prevent some Internet pharmacies from filling prescriptions for citizens

A Sampling of Reliable Medical Web Sites

The staggering number of medical sites on the Internet may at first fluster individuals seeking health-care advice. Web surfers should consider the identity of the site's sponsor and the target audience when considering the reliability and suitability of the information. Generally, sites maintained by governmental institutions, well-established research centers and some health-care provider groups tend to be the most reliable and unbiased. Consumer groups warn users to be skeptical about sites that require the completion of detailed medical-history questionnaires or other personal identifiers, or that offer to sell drugs or medical products without prescriptions or referrals.

Following is a sampling of some sites generally considered reliable, informative and objective that offer different types of medical information aimed at specific audiences:

■ **Medscape (www.medscape.com)** — An all-purpose medical Web site aimed at professionals in health-care, social policy and the media as well as sophisticated consumers. Some material is understandable to consumers without a background in medicine. Its "specialty spotlight" section contains articles on topics such as arrhythmia management and epidemiological studies on such subjects as the connection between pulmonary function and mortality in the population. A "money and management" section recently contained an analysis by social policy expert Lynn Etheredge on reorganizing the oversight of

Medicare, the federal health-care program for the elderly and also features updates from Reuters Medical News.

A search for citations on asthma turned up 268 hits, including journal articles on risk factors for fatal asthma and lifestyle factors that may play a role in pediatric asthma. "Resource centers" for various common conditions contain recent headlines, journal articles, links to professional societies, government sites and consumer information.

■ **National Institutes of Health (www.nih.gov)** — The nation's premiere biomedical research institution maintains a comprehensive home page that links to its 25 constituent institutes and centers. The site provides information about myriad health conditions and diseases as well as information about certain clinical trials. But the site stresses it should not be used for personalized advice, instead urging visitors to cull the data and use it in conjunction with a professional.

The various NIH sites do offer a variety of easily digestible information. The National Heart, Lung and Blood Institute, for example, offers useful primers on lowering blood pressure, controlling cholesterol and information on sleep disorders research and asthma.

■ **CliniWeb International (www.ohsu.edu/cliniweb)** — A Web site maintained by the Oregon Health Sciences University that contains identification and indexing of nearly 10,000 clinically oriented Web pages. The site is designed for health-care professionals and students, with an emphasis on biomedical research. Browsing the biological-sciences

in their states unless they conduct business according to state laws and fill only prescriptions sent by doctors who are licensed in their states.

However, the large number of on-line pharmacies and the borderless nature of the Internet are presenting vexing jurisdictional questions. For instance, it is not clear what authorities in the United States can do about foreign Web sites that sell drugs to U.S. consumers, especially if the drugs in question are legal in the originating country. In Congress, lawmakers appear torn between endorsing tougher enforcement initiatives and being perceived as wanting to add a new layer of regulation to the world of electronic commerce.

"We need to encourage strong enforcement action by the states and

the federal government," House Commerce Committee Chairman Thomas Bliley Jr., said in July. "At the same time, it is important that we do not overreact by piling layers of new regulations onto an emerging marketplace — one that provides great benefits to consumers." Bliley, whose committee would have to approve an expansion of FDA authority, is leery of giving the agency more latitude, believing the responsibility should rest with states.

Because Internet pharmacies are not confined to one state or country, experts say it is likely that states and the federal government will have to coordinate future efforts. "The real challenge lies in dealing with the logistical difficulties of identifying responsible parties and enforcing

laws across state boundaries," says Jodie Bernstein, director of the Federal Trade Commission's Bureau of Consumer Protection.

Is electronic health information reliable?

As with Internet pharmacies, the quality and nature of medical Web sites vary widely. At one end of the spectrum are subscription sites targeted at doctors that are maintained by leading research institutions such as Stanford University. These sites attempt to blend on-line patient records with articles from medical journals, reference materials from textbooks and patient-treatment guidelines. The Stanford site, e-Skolar.com, costs $240 per year and has been hailed for providing a kind

section, one may find 6,208 links to sites that deal with biochemistry and genetics. CliniWeb's features include a link to the National Library of Medicine's PubMed system for accessing scientific journal articles, and a search engine that allows terms to be entered in English, French, German, Spanish and Portuguese.

■ **National Association of Health Data Organizations (www.nahdo.org)** — A not-for-profit organization in Salt Lake City that maintains a site that links to corporate and government Web sites with information about doctors, health plans and hospitals. This resource could prove valuable to consumers who have just moved to a state and need health services, as well as caregivers for family members with debilitating conditions, such as Alzheimer's disease or heart disease. The comparatively low-tech site has a series of general tips for searching medical Web sites that, among other things, urges consumers to question a Web site author's credentials and how his or her affiliation might affect objectivity.

■ **Mayo Clinic (www.mayohealth.org)** — The prestigious facility in Rochester, Minn., operates a consumer Web site that gives visitors a chance to ask staff physicians about various conditions and health concerns. Inquiries on ear, nose and throat conditions, for example, recently took up such issues as cochlear implants and improvements in the design and sound quality of hearing aids.

■ **HCIA-Sachs (www.hcia.com)** — A private firm in Baltimore that studies Medicare beneficiary data and other indicators to compile a Top 100 Hospitals list. The company's criteria include patients' average length of stay, average cost of care and the incidence of postoperative infections and mortality. Lists are broken down by medical specialty.

■ **AMA Health Insight (www.ama-assn.org/consumer.htm)** — This site maintained by the American Medical Association (AMA), the influential physicians trade association, has a stated goal of improving the science and medical literacy of the public. The site has easy-to-digest information about a wide variety of specific conditions and outlines symptoms, treatments and prevention tips with links to journal articles, including those in *JAMA*, the AMA's monthly journal. The site notes that medical reviewers go over all of the content for accuracy and balance before it is posted. The site also boasts a "Doctor Finder" that allows consumers to search for AMA members by name or medical specialty.

■ **www.questionabledoctors.org** — A site maintained by the Ralph Nader-affiliated consumer group Public Citizen that since 1985 has gathered names of physicians and other health-care providers who have been disciplined by state medical boards. The site sells books listing doctors with disciplinary records, noting that disclosure varies state-by-state. The site bills itself as an important alternative to the National Practitioner Data Bank, which contains extensive information on malpractice by doctors but does not provide details of cases to consumers.

of one-stop shopping source for professionals who lack the time to pore through numerous journals to find answers. Using such a site, a physician recently presented with the case of a 9-year-old girl with severe acne identified the likely condition. It turned out to be the hormone imbalance congenital adrenal hyperplasia. The doctor printed out dozens of pages of information and treatment suggestions for treating the condition along with the latest research. [12]

Many medical Web sites tailored more to consumers also provide copious amounts of reliable information. Sites like Medscape, which is supported by advertising, are free and enable patients to read up on common ailments and treatments before they visit a doctor. Another popular site, WebMD.com, offers a consumer section that recently offered an article on the pros and cons of using hormones to reverse the effects of aging, as well as another feature warning about unorthodox treatments touted as cancer cures.

WebMD also has a physicians' section that features an on-line library with more than 40 specialized medical journals, as well as features such as a template for creating customized Web sites for group practices. Additionally, Web sites maintained by prestigious research institutions such as the Mayo Clinic in Rochester, Minn., and Johns Hopkins University in Baltimore give consumers instant access to recent research and advice from staff physicians.

But some Web sites rely heavily on advertising by drug companies, medical-testing firms and other parties, raising questions about whether all of the information presented is unbiased, or whether there are hidden agendas. Experts also warn that on-line information about some medical conditions that merit legitimate concern may resort to fear-mongering or present the condition out of proportion to its significance. [13]

One such condition that is frequently debated is osteoporosis. In recent years, drug and testing companies have spent billions of dollars advertising hormone treatments and bone-mass density screening to women approaching menopause. Others have touted calcium-enriched substances with claims that they reduce the risk of fractures. However, the medical establishment is divided on the efficacy of such measures. The National Institutes of Health (NIH) and the U.S. Preventive Health Services Task Force have declined to endorse bone-mass density screening, noting variations in testing, questioning the accuracy of results and pointing to a lack of evidence the tests are justified in patients without significant risk factors. Moreover, hormone-replacement treatment with estrogen has come under question because estrogen can increase a woman's chances of developing endometrial cancer.

Some experts believe consumers would be better served if Web sites focused on more commonplace preventive measures, such as a balanced diet, exercise, not smoking and not drinking to excess. "Most of what you can do to a patient in later life has nothing to do with taking a drug or test," Mark Helfand, director of the Evidence-Based Practice Center at the Oregon Health Sciences University in Portland, told *The Washington Post*. [14]

Apparent ethical lapses or conflicts of interest have tarnished the reputations of otherwise informative medical Web sites. Former Surgeon General C. Everett Koop, who lends his name to the popular site drkoop.com, in March 1999 failed to reveal a potential conflict of interest when he testified before Congress and criticized claims that gloves containing powdered latex could cause serious and potentially fatal allergic reactions. Koop didn't reveal that he had received substantial payments under a $1 million consulting contract he had with WRP Corp., a manufacturer of latex gloves.

While the federal government polices fraudulent or deceptive Internet marketing, it does not have a fail-safe mechanism for conflicts of interest. The FTC has pushed for more disclosure statements on Web sites' primary

screens and notes that the same consumer-protection laws that apply to commercial activities in other media apply on-line. However, experts say surfing the Internet for health information remains a bit of a crapshoot, with the most reliable sites tending to be those maintained by government agencies, established research institutions and medical centers.

"Some [information] is very good, but it is written in very complex and intricate ways," says Paul Kleeberg, medical adviser to the Web site for Allina Health Systems, a chain of medical centers and clinics in Minnesota and Wisconsin. "Some of it is written by people who are trying to sell something. Some of it is junk. But if a person knows where to go, there is some great information out there." [15]

BACKGROUND

Rise of Computers

Storing and analyzing scientific and medical data actually predates the Internet. In 1969, UCLA, Stanford University, the University of California at Santa Barbara and the University of Utah were linked electronically via ARPANET, a precursor of the Internet commissioned by the Pentagon's Advanced Research Projects Agency. The system allowed researchers to exchange data and communicate via an early form of e-mail. This nascent type of networking was accomplished through a then-new technology called "packet switching," which allowed all of the participating computers to have the same information-routing capabilities, avoiding the need to send all of

the information through one central system. By 1972, 23 research institutions were linked on the system.

Advances in data processing allowed the adapting of computers to more powerful and sophisticated health-related applications. The health-insurance industry in the 1980s and early '90s began using computers to ferret out questionable items in the electronic processing of medical bills. The practice saved more than $250 million per year, according to industry estimates, and put a brake on overall health-care costs during a time of double-digit medical inflation.

Cost-conscious managed-care companies also used computer analysis of patient care to devise performance benchmarks — an innovation both hailed for saving money and harshly denounced for promoting a one-size-fits-all approach to medicine. One aspect that was especially criticized was health plans' unwisely focusing on shortening patients' hospital stays, leading to highly publicized incidents such as mothers being kicked out just one day after delivering their babies. [16]

While computers were rapidly accepted in commercial health situations, clinicians were slower to embrace the technology. Experts tend to attribute this to several factors — the lack of necessary investment on the part of medical schools, a perceived reluctance by practicing physicians to abandon paper records, even excessive control of medical information services by hospital and health-plan bureaucrats, instead of doctors. Another explanation is that doctors think they do not have the time to search computer records while they are diagnosing patients, making decisions and devising treatment plans. [17]

Some innovative medical centers attempted to encourage their doctors to adapt computers to clinical set-

Chronology

1960s-1980s
Early attempts to link research institutions blend scientific and medical data with computers.

1969
UCLA, Stanford University, the University of California at Santa Barbara and the University of Utah are connected on ARPANET, a precursor to the Internet created by the Pentagon. Researchers exchange scientific and medical data via early forms of e-mail.

1981
Computers at more than 200 research sites are linked via ARPANET.

1986
The National Science Foundation launches NSFNet, a regional network of computer routers linked on the Internet backbone to be used by government and academic researchers.

1988
An "Internet worm" disables 6,000 of 60,000 Internet host computers then in operation, in one of the first large-scale electronic breakins. The incident raises security and privacy concerns.

1989
Superceded by the Internet, ARPANET ceases to exist.

———— • ————

1990s *The digital revolution hits full swing, prompting a surge of medical information on the World Wide Web. Advances in computer imaging and transmission*

technology expand the possibilities for telemedicine.

1991
The National Science Foundation lifts restrictions on commercial use of the Internet, ushering in the era of electronic commerce.

1994
The first Internet shopping malls appear.

1995
Early on-line dial-up services, such as Prodigy, CompuServe and America Online, begin providing large numbers of consumers with Internet access.

1996
About 40 million people are connected to the Internet; more than $1 billion of business is transacted on-line. The Health Insurance Portability and Accountability Act of 1996 mandates that Congress develop medical privacy standards by August 1999.

1997
HHS Secretary Donna E. Shalala outlines five principles for protecting the confidentiality of individually identifiable health information.

1998
Yale University plastic surgeons demonstrate the capability of telemedicine by prediagnosing 99 Brazilian patients with congenital abnormalities such as cleft palates, then fly to the Amazon River region to perform operations.

1999
Congress is unable to meet the deadline for developing medical privacy standards. The Department of Health and Human Services (HHS) proposes draft guidelines. An article in the

Journal of the American Medical Association raises the question of doctor liability in the use of telemedicine.

———— • ————

2000s *The federal government moves forward with the development of medical-privacy standards.*

February 2000
After receiving more than 50,000 comments, HHS prepares to issue final medical privacy guidelines set to take effect in 2002. The guidelines call for fines of up to $50,000 and a year in prison for improperly obtaining or disclosing protected health information and up to a $250,000 fine and 10 years in prison if the information was obtained with the intent to use, sell or transfer it for commercial purposes. The guidelines would allow the disclosure of health information without patient authorization for a wide variety of public health and research activities, as well as for law enforcement and by banks and other financial institutions to process health-care payments and premiums.

August 2000
A Gallup survey commissioned by the Institute for Health Freedom finds that more than 90 percent of 1,000 adults polled object to allowing government agencies or other parties to review their medical records without their permission.

February 2002
The HHS medical-privacy guidelines are scheduled to go into effect.

tings. The Center for Evidence-Based Medicine in Oxford, England, built a bulky "evidence cart" consisting of a computer, projector and shelves for textbooks. Doctors wheeled the contraption around while making their rounds in an inpatient clinic, simultaneously consulting medical records while checking patients' vital signs. The cart also contained equipment allowing several people to listen to the same signs on a physical examination, such as a heartbeat.

Tests performed in 1997 showed 90 percent of 79 computer searches surrounding patient care and treatment decisions yielded information that helped the doctors devise a plan of action. Most of the evidence was available in 15 seconds or less.

Physicians at Duke University in Durham, N.C., used computers on a much-larger scale to assess healthcare delivery and make better treatment decisions. The Duke Clinical Research Institute began using computers in the mid-1980s to coordinate clinical trials of drugs and develop protocols for the treatment of certain conditions. A Duke study of more than 217,000 Medicare beneficiaries, for example, demonstrated how deaths after angioplasty (the unblocking of clogged blood vessels in patients with heart conditions) were higher at hospitals that performed fewer of the procedures. Researchers said the findings pointed to the need for expanding the availability of the procedures to more regional medical centers.

Regulating Telemedicine

Advances in computer imaging and transmission technology, meanwhile, expanded the possibilities for telemedicine -diagnosing and treating patients over long distances through the use of computers, video cameras and an Internet connection. Yale University plastic surgeons demonstrated the capability in 1998 by prediagnosing 99 Brazilian patients with congenital abnormalities such as cleft palates. Armed with the information, the surgeons then flew to the Amazon River region to perform operations under the auspices of Interplast, a pro bono plastic surgery program. The prediagnoses cut treatment times by 20 percent by eliminating the need for extensive on-site screening. Such capabilities are expected to be a boon for rural medical centers in the United States, which have struggled due to lower government reimbursements for programs such as Medicare and — in many cases — cannot afford to keep specialists on staff. [18]

Some believe the entire healthcare industry should adopt standards for medical language and database structures to allow information such as the Duke angioplasty study to be shared by the largest number of clinicians. Those standards would also include appropriate security measures.

"The health-care industry needs information systems that support the core business of health care — patient care," says Lewis Lorton, administrator of The Forum on Privacy and Security in Health Care, a government-industry partnership in Columbia, Md., that promotes industry standards to protect electronic medical information. "Today health-care is everywhere, health-care information is everywhere and the public is no longer just the provider of information but an active participant in the health-care information sphere."

However, many believe that the legal implications of digital medicine must be addressed before a nationwide system can be created. As data storage becomes more widespread, the medical world is confronting questions about the how to protect personally identifiable health data with the patchwork of state privacy laws and the lack of comprehensive federal standards. For instance, doctors in the coming years may be forced to deal with questions about whether transmitting certain patient information via e-mail could be deemed a privacy violation without the patient's prior consent. Another uncharted area is whether doctors somehow have the obligation to use medical information on line — and whether they could be liable for failing to use readily available databases.

Telemedicine poses its own set of murky legal issues. Writing in the *Journal of the American Medical Association*, James G. Hodge Jr. and Lawrence Gostin of Georgetown University Law Center and Peter D. Jacobson of the University of Michigan School of Public Health consider the borderless nature of cyberspace and the jurisdictional problems it could create for telemedicine regulations. The legal scholars ask at what point does the physician-patient relationship arise in a telemedicine encounter, and at what point could a doctor be liable for negligent care?

Another issue is how to legally resolve errors of omission, such as when the treating physician fails to use telemedicine when needed, and errors of commission, such as the failure to use the technology properly. [19]

Most scholars agree the most direct way to confront such difficult questions is for HHS and Congress to establish a "floor" of health-data privacy protections with defined civil penalties for inappropriate disclosure of confidential information. Lawmakers then can assess the evolving marketplace, consider the positive aspects of computers in medicine and supplement and toughen the laws when necessary.

Remote Medical Consultation

Telepathology, the science of remote diagnosis, allows medical experts to consult on information using sophisticated technology from anywhere in the world.

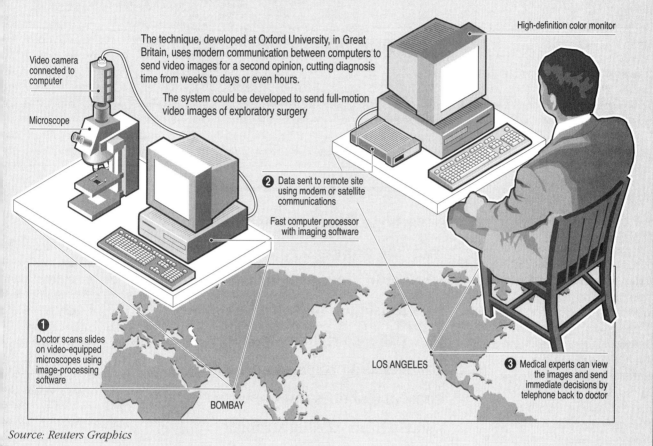

High-definition color monitor

Video camera connected to computer

The technique, developed at Oxford University, in Great Britain, uses modern communication between computers to send video images for a second opinion, cutting diagnosis time from weeks to days or even hours.

The system could be developed to send full-motion video images of exploratory surgery

Microscope

❷ Data sent to remote site using modem or satellite communications

Fast computer processor with imaging software

❶ Doctor scans slides on video-equipped microscopes using image-processing software

LOS ANGELES

❸ Medical experts can view the images and send immediate decisions by telephone back to doctor

BOMBAY

Source: Reuters Graphics

CURRENT SITUATION

Privacy Initiatives

Critics have noted that today's patchwork privacy laws guard the confidentiality of an American consumer's video rentals, but do not necessarily offer the same safeguards for his health records. The 106th Congress spent the better part of 1999 and 2000 considering various proposals to toughen medical privacy standards, but could not arrive at a consensus. As a result, under the provisions of the Health Insurance Portability and Accountability Act, HHS was left with the task of drafting regulations to protect personally identifiable medical information that is stored or transmitted electronically. The regulations are due out this fall, though the release of new rules on the sensitive topic could be delayed until after the presidential election.

The congressional deliberations got hung up over several issues, including whether new federal standards would pre-empt existing state privacy laws, and what kind of prior consent patients need to give to allow third parties to review their records. Most of the proposals guaranteed that patients could see and have the right to amend their medical records, and required record-keepers to tell patients who is viewing the records. The proposals also prescribed penalties for misusing records. [20]

One much-discussed proposal by Sens. Patrick J. Leahy, D-Vt., and Edward M. Kennedy, D-Mass., and backed by privacy groups would place tough restrictions on which parties can see medical records and require patients to give their consent each time a third party — whether a medical researcher or an insurance company — wants to look at their medical records. The measure also would limit how much access law enforcement gets to the records and allow states to pass new and tougher privacy laws.

A rival plan proposed by Sens. James M. Jeffords, R-Vt., and Christopher J. Dodd, D-Conn., and supported by many in the health-care industry would allow patients to give a single, blanket authorization for insurance companies to review their records for treatment decisions, payment histories and audits of the quality of care. The bill would grandfather existing state laws that are tougher than the federal standards and give remaining states 18 months to bring their laws up to the federal minimum.

More narrowly tailored provisions proposed during the 106th Congress included language that would require banks and insurance companies to obtain consumers' prior consent before sharing medical records with third parties. Another provision would have prohibited insurance companies from discriminating against customers based on genetic information, which could yield important clues about predisposition to certain inherited diseases.

However, Republican leaders expressed skepticism that specific medical-privacy legislation was needed and questioned whether Democrats were using the issue to score political points in advance of the presidential election. Heavy lobbying by the insurance industry, banks and health-care groups such as the American Medical Association (AMA) helped fragment the debate, making it more difficult for lawmakers to arrive at a compromise.

New HHS Rules

The HHS medical privacy guidelines, thus, are the only federal rules likely to go into effect — and even those will not be effective until February 2002. The department issued draft guidelines in the fall of 1999 and received more than 50,000 written comments, reflecting the strong interest in the issue. While the final rules have not been issued, draft guidelines call for allowing patients to see copies of their records and request corrections and require health-care providers to explain how the information will be used.

The guidelines call for fines of up to $50,000 and a year in prison for improperly obtaining or disclosing protected health information, up to $100,000 and five years in prison for obtaining protected health information under false pretenses and up to $250,000 and 10 years in prison if the information was obtained with the intent to use, sell or transfer it for commercial purposes.

The guidelines would allow the disclosure of health information without patient authorization for a wide variety of public health and research activities, as well as for law enforcement and by banks and other financial institutions to process health-care payments and premiums. State laws tougher than the federal regulations generally would continue to apply.

Though HHS Secretary Donna E. Shalala calls the draft rules "an important step forward in protecting the privacy of some of our most personal information," parties on both sides of the debate appear unhappy with the rules. The AMA says the department's initiative "unacceptably increases administrative burdens for physicians" by imposing unreasonable patient-consent requirements.

"Informed consent should be obtained, where possible before personally identifiable health information is used for any purpose," the AMA says in a position paper. "However, this is clearly not practical or even possible in some instances. In those situations in which patient consent is not feasible, either a) the information should have identifying information stripped from it o

> 'We hope that Congress will view the proposed regulations as minimal protections and pass legislation that establishes the patient's right to privacy, restores and protects informed consent and does not pre-empt states from passing stronger protection in the future.'
>
> — *Peter Kane,*
> *Executive Director*
> *National Coalition for*
> *Patient Rights*

At Issue:

Is government action necessary to ensure privacy on the Internet?

ANDREW SHEN

POLICY ANALYST, ELECTRONIC PRIVACY INFORMATION CENTER

FROM TESTIMONY BEFORE HOUSE COMMERCE SUBCOMMIT-
TEE ON TELECOMMUNICATIONS, TRADE AND CONSUMER
PROTECTION, OCT. 11, 2000

*i*n the years between our first and last reports, we have documented the lack of protections for consumer privacy in these crucial early years of e-commerce. . . . If anything, recent developments such as on-line profiling indicate that the current approach of self-regulation may be putting consumer privacy at increasing risk. . . .

We support efforts to strengthen the privacy safeguards for federal Web sites. History has proven that such restrictions are necessary to curtail possible governmental abuses of power. Events like Watergate spurred laws such as the Privacy Act of 1974. . . .

Since the beginning of the on-line privacy debate, [the Electronic Privacy Information Center] has urged the wide adoption of privacy-enhancing technologies to protect consumers. However, I would like to point out what makes a technology one that enhances rather than invades privacy. Privacy-enhancing technologies make it easier to take advantage of rights as provided through fair information practices and minimize or eliminate the collection of personal data.

Without legal guarantees that data is collected for limited, specific purposes, is collected only with consent, is accessible to the consumer, is securely stored and transmitted, privacy technologies can currently do little to help consumers utilize their rights. Only when existing law provides those rights will technologies develop to help consumers take advantage of them. . . .

There is, however, one area in which technology can address privacy in the absence of laws. That is in the promotion of anonymity and elimination of the need to collect personal data. Most of the activities conducted on-line, such as reading news, shopping for products, searching for information, can be done without the collection of information from consumers. However, the current trend toward "personalization" results in the increased storage and analysis of these basic on-line activities.

Infomediaries that seek to provide information according to user preferences do not provide this anonymity. [T]hey seek to encourage more information collection by making it easier than ever for personal data to be disclosed.

Congress has a critical role to play in safeguarding on-line privacy. It should build on the legal framework for privacy protection, consistent through many federal laws protecting personal information. . . . Consumers should not be left without legal rights in the on-line world.

GLEE HARRAH CADY

VICE PRESIDENT FOR GLOBAL PUBLIC POLICY, PRIVADA

FROM TESTIMONY BEFORE HOUSE COMMERCE SUBCOMMIT-
TEE ON TELECOMMUNICATIONS, TRADE AND CONSUMER
PROTECTION, OCT. 11, 2000

*t*oday's privacy debate has been fueled by two very opposing views — one side advocates exploitation of personal information for any and all purposes, and the other wishes to prohibit the use of personal information for any and all purposes. As the debate acknowledges, we fear intrusion into our private lives by both government and business. We all want the benefits of personal services but fear the possibly unpleasant surprise of someone we don't know knowing too much about us.

This is why digital privacy is so important to us. With Internet access we have grand opportunities to gain knowledge, improve communication and have products and services delivered to us wherever we are, whenever we want them. But we know we are being watched, and we don't like it.

Privacy is an intensely individual matter. The choices I make about my personal information will not necessarily match yours. For example, I don't mind if you know that I am a proud parent — if you give me a chance I will certainly boast about my wonderful children. But in fear of predators, some people don't want others to know they have children.

I don't mind if you know what kind of car I drive — certain of my friends say that I sound like a car commercial. Others don't want that information to be available unless you are the car manufacturer and there is a product recall. I don't want you to have access to my financial information unless I give you that permission so you can help me with a financial transaction. I don't want intimate details of my medical records in the public domain. Unless I know you well, I am unlikely to share a list of the e-mail addresses of my fellow Privada employees. . . .

Because we don't yet have consensus about privacy among individuals, businesses, and government, and because the technology is changing almost daily, governmental solutions necessarily lag behind. Laws take an even longer time than computer programs to define, construct, test and implement. Here is where technologies play a significant role. While committees like this one strive to determine the best way to provide legal protection, technology can provide tools for individuals to use to protect themselves. With each of us in control of our individual information, the rewards of the digital economy can reach more people. This is a win for individuals; for business, with more consumer confidence; and for government, with one less area to track. Privacy-enhancing technologies can benefit everyone.

b) an objective, publicly accountable entity must conclude that patient consent is not required after weighing the risks and benefits of the proposed use."

Privacy groups, meanwhile, believe the new rules are too permissive and are urging Congress to try again when it reconvenes in January. "We hope that Congress will view the proposed regulations as minimal protections and pass legislation that establishes the patient's right to privacy, restores and protects informed consent and does not pre-empt states from passing stronger privacy protection in the future," says Peter Kane, executive director of the National Coalition for Patient Rights. ■

OUTLOOK

Cutting-Edge Tools

E ven as policy-makers debate how to regulate and reconcile computer technology and medicine, the information-technology industry is forging ahead with innovations that promise to change the way the most basic health services are delivered. Many experts believe that by 2010, health-care providers will be using powerful hand-held computers, Internet links and databases in the most routine tasks — and that patients will use on-line information to come to their appointments armed with information and increasingly technical questions. For example, a doctor may use a device similar to a Palm Pilot to track patient information and lab test results and, perhaps, link to a hospital's computerized medical records.

Writing in the medical journal *Hippocrates*, computer engineer Ray

Kurzweil, author of *The Age of Spiritual Machines: When Computers Exceed Human Intelligence*, outlines some even more sophisticated developments. Computerized virtual-reality systems gradually are being used to train surgeons' sense of touch for certain procedures. The virtual environment is allowing physicians to interact both with simulated patients and real people in physically remote locations. In the case of simulated patients, doctors can examine the patient, diagnose the treatment, then "fast forward" to the patient's next visit — or years later — to determine whether their approach worked. The system also can teach nurses basic procedures, such as how to properly insert a needle into a vein, without having to rely on old plastic arm models. [21]

Another innovation is microchip-based gene analysis, a system perfected at the Palo Alto, Calif., technology firm Affymetrix. The "gene chip" is similar to the silicon wafers found in electronics but contains molecules of DNA instead of transistors. By inserting molecules of DNA programmed for the gene sequence of whatever the researchers want to target, researchers can measure gene expression and pinpoint mutations that may trigger dispositions to cancer or other conditions. The technology works because the DNA on the chip chemically recognizes a real gene and can highlight the mutations it carries while offering clues about how it is working. The DNA sequence on the chip is downloaded from a computer data bank, after which the chip is designed to study all of the target genes. [22]

Yet another cutting-edge discipline, biomedical nanotechnology, uses microcircuitry to create "smart" implants that dispense drugs, such as insulin for diabetics. Researchers at Ohio State University this year reported they created tiny capsules with sensors that can

be implanted under a patient's skin. The sensors can detect concentrations of certain chemicals in a patient's bloodstream and trigger the release of appropriate medicines. Microsensors equipped with radioactive substances or chemotherapy agents also may be used to home in on and kill cancerous tumors in hard-to-reach parts of the body, where surgery is inappropriate.

Government may play an active role in developing more devices and technologies. The Clinton administration's fiscal 2001 budget request called for $2.9 billion in new spending for a variety of civilian research and development initiatives, many of which have biomedical science applications. The administration regards basic, university-based research as essential for developing supercomputers, microsensors and other technologies with the potential for commercial spinoffs.

However, that may represent a departure from recent congressional funding priorities. Lawmakers in the House and Senate have preferred to bestow large funding increases on biomedical research institutions, such as the NIH, believing that its activities identifying gene-based treatments for a variety of afflictions should receive the lion's share of new spending. While the 106th Congress pressed ahead with plans to double NIH's budget over five years, it also appeared to heed calls to increase the budgets of such agencies as the National Science Foundation, the government's prime supporter of basic scientific research.

"From the basic research come the magnetic resonance imaging (MRI), the advances in being able to devise drug treatments tailored to an individual . . . and being able to have prescriptions in the future that are not just a general prescription but prescription for you as an individual based on your metabolism, your specific genetic traits," National Sci ence Foundation Director Rita Colwell said in February, as the White House outlined its spending plan. "It's the basic research in physics, in math, in chemistry and in biology that leads to the medical advances." ∎

Notes

[1] See Robert O'Harrow, "Firm Tracking Consumers on Web for Drug Companies," *The Washington Post*, Aug. 15, 2000, p. E1.

[2] For background, see *The CQ Researcher*,

[3] See John Hanchette, "Poll Finds Public Concerned With Assaults on Private Medical Records," Gannett News Service, Aug. 27, 2000.

[4] For background, see Laura Bell and Charles Ornstein, "Patients' Data Not So Private: New Rules to Limit Disclosure," *The Dallas Morning News*, Sept. 17, 2000, p. 1A

[5] See "Best Principles for Health Privacy," Health Privacy Project, Georgetown University Institute for Health Care Research and Policy, 1999.

[6] "The State of Health Privacy: An Uneven Terrain," Health Privacy Project, Georgetown University Institute for Health Care Research and Policy, 1999.

[7] See Jim Abrams, "Congress Urged to Try Again on Medical Privacy," The Associated Press, April 27, 2000.

[8] For background, see Amy J. Oliver, "Internet Pharmacies: Regulation of a Growing Industry," *Journal of Law, Medicine and Ethics*, Vol. 28, No. 1 (2000), pp. 98-101.

[9] See Adriel Bettelheim, "Drugmakers Under Siege," *The CQ Researcher*, Sept. 3, 1999, pp. 753-776.

[10] See Alicia Caldwell, "Herbal Diet Product Suspected in Death," *The Plain Dealer*, May 22, 2000, p. 2F.

[11] See Robert Pear, "On-line Sales Spur Illegal Importing of Medicine to U.S.," *The New York Times*, Jan. 10, 2000, p. A1.

[12] See Milt Freudenheim, "New Web sites

FOR MORE INFORMATION

Center for Democracy and Technology, 1633 I St. N.W., Suite 1100, Washington, D.C. 20006; (202) 637-9800; www.cdt.org. Promotes civil liberties and democractic values in new computer and communications media, with special interest in privacy and freedom of information.

Department of Health and Human Services, 200 Independence Ave. S.W. Suite 615F; Washington, D.C. 20201; (202) 690-7000; www.os.dhhs.gov. The department is now implementing regulations to protect personal health information.

Electronic Privacy Information Center, 666 Pennsylvania Ave. S.E., Suite 301, Washington, D.C. 20003; (202) 544-9240; www.epic.org. A public interest research center focusing on domestic and international civil liberties issues, including privacy, free speech and information access and computer security. Affiliated with the Fund for Constitutional Government.

Forum on Privacy and Security in Health Care, Columbia, Md., healthcaresecurity.org. A government-industry partnership that promotes industry standards to protect medical information.

Health Privacy Project, Institute for Health Care Research and Policy, Georgetown University, 2233 Wisconsin Ave. N.W., Suite 525, Washington, D.C. 20007; (202) 687-0880; www.healthprivacy.org. Dedicated to raising public awareness of the importance of ensuring health privacy in order to improve health care access and quality.

National Coalition for Patient Rights, 9 Bartlet St., Box 144, Andover, Mass. 01810-3884; (888) 44-PRIVACY; www.nationalcpr.org. A nonprofit organization "dedicated to the premise that patients have the right to privacy when they consult a health-care professional."

Altering Visits to Physicians," *The New York Times*, May 30, 2000, p. A1.

[13] For background, see Craig Stoltz, "What You Get Depends on Who Owns the Web Site Technology," *The Los Angeles Times*, May 29, 2000, p. S5.

[14] Quoted in Sandra G. Boodman, "Hard Evidence," *The Washington Post*, Sept. 26, 2000, p. Z12.

[15] See Tom Majeski, "Millions of Americans Regularly Use Web for Medical Information, Survey Says," Knight-Ridder Tribune Business News, Oct. 10, 2000.

[16] See Adriel Bettelheim, "Managing Managed Care," *The CQ Researcher*, April 16, 1999, pp. 305-328.

[17] See David C. Classen, "Clinical Decision Support Systems to Improve Clinical Practice and Quality of Care," *JAMA*, Oct. 21, 1998, Vol. 280, No. 15, pp. 1360-1361.

[18] See Leo R. Otake *et al.*, "Telemedicine: Low-Bandwidth Applications for Intermittent Health Services in Remote Areas," *JAMA*, Oct. 21, 1998, Vol. 280 No. 15.

[19] See James G. Hodge *et al.*, "Legal Issues Concerning Electronic Health Information," *JAMA*, Oct. 20, 1999, Vol. 282, No. 15, pp. 1466-1471.

[20] See Karen Foerstel, "Protecting Medical Records: Privacy vs. Progress," *CQ Weekly*, March 13, 1999, p. 593.

[21] See Ray Kurzweil, "Computers and Medicine: Real Virtual Medicine," *Hippocrates*, March 2000, serial on-line at 222.hippocrates.com.

[22] See Adriel Bettelheim, "Biology and Behavior," *The CQ Researcher*, April 3, 1998, pp. 289-312.

Bibliography

Selected Sources Used

Books

Slack, Werner V., *Cybermedicine: How Computing Empowers Doctors and Patients for Better Health Care*, Jossey-Bass, 1997.

A physician and passionate advocate for increased use of computers in medicine explains how the devices have been used to humanize medicine since the 1950s. Pleas for expanded use in settings such as clinics and examination rooms are tempered with concerns over privacy of patients' records.

Wood, M. Sandra, ed., *Health Care Resources on the Internet: A Guide for Libraries and Health-Care Consumers*, Haworth Press, 1999.

A practical guide for how to search for medical information on the Internet.

Hersh, William R., *Information Retrieval: A Health Care Perspective*, Spring Verlag, 1995.

An early book on how to design information-retrieval systems to make on-line health-information searching quicker.

Articles

Bell, Laura, and Charles Ornstein, "Patients' Data Not So Private: New Rules to Limit Disclosure," *The Dallas Morning News*, Sept. 17, 2000, p. 1A.

No federal law makes medical information private, and state protections are piecemeal at best. However, the landscape may soon change with the introduction of new federal medical-privacy rules this fall.

Stoltz, Craig, "What You Get Depends on Who Owns the Web Site Technology," *Los Angeles Times*, May 29, 2000, p. S5.

Health Web sites vary significantly in quality and ambition, and it's sometimes hard to tell who is providing information, how good it is and what the provider's ulterior motives might be.

Oliver, Amy J., "Internet Pharmacies: Regulation of a Growing Industry," *Journal of Law, Medicine and Ethics*, Vol. 28, No. 1 (2000), pp. 98-101.

The rapidly growing business of dispensing drugs on-line represents one of the most robust sectors of e-commerce, but also is giving regulators headaches. This article examines different types of Internet pharmacies and how some dispense drugs of questionable quality or without a valid prescription.

Freudenheim, Milt, "New Web Sites Altering Visits to Physicians," *The New York Times*, May 30, 2000, p. A1.

New medical Web sites reinforce doctors' knowledge, suggest diagnoses and give patients on-the-spot answers about their symptoms. In the process, they are changing the nature of visits to physicians.

Hodge, James, et al., "Legal Issues Concerning Electronic Health Information," *JAMA*, Oct. 20, 1999, Vol. 282, No. 15, pp. 1466-1471.

Computer technology may be transforming the way health information is stored and analyzed, but it also is creating new legal questions about privacy, quality and reliability of medical information and tort-based liability, the authors argue.

Luetkemeyer, Annie, "Practicing Medicine in the Internet Age," Risk Management Foundation of the Harvard Medical Institutions, May 1998 (serial online at www.rmf.harvard.edu/publications).

A third-year medical student's perspectives of how innovations on the World Wide Web are changing the way doctors practice medicine.

Reports

Goldman, Janlori, and Zoe Hudson, "Privacy: Report on the Privacy Policies and Practices of Health Web Sites," California HealthCare Foundation, January 2000.

Health-care Web sites have access to an unprecedented amount of personal information about consumers. But they have inconsistent policies about the privacy of that information, this study concludes.

Health Privacy Project, "Best Principles for Health Privacy," Georgetown University Institute for Health Care Research and Policy, 1999.

A thorough background paper on the benefits and concerns surrounding the computerization of medical information and storing large amounts of patient information in electronic form.

Health Privacy Project, "The State of Health Privacy: An Uneven Terrain," Georgetown University Institute for Health Care Research and Policy, 1999.

A review of states' medical privacy laws, how they do and do not deter the release of sensitive personal information and what prohibitions exist on sharing such information.

Credits

Index

2361